W9-BVW-297

'9-95
J-OP BOOKSTORE
TEXT
$19.95

A primer of
DRUG
ACTION

A Concise,

Nontechnical Guide

to the Actions,

Uses, and

Side Effects of

Psychoactive Drugs

SEVENTH EDITION

A primer of
DRUG
ACTION

A Concise,

Nontechnical Guide

to the Actions,

Uses, and

Side Effects of

Psychoactive Drugs

SEVENTH EDITION

Robert M. Julien, M.D., Ph.D.
St. Vincent Hospital and Medical Center
Portland, Oregon

W. H. Freeman and Company
New York

Library of Congress Cataloging–in–Publication Data
Julien, Robert M.
    A primer of drug action : a concise, nontechnical guide to the actions, uses, and
side effects of psychoactive drugs / Robert M. Julien. —7th ed.
        p.   cm.
    Includes bibliographical references and index.
    ISBN 0–7167–2388–3 (hard cover). — ISBN 0–7167–2619–X (soft cover)
    1. Psychotropic drugs. 2. Psychopharmaciology. I. Title.
    [DNLM: 1. Psychopharmacology. 2. Psychotropic Drugs. QV 77 J94p 1995]
RM315.J75 1995
615'.78—dc20
DNLM/DLC
for Library of Congress   94–33612
                                                                                CIP

© 1995, 1992, 1988, 1985, 1981, 1978, 1975 by W. H. Freeman and Company
No part of this book may be reproduced by any mechanical, photographic, or elec-
tronic process, or in the form of a phonographic recording, nor may it be stored in
a retrieval system, transmitted, or otherwise copied for public or private use, without written permission from the publisher.

Printed in the United States of America
  2 3 4 5 6 7 8 9 0 VB 9 9 8 7 6 5

    Second printing

CONTENTS

In the 20 years since the publication of the first edition of *A Primer of Drug Action* there has been an explosion of knowledge about psychoactive drugs, their use in the treatment of mental dysfunction, and their potential for misuse. In 1975, drug abuse was generally of more interest than was psychopharmacotherapy (the use of drugs to treat psychological disorders). Today, however, although drug abuse remains a continuing problem of great importance, many psychological disorders formerly resistant to drug treatment are increasingly the targets of drug therapy. Such disorders include bipolar illness, anxiety, panic disorder, phobias, and obsessive-compulsive disorder.

In the first edition of this text, the primary goal was to provide pharmacological information that was concise, accurate, and timely. The discussion was presented in clear language, as free of technical jargon as was possible, so that it could be easily understood by students and general readers with minimal background in the biological sciences.

This philosophy continues in this 20th anniversary edition. Yet recent research has dictated major content changes:

•Added to the detailed discussion of the drugs of abuse are new discussions of the anabolic-androgenic hormones, inhalants of abuse, and free-based methamphetamine (ICE).

•The many new psychotherapeutic agents are presented, along with their uses in treating bipolar illness, anxiety, panic disorder, specific and social phobias, and obsessive- compulsive disorder.

•The recent research in molecular biology of drug receptors has allowed new and much more sophisticated discussion of the receptors on which psychoactive drugs act. Although such presentation is technical, I think that its inclusion greatly demystifies drug action. Indeed, it allows the reader to visualize the receptors on which drugs act, and it provides introductory insights into how the process of receptor occupancy by a drug is translated into alterations in the intracellular chemistry of a neuron (the so-called process of signal transduction by intracellular second-messenger enzymes).

•The pharmacological intervention and treatment of psychological disorders that formerly were not amenable to drug therapy necessitate discussion of the interface between psychopharmacotherapy and the various professions of counseling, psychology, and psychotherapy. Those entering these and related professions now must be knowledgeable about and conversant in the pharmacology of the drugs their clients or patients may be taking. To this end, each chapter contains brief discussion of this interface, and a new chapter, cowritten by a clinical psychologist, is totally devoted to this topic.

Features of the Seventh Edition

In its first two decades of publication, *A Primer of Drug Action* helped shape courses in psychopharmacology, drug abuse, and drug education. As it enters its third decade of publication, I have again completely revised and updated the book with the aim of continuing its history as the most current and most understandable drug education text available.

Two new chapters have been added to this edition (Chapter 9, "Drugs Used in the Treatment of Bipolar Disorder," and Chapter 16, "Psychology and Psychopharmacotherapy"). All other chapters have been extensively revised to update each topic of discussion. I have updated literature citations, and most are from 1993 and 1994. Included are discussions of both current and future directions in drug research (including new drugs that are, as of this date, on the horizon but not yet available for clinical use). The new material included in this edition includes

•New topics of drugs of abuse. These include the anabolic-androgenic steroids, inhalants of abuse, and ICE
•New focus on the mechanisms of drug-induced "reward" and how such mechanisms relate to a drug's potential for abuse
•Molecular biology of drug receptors, including

—*the cannabinoid receptor and the endogenous neurotransmitter, anandamide*
—*the GABA$_A$ receptor and the action of benzodiazepines*
—*the presynaptic dopamine transporter and the action of cocaine*
—*the adenosine receptor and the action of caffeine*
—*the NMDA-glutamate receptor and the action of phencyclidine*
—*the presynaptic serotonin transporter and the action of antidepressants*
—*GABA$_A$ and GABA$_B$ receptor antagonists and partial agonists as cognitive enhancers.*
—*Serotonin$_2$ receptors and the action of psychedelic drugs*

•New discussions on the treatments of mental disorders including bipolar illness, obsessive-compulsive disorder, panic disorder, and the anxieties

•New drugs, including

—*clozapine*
—*risperidone*
—*remoxipride*
—*venflaxatine and other serotonin-specific antidepressants*
—*flumazenil*
—*zolpidem*
—*buspirone*
—*carbamazepine, valproic acid, and other drugs for treating*
bipolar illness
—*reversible MAO inhibitors*
—*Depo-Provera, Norplant, and mifepristone as contraceptives*

As in previous editions, I hope that this expanded and rewritten text will continue to serve the needs of all those who desire a concise, clearly presented introduction to the fields of psychopharmacology, drug education, and psychopharmacotherapy.

Acknowledgments

I would like to sincerely thank Dr. Donald Lange (Clinical Psychologist, Portland, Oregon) for his generous contribution of Chapter 16. I also offer my thanks to Dr. Jack Elder (Professor of Pharmacology, Creighton University, Omaha, Nebraska) for his review of the manuscript, and to Dr. Jerrell Driver (Clinical Psychologist, Southeast Missouri Hospital, Cape Girardeau, Missouri) for his review of Chapter 16.

Robert M. Julien, M.D., Ph.D.
November 1994

CHAPTER 1

CLASSIFICATION OF PSYCHOACTIVE DRUGS

Psychoactive drugs are defined as substances that act to alter mood, thought processes, or behavior, or that are used to manage neuropsychological illness. Because the etiology of neuropsychological illness is often unknown and because the actions of drugs that are effective in treating such illness are complex, the classification of psychoactive drugs is not a straightforward task.

Several methods of classification have been formulated, but each has limitations. Certainly, an ideal method of classification would be based on a drug's mechanism of action. However, there is still too much that we don't know about those mechanisms to synthesize a comprehensive scheme.

Another possible classification scheme is based on the chemical structures of drugs; in this approach, it is assumed that drugs with similar chemical structures have similar effects. However, too many drugs with similar structures induce different pharmacological activity, and too many drugs with dissimilar chemical structures induce pharmacological activity that is nearly identical. Thus, the chemical structure of a drug does not produce a reliable guide to its pharmacological effects.

Perhaps the most useful classification of drugs is based on their most characteristic behavioral effects or the widest clinical use. A classification of drugs using these criteria is presented in Table 1.1.

TABLE 1.1   Classification of drugs and representative agents.

I. Traditional, nonselective CNS depressants
   A. Barbiturates: phenobarbital (Luminal), amobarbital (Amytal),
      pentobarbital (Nembutal), thiopental (Pentothal)
   B. Nonbarbiturate, nonbenzodiazepine hypnotics: meprobamate (Equanil),
      glutethimide (Doriden), methyprylon (Noludar), methaqualone,
      chloral hydrate
   C. Ethyl alcohol
   D. General anesthetics
   E. Inhalants of abuse

II. Antianxiety agents
   A. Benzodiazepines: diazepam (Valium), lorazepam (Ativan),
      triazolam (Halcion), others
   B. Nonbenzodiazepine, GABA-agonist hypnotic: zolpidem (Ambien)
   C. Nonbenzodiazepine, "second-generation" anxiolytic: buspirone (BuSpar)

III. Antiepileptic drugs
   A. Traditional agents: phenytoin (Dilantin), primidone (Mysoline)
   B. Benzodiazepines: clonazepam (Clonopin), clorazepate (Tranxene)
   C. Newer agents used in treating psychological disorders: carbamazepine
      (Tegretol), valproic acid (Depakene), alprazolam (Xanax)
   D. Newer meprobamate derivative: felbamate (Felbatol)

IV. Psychomotor stimulants (psychostimulants)
   A. Dopamine reuptake blocker: cocaine
   B. Dopamine-releasing agents
      1. Amphetamines: *d*-amphetamine (Dexedrine), methamphetamine
      2. Amphetamine derivatives: methylphenidate (Ritalin), pemoline (Cylert)
   C. Adenosine receptor blocker: caffeine
   D. Acetylcholine receptor stimulant (agonist): nicotine

V. Antidepressants
   A. Tricyclic antidepressants (TCAs): imipramine (Tofranil), amitriptyline (Elavil),
      others

Assumptions about Classification

There are several caveats to the classification scheme used in Table 1.1. First, the action of psychoactive drugs is not usually restricted to any one functional or anatomical subdivision of the brain. There are exceptions, of course (such as the use of levodopa for treating Parkinson's disease), but a psychoactive drug usually affects several parts of the brain simultaneously. This factor complicates the classification of drugs, because different behavioral effects may predominate at different doses. Some compromises must therefore be made.

TABLE 1.1 Classification of drugs and representative agents *(continued).*

      B. Second-generation antidepressants: maprotiline (Ludiomil), amoxapine (Asendin), trazodone (Desyrel), bupropion (Wellbutrin)

      C. Serotonin-specific reuptake inhibitors: fluoxetine (Prozac), paroxetine (Paxil), sertraline (Zoloft), clomipramine (Anafranil), venlafaxine (Effexor)

      D. Monoamine oxidase (MAO) inhibitors: tranylcypromine (Parnate), phenelzine (Nardil), isocarboxazid (Marplan)

  VI. Mood stabilizers

      A. Lithium

      B. Carbamazepine (Tegretol)

      C. Valproic acid (Depakene)

      D. Adjunctive, nonspecific antimanic drugs

         1. Benzodiazepines: clonazepam (Klonopin), lorazepam (Ativan)

         2. Calcium-channel-blocking agents: Verapamil (Calan), nimodipine

         3. Clonidine (Catapres)

 VII. Narcotic analgesics: opioids

      A. Pure opioid agonists (e.g., morphine, codeine, heroin)

      B. Partial opioid agonists (e.g., nalbuphine, pentazocine)

      C. Opioid antagonists (e.g., naloxone, naltrexone)

VIII. Antipsychotic agents

      A. Phenothiazines: chlorpromazine (Thorazine)

      B. Butyrophenones: haloperidol (Haldol)

  IX. Psychedelics and hallucinogens

      A. Anticholinergic psychedelics: scopolamine

      B. Norepinephrine psychedelics: mescaline, DOM (STP), MDA, MMDA, TMA, DMA, Myristin

      C. Serotonin psychedelics: lysergic acid diethylamide (LSD); dimethyltryptamine (DMT); psilocybin, psilocin, bufotenine; ololiuqui (morning glory seeds); harmine

      D. Psychedelic anesthetics: phencyclidine (Sernyl), ketamine (Ketalar)

      E. Tetrahydrocannabinol: marijuana, hashish, cannabis

This table classifies drugs that alter mood or behavior, are useful in treating neuropsychological disorders, or are subject to compulsive abuse.

Second, the ultimate action of any given psychoactive drug may be explained by its effects on a specific neurotransmitter chemical. (The neurochemical processes that mediate transmission of information between neurons are discussed at some length in Appendix III.) Further, the same neurotransmitter chemical may be involved in many different activities of the brain (norepinephrine, for example, may be involved in temperature regulation, behavioral arousal, satiety, or rage). Thus, although a psychoactive drug might ultimately exert a single effect on a specific neurotransmitter chemical, a variety of behavioral effects might follow if the neurotransmitter is involved in many different functions.

Third, it is important to understand that psychoactive drugs do not create new behavioral or physiological responses; they simply modify ongoing processes. The current view is that the behavioral effects induced by psychoactive drugs are secondary to their effects on biochemical and physiological processes, particularly those processes involved in the synaptic transmission in the brain.

Fourth, the classification of psychoactive drugs listed in Table 1.1 is not rigid. As noted, drugs ingested at different doses provoke different behavioral responses. Alcohol, for example, is classified as a general nonselective depressant despite the fact that, at low doses, it may cause behavioral excitation. Thus, classification alone does not clearly describe the pharmacology of a drug. It does, however, serve as a starting point for comparing compounds.

Fifth, certain factors that predispose persons to compulsive misuse of a drug must be considered when classifying centrally acting drugs. Such factors include physiological and psychological dependence and tolerance. Psychoactive drugs differ in their potential to induce such hazards. Clearly, any drug that can favorably alter a person's mood or behavior can induce psychological dependence—that is, a compulsion to use the drug for a favorable effect.

Further Discussion

In subsequent chapters, we describe specific agents within each class of psychoactive agents listed in Table 1.1. Alcohol and marijuana are discussed separately (in Chapters 5 and 13, respectively). Although both agents could be included in the chapter on sedative-hypnotic compounds (Chapter 3), they deserve separate discussions because of their wide range of use, ready availability, and social and legal implications. Similarly, the benzodiazepine and other more modern anxiolytic (antianxiety) compounds deserve their own discussion (Chapter 4), although their behavioral effects superficially resemble those of the barbiturates.

Chapter 8 discusses the antidepressant compounds, including those compounds likely to become available in the future. Chapter 9 presents a discussion of the mood stabilizers, which are compounds used to treat bipolar disorder (manic-depressive illness). The antidepressants (and lithium) have become widely used, and their unique properties clearly separate them from the psychomotor stimulants (Chapter 6).

Chapter 14 discusses drugs (in particular, oral contraceptives, fertility agents, and anabolic steroids) affecting the body hormones that influence the brain and behavior. Although these compounds are not psychoactive drugs, the wide interest in these drugs warrants the inclusion of this material.

Finally, Chapter 15 addresses the sociological issues of drug abuse, dependence, and addiction. Chapter 16 discusses individuals who are specifically involved in (or who are studying) the clinical interface between pharmacology and human neurophysiological dysfunction, bringing together the pharmacological and the nonpharmacological treatments of individuals with neuropsychological illness.

Before we discuss the individual classes of psychoactive drugs, however, we first look at the basic principles of drug action. This discussion (Chapter 2) lays the foundation for our later descriptions of psychoactive drugs.

PRINCIPLES OF DRUG ACTION

When we have a headache, we take for granted that after taking some aspirin, our headache will probably disappear within 15 to 30 minutes. We also take for granted that, unless we take more aspirin later, the headache may recur within a few hours.

This familiar scenario reveals the primary events of pain relief. The first is the *administration and absorption* of the drug into the body; the second is the *distribution* of the drug throughout the body; the third is the *interaction* of the drug with its "receptors" in the body, which are responsible for the drug's actions; and the fourth is the *elimination* of the drug from the body.

Pharmacodynamics, the study of these drug–receptor interactions, will be discussed later in this chapter. First, however, we will discuss *pharmacokinetics*, the study of how drugs move through and affect the body.[1]

PHARMACOKINETICS: HOW DRUGS MOVE THROUGH THE BODY

Pharmacokinetics, in its simplest form, describes the time course of a particular drug's actions—the time to onset and the duration of a drug's effects. Usually the time course simply reflects the amount of time required for the rise and fall of the drug's concentration at the target site. Simple though this may sound, the process of transporting a

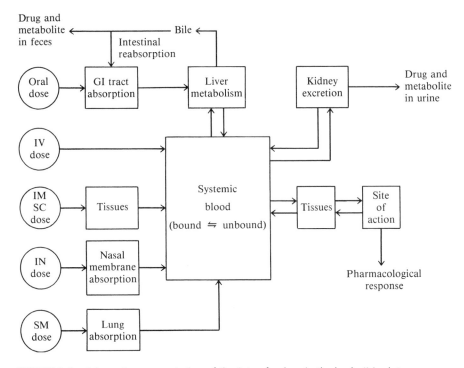

FIGURE 2.1 Schematic representation of the fate of a drug in the body. IM = intramuscular; IV = intravenous; IN = intranasal; SC = subcutaneous; SM = smoked. [Adapted from C. N. Chiang and R. L. Hawks, "Implications of Drug Levels in Body Fluids: Basic Concepts," in R. L. Hawks and C. N. Chiang, eds., *Urine Testing for Drugs of Abuse,* NIDA Research Monograph No. 73 (Rockville, Md.: National Institute on Drug Abuse, 1986), p. 63.]

drug from outside the body to its ultimate site of action inside the body is complex; a detailed picture of the process is given in Figure 2.1. Below we will briefly described the processes.

Drug Absorption

The phrase *drug absorption* refers to mechanisms by which drugs pass from the point of entry into the bloodstream. When administering any drug, one must select a *route* of administration, a *dose* of the drug, and a *dosage form* (liquid, tablet, capsule, or injection) that will both place the drug at its site of action in a pharmacologically effective concentration and maintain the concentration for an adequate period of time.

Drugs are most commonly administered in one of five ways: orally (through the mouth), rectally (into the rectum), parenterally (by injection), by inhalation through the lungs, and by absorption through mucous membranes. Let us consider these methods of administration and absorption in more detail.

Oral Administration

Drugs are most commonly taken by mouth and swallowed. To be effective when administered orally, the drug must be soluble and stable in stomach fluid, enter the intestine, penetrate the lining of the intestine, and pass into the bloodstream.

Because they are already in solution, drugs that are administered in liquid form tend to be absorbed more rapidly than those given in tablet or capsule form. Alcohol, for example, is taken in liquid form. As a result, about one-fourth to one-third of the alcohol that is ingested is absorbed directly from the stomach into the bloodstream. Thus, absorption is rapid and the effects of the alcohol can be felt rapidly, especially if no food is present in the stomach. When a drug is taken in solid form, both the rate at which it dissolves and its chemistry limit its rate of absorption.

After a drug dissolves in the stomach, it is absorbed into the bloodstream after its passive transfer across the stomach or intestinal lining. This process occurs against a developing concentration gradient of drug at a rate that is determined by the ratio of water solubility to lipid solubility of the drug molecules. Indeed, once they are in the body, drugs exist as a mixture of two interchangeable forms: one that is water soluble (the ionized, or electrically charged, form) and one that is lipid soluble (the nonionized, or uncharged, form). When the drug molecule is in the water-soluble form, it does not readily cross lipid membranes; in the lipid-soluble form, it can freely permeate the membrane.

The relative concentrations of the two forms of a drug depends on the relative acidity (pH) of the fluid in which it is dissolved and on a characteristic of the drug molecule itself (its pK_a—the pH at which 50 percent of the drug is ionized).* Gastric juice is very acidic; intestinal

---

*The ratio of lipid-soluble (nonionized) drug to water-soluble (ionized) drug at each pH (and, therefore, in each body compartment) can be calculated from the Henderson-Hasselbalch equation:

$$pH = pK_a + \log \text{ of base or acid}$$

For drugs that are weak acids, the acid form of the drug is the nonionized form; for drugs that are weak bases, the base form is nonionized. The reader interested in a more in-depth discussion of this chemistry should consult any of the several textbooks of pharmacology listed in the bibliography.

contents are less acidic; and plasma (the noncellular component of blood) is slightly alkaline. As we have already stated, only lipid-soluble molecules diffuse readily across cell membranes; thus the level of lipid solubility is the factor that determines how quickly a drug passes across a lipid membrane.

If the pH is different on the two sides of a membrane (as, for example, between the stomach and the bloodstream), the ratios of water-soluble drug to lipid-soluble drug also are different on the two sides. At equilibrium, the concentration of the lipid-soluble drug is equal on both sides of the membrane (because, as we have said, the lipid-soluble form of the drug can freely permeate the membrane), but the total quantity of drug is higher on the side where the ratio of water-soluble drug to lipid-soluble drug is greater (because the water-soluble drug molecules cannot cross the membrane). Thus, a drug is absorbed along its concentration gradient by passive transfer without the expenditure of energy that would be necessary to maintain an active pump to move molecules against a concentration gradient.

Although oral administration of drugs is common, it does have disadvantages. First, it may lead to occasional vomiting and stomach distress. Second, although the amount of a drug that is put into a tablet or capsule can be calculated, how much of it will be absorbed into the bloodstream cannot always be accurately predicted because of unexplained differences between individuals and differences in the manufacturing of the drugs. (Indeed, different brands of the same drug may be absorbed at widely differing rates.) Third, some drugs, such as the local anesthetics and insulin, when administered orally, are destroyed by the acid in the stomach before they are absorbed. To be effective, such drugs must be administered by injection.

Despite the disadvantages, about 75 percent of an orally administered drug is absorbed by the body within about 1 to 3 hours. This figure can vary widely, however, because of factors such as particle size, formulation, and blood flow to the stomach.

Rectal Administration

Although the primary route of drug administration is oral, some drugs are administered rectally (usually in suppository form) if the patient is vomiting, unconscious, or unable to swallow. However, absorption is often irregular, unpredictable, and incomplete; furthermore, many drugs irritate the membranes that line the rectum.

Inhalation

Inhalation is an increasingly popular method of drug administration, because it avoids the unpredictability of administration through the gastrointestinal tract. Drugs that are administered as gases or aerosols penetrate the cell linings of the respiratory tract easily and rapidly. For example, anesthetic gases (such as nitrous oxide or halothane) consist of small, highly lipid-soluble molecules that are absorbed across the membranes of the lungs into the bloodstream nearly as fast as they are inhaled. They are absorbed promptly because of the close contact between the blood and the membranes of the lung.

In a novel variation of pulmonary absorption, some drugs that act directly on lung tissue can be formulated so that they are not absorbed into the bloodstream, thereby eliminating or at least minimizing side effects. For example, patients with asthma often require cortisone-like, anti-inflammatory steroids to control their attacks of asthma. Steroids (including glucocorticoids) produce undesirable side effects on the body when taken orally in the doses necessary to control asthma. However, by formulating the steroid as large, poorly soluble, and poorly absorbed particles suspended in a carrier gas, the drug can be inhaled through the mouth (on a metered dose of carrier gas) and carried into the trachea and lungs with a deeply inspired breath. The particles sit on the lung tissue and exert their action. Any particles remaining in the mouth are swallowed but not absorbed because of their large size and poor solubility.

To date, little is known about the pulmonary absorption of non-gaseous drugs, especially those used as drugs of abuse. Such drugs, including nicotine, cocaine, and marijuana, are administered as very small particles that are carried in a gas or smoke. The pharmacological effects of these drugs are discussed in later chapters.

It is also well known that inhalation of substances that are not volatile, such as tars, which are abundant in inhaled cigarette smoke, can injure the sensitive tissues of the lung. Lung cancer, which can be induced by long-term inhalation of cigarette smoke, is thought to be fatal in more than 90 percent of cases and is estimated to result in more than 75,000 deaths a year in the United States.

Administration through the Mucous Membranes

Occasionally drugs are administered through the mucous membranes of the mouth or nose. A heart patient taking nitroglycerin, for instance, places the tablet under the tongue, where the drug is absorbed into the bloodstream directly from the mouth. Cocaine powder, when sniffed, adheres to the membranes on the inside of the nose and is absorbed directly into the bloodstream. Nasal decongestants are sprayed directly onto mucous membranes. Nicotine in snuff or gum (for example, Nicorette gum) is absorbed by the buccal membranes directly into the bloodstream.

Aministration through the Skin

Recently several prescribed medications have been incorporated into patches that adhere to the skin; the pharmacologically active ingredient is slowly absorbed into the bloodstream at the area of contact. Examples include nicotine (used to deter smoking), fentanyl (used to treat chronic, unrelenting pain), nitroglycerin (used to prevent the symptoms of angina pectoris in patients with coronary artery disease), clonidine (used to treat hypertension), and estrogen (used to replace hormones in postmenopausal women). In each case, the drug is released and absorbed over a period of days, allowing the levels of drug in plasma to remain relatively constant.

Injection

Administration of drugs by injection can be *intravenous* (directly into a vein), *intramuscular* (directly into a muscle), or *subcutaneous* (just under the skin). Each of these routes of administration has its advantages and disadvantages (Table 2.1), but some features are shared by

TABLE 2.1   Some characteristics of drug administration by injection.

Route	Absorption pattern	Special utility	Limitations and precautions
Intravenous	Absorption circumvented Potentially immediate effects	Valuable for emergency use Permits titration of dosage Can administer large volumes and irritating substances when diluted	Increased risk of adverse effects Must inject solutions slowly as a rule Not suitable for oily solutions or insoluble substances
Intramuscular	Prompt action from aqueous solution Slow and sustained action from repository preparations	Suitable for moderate volumes, oily vehicles, and some irritating substances	Precluded during anti-coagulant medicine May interfere with interpretation of certain diagnostic tests (e.g., creatine phosphokinase)
Subcutaneous	Prompt action from aqueous solution Slow and sustained action from repository preparations	Suitable for some insoluble suspensions and for implantation of solid pellets	Not suitable for large volumes Possible pain or necrosis from irritating substances

Modified from L. Z. Benet, J. R. Mitchell, and L. B. Sheiner,[1] p. 6.

all. In general, administration by injection produces a more prompt response than does oral administration because absorption is faster. Also, injection permits a more accurate dose because the unpredictable processes of absorption through the stomach and intestine are bypassed.

Administration of drugs by injection, however, has several drawbacks. First, the rapid rate of absorption leaves little time to respond to an unexpected drug reaction or accidental overdose. Second, administration by injection requires the use of sterile techniques. The ongoing AIDS crisis is a vivid example of the drastic consequences of unsterile injection techniques. Third, once a drug is administered by injection, it cannot be recalled.

Intravenous Administration   In an intravenous injection, a drug is introduced directly into the bloodstream. This technique avoids all the variables related to oral absorption. The injection can be made slowly, and it can be stopped instantaneously if untoward effects develop. Finally, the dosage amount can be extremely precise, and the practitioner can dilute and administer in large volumes drugs that at higher concentrations would be irritants to the muscles or blood vessels.

The intravenous route has several important drawbacks, however. First, it is the most dangerous of all routes of administration, because it has the fastest speed of onset of pharmacological action. Second, a normally safe dose may be given too rapidly, causing catastrophic, life-threatening reactions (such as collapse of respiration or of heart function). Third, allergic reactions may be mild to a drug administered orally, but they may be extremely severe when the same drug is administered intravenously. Fourth, drugs that are not soluble in the blood or drugs that are dissolved in oily liquids cannot be given intravenously because of the danger of blood clots forming. Finally, infection by bacterial contaminants is a danger, and infectious diseases can be transmitted or abscesses induced when sterile techniques are not employed.

Intramuscular Administration   Drugs that are injected into skeletal muscle (usually in the arm, thigh, or buttock) are generally absorbed fairly rapidly. Absorption of a drug from muscle is more rapid than absorption of the same drug from the stomach but slower than absorption of the drug administered intravenously. The absolute rate of absorption of a drug from muscle varies, depending on the rate of blood flow to the muscle, the solubility of the drug, the volume of the injection, and even the vehicle in which the drug is injected.

In general, most of the precautions that apply to intravenous administration also apply to intramuscular injection. However, drugs that are intended for intramuscular administration should not be given intravenously as a rule; consequently, one must be careful to avoid hitting a blood vessel when inserting a needle into muscle.

Subcutaneous Administration Absorption of drugs that have been injected under the skin (subcutaneously) is rapid. The exact rate depends mainly on the ease of blood vessel penetration and the rate of blood flow through the skin. Irritating drugs should not be injected subcutaneously because they may cause severe pain and damage to local tissue. The usual precautions to maintain sterility apply.

Self-administration of any drug by injection is to be discouraged except when oral administration is not effective or when the drug is being taken therapeutically under the direction of a physician (injection of insulin by a diabetic is a prominent example). The risks associated with injection of a drug (infection, overdose, allergic responses, and transmission of the AIDS virus) are far greater than those associated with oral administration of the same drug.

Drug Distribution

Once absorbed, a drug is distributed throughout the body by the circulating blood, passing across various barriers to reach its site of action. At any given time, only a very small portion of the total amount of a drug that is in the body is in contact with its receptors. Most of the administered drug is found in areas of the body that are remote from the drug's site of action. For example, in the case of a psychoactive drug (a drug that alters mood or behavior as a result of its effect on the central nervous system [CNS]), most of the drug circulates outside the brain and therefore does not contribute directly to its pharmacological effect. Indeed, this wide distribution often accounts for many of the side effects of a drug. *Side effects* are results that are different from the primary, or therapeutic, effect for which a drug is taken. Importantly, it is the total amount of a drug in the body that (1) governs the movements of that drug through the tissues and its ultimate elimination, (2) determines both the duration and the intensity of the drug's effect, and (3) underlies many of the drug's side effects.

Action of the Bloodstream

In the average-size adult, each minute the heart pumps approximately 5 liters (1 liter = 2.1 pints) of blood, which is roughly equal to the total

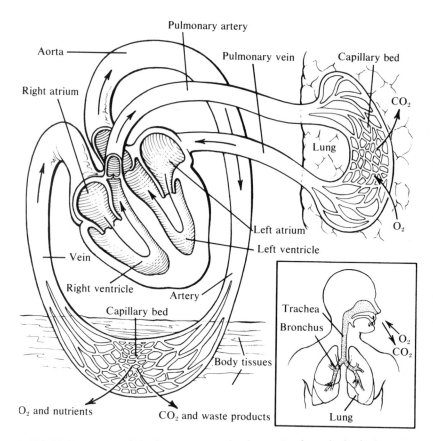

FIGURE 2.2   Heart and circulatory system. Blood returning from the body tissues to the heart via the veins passes through the right atrium into the right ventricle and, with the contraction of the heart, is pumped into the arteries leading to the lungs. In the lungs, carbon dioxide (CO_2) is lost and replaced by oxygen. This oxygenated blood returns to the heart through the left atrium, is pumped out of the left ventricle into the aorta, and is carried to the body tissues, where oxygen and nutrients are exchanged in the capillary beds. Oxygen and nutrients are supplied to the body tissues through the walls of the capillaries; CO_2 and other waste products are returned to the blood. The CO_2 is eliminated through the lungs, and the other waste products are excreted through the kidneys.

amount of blood in the circulatory system. Thus, the entire blood volume circulates in the body about once every minute. Therefore, once a drug is absorbed into the bloodstream it is rapidly (usually within this 1-minute circulation time) distributed throughout the circulatory system.

A schematic diagram of the circulatory system is presented in Figure 2.2. Blood returning to the heart through the veins is first pumped into the pulmonary (lung) circulation system, where carbon dioxide is removed and replaced by oxygen. The oxygenated blood then returns to the heart and is pumped into the great artery (the aorta). From there blood flows into the smaller arteries and finally into the capillaries, where nutrients (and drugs) are exchanged between the blood and the cells of the body.

To perform this exchange, the body has an estimated 10 billion capillaries, which have a total surface area of more than 200 square meters. Probably no single functioning cell of the body is more than 20 to 30 micrometers away from a capillary (1 micrometer = 0.0004 inch). After the blood passes through the capillaries, it is collected by the veins and returned to the heart to circulate again.

Thus, drugs are fairly evenly distributed throughout the bloodstream. The body of a normal, lean, 150-pound man contains approximately 41 liters of the water (equivalent to 60 percent of the total body weight). About 5 liters of water are in his circulating blood, and about 35 liters are in his body tissues. However, that 35 liters of water is not isolated from his blood, because fluids (and most drugs) are freely exchanged, or equilibrated, between the blood, other body fluids, and most cells of the body. Thus, drugs are diluted not only by the blood but also by the total amount of water contained in the body.

In addition to solubility, another factor often limits drug distribution: the reversible binding of drugs to proteins present in the blood plasma. Protein-bound drug exists in equilibrium with free (unbound) drug, as shown in Figure 2.1. Because plasma proteins (albumin, for example) are quite large, they are unable to leave the bloodstream. Thus, the amount of drug that is bound to plasma proteins remains confined within the blood vessels, markedly affecting drug distribution.

The unequal distribution of three drugs in the different body compartments is illustrated in Figure 2.3. Drug 1 becomes almost completely protein-bound and is largely confined to the bloodstream. Drug 2 does not bind to blood proteins and passes easily out of the bloodstream into tissue fluid, but it is unable to pass into cells. Drug 3 is a compound that passes easily from the bloodstream and readily penetrates cell membranes into the fluid inside the cell. An example of this drug is thiopental (Pentothal), a commonly used anesthetic that induces anesthesia within a matter of seconds after i.v. injection. Because thiopental is extremely soluble in the fat of cell membranes, it can leave the bloodstream rapidly and pass into brain cells, where it acts quickly to abolish consciousness.

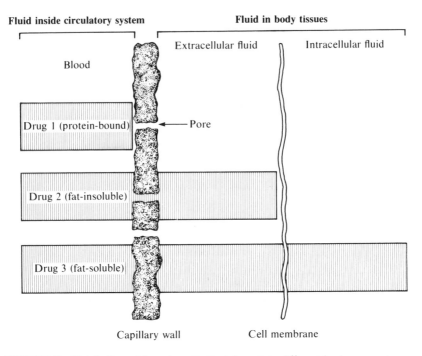

FIGURE 2.3 Distribution of three hypothetical drugs into different body compartments. Drug 1 is bound to blood proteins; drug 2 is unbound, soluble in water, but insoluble in fat; drug 3 is unbound and soluble in both water and fat. Note that drug 1 is largely restricted to the bloodstream; drug 2 is distributed in the blood and in the fluid outside the body cells; and drug 3 is distributed through all the body compartments and readily passes into the brain, easily crossing the blood–brain barrier.

Body Membranes That Affect Drug Distribution

Various types of membranes in the body affect drug distribution. The four most important are (1) the cell membranes, (2) the walls of the capillary vessels in the circulatory system, (3) the blood–brain barrier, and (4) the placental barrier.

Cell Membranes To be absorbed from the intestine or to gain access to the interior of a cell, a drug must penetrate the cell membranes. What, then, is known of the structure and properties of such membranes that determine their permeability to drugs? In Figure 2.4, the two layers of circles represent the water-soluble head groups of complex lipid molecules called *phospholipids*. These phospholipid heads form a rather continuous layer on both the inside and the outside of the cell membrane. The wavy lines that extend from the heads

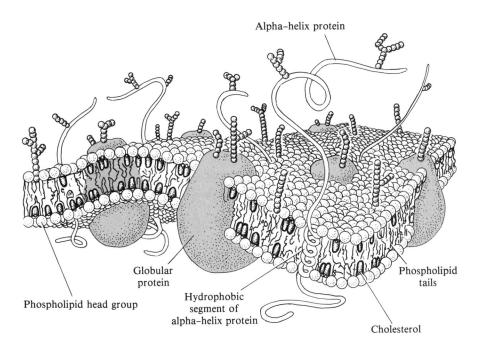

Alpha-helix protein

Globular protein

Phospholipid head group

Hydrophobic segment of alpha-helix protein

Phospholipid tails

Cholesterol

FIGURE 2.4   Diagrammatic representation of the cell membrane, a phospholipid bilayer in which cholesterol and protein molecules are embedded. Both globular and helical kinds of protein traverse the bilayer. Cholesterol molecules tend to keep the tails of the phospholipids relatively fixed and orderly in the regions closest to the hydrophilic phospholipid heads; the parts of the tails closer to the core of the membrane move about freely. [From M. S. Bretscher, "The Molecules of the Cell Membrane," *Scientific American* 253 (1985): 104.]

into the membrane are the lipid chains of the phospholipid molecules. Therefore, for our present purposes, the interior of the cell membrane can be considered to consist of a sea of liquid lipid in which large proteins are suspended. This structure has been named the *fluid mosaic model.*

Notice in Figure 2.4 that several large globules and spiral strands appear to be situated on the outer layer of the membrane and extend either into or through the three layers of the membrane, the total thickness of which is about 80 angstroms. (The angstrom is equal to 0.0001 micrometer, or 0.00000004 inch.) These globules and spirals represent protein structures, at least some of which are sites of drug action (i.e., these may be the transmembrane receptor proteins upon which certain psychoactive drugs act).

This membrane, consisting of protein and fat, provides a barrier that is permeable to many drug molecules but impermeable to others. Given this model, it is not surprising to find that the penetration of a drug molecule through the membrane, and thus into a cell, is determined by the solubility of that drug in oil (oil is a fat, and the core of this membrane consists of fat molecules). In addition to this layered structure of protein and fat, the membrane also appears to contain small pores (about 8 angstroms in diameter) that permit small water-soluble molecules to pass, such as alcohol and water.

These cellular membranes (as barriers to the absorption and distribution of drugs) are important for the passage of drugs (1) from the stomach and intestine into the bloodstream, (2) from the fluid that closely surrounds tissue cells into the interior of cells, (3) from the interior of cells back into the body water, and (4) from the kidneys back into the bloodstream.

Capillaries Within a minute or so of entering the bloodstream, a drug is distributed fairly evenly throughout the entire blood volume. However, most drugs are not confined to the bloodstream because they are exchanged back and forth between blood capillaries and tissues.

Figure 2.5 is a cross-sectional diagram of a capillary. Capillaries are tiny, cylindrical blood vessels with walls that are formed by a thin, single layer of cells packed tightly together. Between the cells are small passageways (pores) that connect the interior of the vessel (the capillary) with the exterior (the body tissues). The diameter of the pores is between 90 and 150 angstroms, which is larger than most drug molecules. Thus, most drugs freely leave the blood through these pores in the capillary membranes, passing along their concentration gradient until equilibrium is established between the concentrations of drug in the blood and in body water.

Therefore, the transport of drug molecules out of blood capillaries and into tissues (and, conversely, from tissues back into the blood through the capillaries) is independent of lipid solubility, because the membrane pores are large enough for even fat-insoluble drug molecules to penetrate. However, the pores in the capillary membrane are not large enough to permit the red blood cells and the plasma proteins to leave the bloodstream. Thus, the only drugs that do not readily penetrate capillary pores are those rare drugs that are composed of proteins and those that bind to plasma proteins. Thus, protein-bound drugs essentially become trapped in the bloodstream and do not diffuse into the tissues.

The rate at which drug molecules enter specific body tissues depends on two factors: the rate of blood flow through the tissue and the

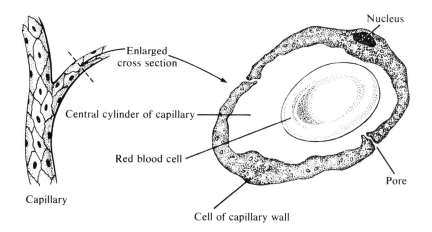

FIGURE 2.5 Cross section of a blood capillary. Within the capillary are the fluids, proteins, and cells of the blood, including the red blood cells. The capillary itself is made up of cells that completely surround and define the central cylinder (or lumen) of the capillary. Water-filled pores form channels, allowing communication between the lumen and the fluid outside the capillary.

ease with which drug molecules pass through the capillary membranes. Because blood flow is greatest to the brain and much poorer to the bones, joints, and fat deposits, drug distribution generally follows a similar pattern. However, some capillaries (such as those in the brain) have special structural properties that can further limit the diffusion of a drug into the brain.

Blood–Brain Barrier The brain requires a protected environment in which to function normally, and a specialized structural barrier, called the *blood–brain barrier,* plays a key role in maintaining this environment.[2] The blood–brain barrier involves specialized cells in the brain that affect nearly all its blood capillaries (Figure 2.6). In most of the rest of the body, the capillary membranes have pores; in the brain, however, the capillaries are tightly joined together and covered on the outside by a fatty barrier called the glial sheath, which arises from nearby astrocyte cells.

Thus, a drug leaving the capillaries in the brain has to traverse both the wall of the capillary itself (because there are no pores to pass through) and the membranes of the astrocyte cells in order to reach the cells in the brain. Therefore, as a general rule, the rate of passage of a drug into the brain is determined by the lipid (fat) solubility of the

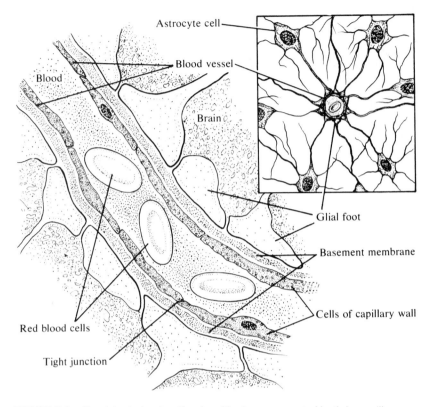

FIGURE 2.6 Blood–brain barrier. Blood and brain are separated both by capillary cells packed tightly together and by a fatty barrier called the *glial sheath,* which is made up of extensions (glial feet) from nearby astrocyte cells (see inset). A drug diffusing from the blood to the brain must move through the cells of the capillary wall because there are tight junctions rather than pores between the cells; the drug must then move through the fatty glial sheath.

particular drug. Highly ionized drugs (penicillin, for example) penetrate poorly, while fat-soluble drugs penetrate rapidly. Drugs are often classified by their ability or inability to penetrate the blood–brain barrier. By definition, psychoactive drugs (those discussed in this book) are lipid soluble, since they exert their actions only after crossing the blood–brain barrier. Drugs whose actions are predominantly outside the CNS are usually more highly ionized (less lipid soluble) and therefore their CNS actions are usually not of major significance.

Placental Barrier   Among all the membrane systems of the body, the placenta membranes are unique. They separate two distinct human beings with differing genetic compositions, physiological responses, and sensitivities to drugs. The fetus obtains essential nutrients and eliminates metabolic waste products through the placenta without depending on its own organs, many of which are not yet functioning. This dependence of the fetus upon the mother, however, places the fetus at the mercy of the placenta when foreign substances (such as drugs or toxins) appear in the mother's blood.

A pregnant woman in the United States regularly takes both prescription and nonprescription drugs, and she routinely exposes the fetus to potentially toxic substances in food, cosmetics, household chemicals, and the general environment. The extent to which these substances affect the fetus is not yet known. The consequences of maternal alcohol ingestion and cigarette smoking on fetal growth and development are now well documented and will be discussed in Chapters 5 and 7. Cocaine use also has resulted in severe effects on the developing fetus.

Early in pregnancy, when the limbs and organ systems of the fetus are forming, drugs may induce structural abnormalities (called *teratogenesis*). Thalidomide was the most dramatic example of a teratogenic compound. This tranquilizer was marketed in several countries during the early 1960s; the fetuses of women who were given the drug in the fifth through seventh weeks of pregnancy had a high incidence of abnormal limb growth.

Later in pregnancy and during delivery, drugs such as cocaine (Chapter 5) may induce respiratory depression in the newborn because the baby is unable to metabolize or excrete the drugs. Problems can follow from the intense vasoconstriction cocaine produces and the consequent reduction in placental blood flow. This can result in fetal hypoxia (reduced availability of oxygen), which can have deleterious effects.

Schematic representations of the placental network, which transfers substances between the mother and the fetus, are shown in Figures 2.7 and 2.8. In general, the mature placenta consists of a network of vessels and pools of maternal blood into which protrude treelike or fingerlike villi (projections) that contain the blood capillaries of the fetus (see Figure 2.8). Oxygen and nutrients travel from the mother's blood to that of the fetus, while carbon dioxide and other waste products travel from the fetus's to the mother's blood.

The membranes that separate fetal blood from maternal blood in the intervillous space resemble, in their general permeability, the cell membranes that are found elsewhere in the body. In other words,

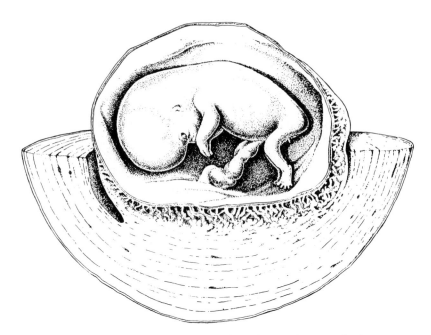

FIGURE 2.7 Placenta, embryo, and section through part of a uterus [Redrawn from W. J. Hamilton, J. D. Boyd, and H. W. Mossman, *Human Embryology: Prenatal Development of Form and Function* (Baltimore: Williams & Wilkins, 1962), fig. 86, p. 85.]

drugs cross the placenta primarily by passive diffusion. Fat-soluble substances (including all psychoactive drugs!) diffuse across readily, rapidly, and without limitation. That drugs profoundly affect the fetus is illustrated by the withdrawal symptoms observed in infants born of alcohol-, narcotic-, and cocaine-addicted mothers.

Tranquilizing and sedating drugs also cross the placenta readily. The blood levels of a barbiturate administered intravenously to mothers during labor are plotted in Figure 2.9. The blood concentrations of the drug were determined in both maternal and fetal blood. One can see from this figure that significant amounts of the barbiturate are distributed to the infant and that blood levels in the mother and the newborn baby are almost identical about 10 minutes after injection.

The view that the placenta is a barrier to psychoactive drugs is inaccurate. In contrast, the fetus receives (and is therefore exposed to) all psychoactive drugs taken by the mother, with fetal levels of drug usually equaling those achieved in the mother.

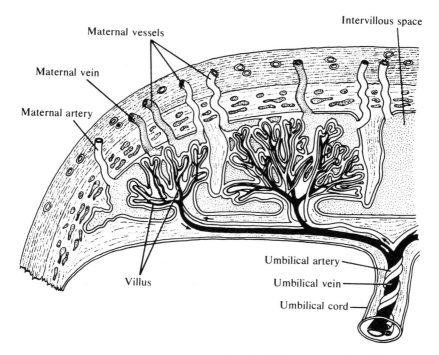

FIGURE 2.8 Placental network separating the blood of mother and fetus. [From C. M. Goss, ed., *Gray's Anatomy of the Human Body,* 29th ed. (Philadelphia: Lea and Febiger, 1973), fig. 2.51, p. 40.]

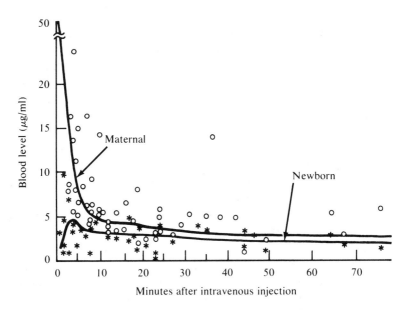

FIGURE 2.9 Effect of barbiturate on mothers in labor. Blood levels of secobarbital in mothers and their newborn infants after intravenous administration of the drug to the mothers . Each point represents one subject (*circles,* mothers; *asterisks,* infants). [From B. Root, E. Eichner, and I. Sunshine, "Blood Secobarbital Levels and Their Clinical Correlation in Mothers and Newborn Infants," *American Journal of Obstetrics and Gynecology* 81 (1961): 948.]

Termination of Drug Action

The main routes through which drugs leave the body are (1) the kidneys, (2) the lungs, and (3) the bile. Excretion through the lungs occurs only with highly volatile or gaseous agents such as the general anesthetics and, in small amounts, alcohol ("alcohol breath"). Drugs that are passed through the bile and into the intestine are usually reabsorbed into the bloodstream from the intestine. Thus, the majority of drugs leave the body in urine. More correctly, as we shall see next, the major route of drug elimination from the body is *renal excretion of drug metabolites following the hepatic (liver) biodegradation of the drug into drug metabolites.*

In general, the same lipid-soluble properties of psychoactive drugs that facilitate rapid transport across cellular membranes into the brain also impair their subsequent excretion by the kidneys. In order for the drug to be eliminated, it must be metabolically transformed (by enzymes located in the liver) into a form that can be excreted rapidly and reliably. Such biotransformation relieves the body of the burden of foreign chemicals and is essential to our survival.[1]

Elimination of Drugs by the Kidneys and Liver

Physiologically, our kidneys perform two major functions. First, they excrete most of the products of body metabolism; second, they closely regulate the levels of most of the substances found in body fluids. The kidneys are a pair of bean-shaped organs (Figure 2.10), each a little smaller than a fist and weighing about a quarter of a pound. They lie at the rear of the abdominal cavity at the level of the lower ribs.

The outer portion of the kidney is made up of over a million functional units, called *nephrons* (Figure 2.11). Each unit consists of a knot of capillaries (the glomerulus) through which blood flows from the renal artery to the renal vein. The glomerulus is surrounded by the opening of the nephron (Bowman's capsule), into which fluid flows as it filters out of the capillaries. Pressure of the blood in the glomerulus causes fluid to leave the capillaries and flow into Bowman's capsule, from which it flows through the tubules of the nephrons and, finally, into a duct that collects fluid from several nephrons. This fluid from the collecting ducts is eventually passed through the ureters and into the urinary bladder, which is emptied periodically.

In an adult, about one liter of plasma is filtered into the nephrons of the kidneys each minute. Left behind in the bloodstream are blood cells, plasma proteins, and the remaining plasma. As the filtered fluid flows through the nephrons, substances that are not reabsorbed pass into the urinary bladder for excretion later.

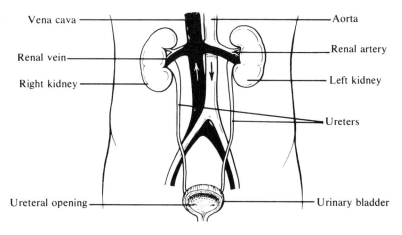

FIGURE 2.10 Architecture of the kidneys.

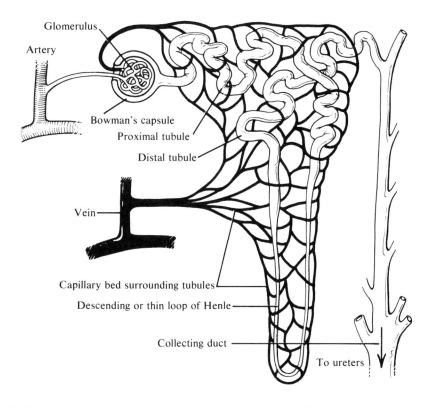

FIGURE 2.11 Nephron within a kidney. Note the complexity of the structure and the intimate relation between the blood supply and the nephron. Each kidney is composed of more than a million such nephrons.

Because drugs are small particles, they are filtered into the kidneys and then reabsorbed into the bloodstream. As the drug become concentrated inside the nephrons (as a result of water reabsorption), the drugs are themselves reabsorbed into plasma. Thus, the kidneys alone cannot eliminate drugs from the body. Some other mechanism must therefore overcome this process of drug reabsorption. What occurs is that the drug is enzymatically biotransformed in the liver into a compound that is less fat soluble and therefore less capable of being reabsorbed (Figure 2.12). This process of *hepatic biotransformation* results in the conversion of fat-soluble drugs into water-soluble *metabolites* that are poorly reabsorbed once they are filtered into the renal tubules.

Free drug (that is, drug not bound to plasma proteins) is carried to the liver (by blood flowing in the hepatic artery and portal vein), and a portion is "cleared" from the blood by the liver cells and metabolized to by-products (metabolites), which are returned to the bloodstream (see Figure 2.12). These metabolites are then transported in the bloodstream to the kidneys for excretion.

Usually (but not always) this process of metabolism decreases the pharmacological activity of the drug. Thus, even though a metabolite might persist in the body, it is usually in a pharmacologically inactive

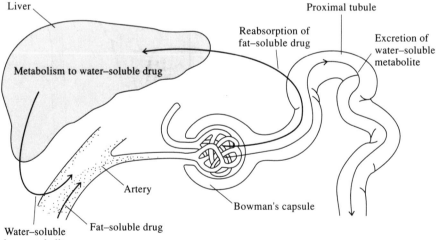

FIGURE 2.12 How liver and kidneys eliminate drugs from the body. Drugs may be filtered into the kidney, reabsorbed into the bloodstream, and carried to the liver for metabolic transformation to a more water-soluble compound that, having been filtered into the kidney, cannot be reabsorbed and is therefore excreted in urine.

form and does not produce the effects of the parent drug. Sometimes, however, the metabolite is pharmacologically active (in some instances, even more active than the parent drug); in such cases the metabolite is usually further metabolized to an inactive compound. Examples of this phenomenon are presented later in this text.

A description of the exact mechanisms by which the liver alters a drug's chemical structure is beyond the scope of our discussion, but suffice it to state that the reactions are carried out by a special system of enzymes in the liver cells. Many psychoactive drugs have the ability to increase the rate at which this enzyme system metabolizes a variety of such drugs, including themselves, thereby increasing the speed with which the drugs are eliminated. Drugs increase both the enzymatic activity of these cells and the total amount of drug-metabolizing enzymes present in the liver. This enzyme-induction process is one mechanism for producing pharmacological tolerance, whereby increasing doses of a drug must be administered to maintain the same level of drug in plasma and thus produce the same effect that smaller doses produced earlier.

Because these enzymes have a low specificity for drugs (that is, one enzyme may metabolize many different types of drugs), an increase in the metabolizing enzymes induced by one drug will increase the enzymes' rate of metabolizing not only that particular drug but also a variety of others. This process of *cross-tolerance* will be elaborated on later in this chapter.

Earlier, we discussed how drugs from the mother are distributed to the fetus through the placenta. While the fetus is attached to the mother, those drugs may be excreted through the umbilical cord back into the mother's bloodstream. The mother can then eliminate the drug through her liver and kidneys. After delivery, however, the newborn baby must get rid of the drug by itself. Unfortunately, the newborn (especially the premature infant) has few drug-metabolizing enzymes in its liver, and its kidneys may not yet be fully functional. Therefore, the infant has great difficulty metabolizing and excreting drugs. If it has received a high concentration of depressants (anesthetics, narcotics, and so on) from the mother, the infant may be depressed for a long time after delivery.

Other Routes of Drug Elimination

Other routes for excreting drugs include the lungs, bile (both discussed already), sweat, saliva, and breast milk. Many drugs and drug metabolites may be found in the latter three secretions; however, their concentrations are usually low, and these routes are not usually considered primary paths of drug elimination. Occasionally, however, concern arises over the transfer of psychoactive drugs (such as nicotine) from mothers to their breast-fed babies. Similarly, concern has been expressed about the secretion of antibiotics, administered to cows, into milk that is ultimately consumed by humans. These topics are of obvious importance to the pharmacologist and to the Food and Drug Administration, especially because guidelines for such uses of drugs are needed to minimize danger to the public.

Time Course of Drug Distribution and Elimination

Concept of Drug Half-Life

Knowledge about the relationship between the initial concentration of a drug in the body and the concentration at some time after its administration is essential for (1) predicting the optimal dosages and dose intervals needed to reach a therapeutic effect, (2) maintaining a therapeutic drug level for the desired period of time, and (3) determining the time needed to eliminate the drug. Indeed, it is a fundamental of pharmacology that there is a relationship between the pharmacological or toxic response to a drug and its concentration at a readily measurable site in the body (for example, in blood). Furthermore, the therapeutic drug level (as measured in blood) correlates with the level of drug at the "receptor site" (see Figure 2.1).

Figure 2.13 illustrates this time-concentration relationship for a drug administered intravenously to a rat. Note that after injection, the drug concentration in plasma peaked, fell rapidly, and then declined more slowly. The rapid fall reflects distribution of the drug throughout the body after intravenous injection. The steeply sloped line in Figure 2.13 (tangent line A) represents the blood-flow-independent, rapid-distribution phase. The rapid-distribution phase is represented by a *distribution half-life*, which indicates the time it takes for distribution to reduce the initial peak level of the drug by 50 percent. If the distribution process were to lower the plasma drug level below that required for a pharmacological effect (indicated by the dotted horizontal line), the therapeutic effect would be quite short-lived; more of the drug would have to be administered to continue the effect.

The slower decrease (tangent line B) represents the time required for the body to eliminate the drug through metabolism (by the liver) and the excretion of metabolites (by the kidneys). The calculated elimination half-life is a measure of this process, and it allows the time course of drug action to be calculated.

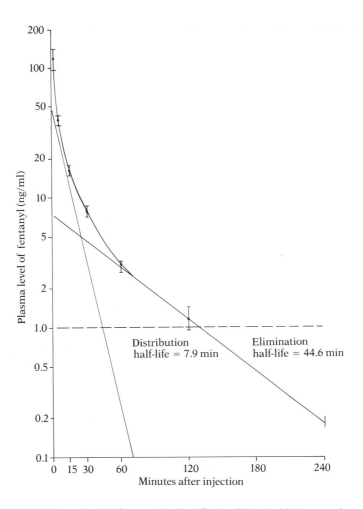

FIGURE 2.13   Plasma levels of a narcotic drug (fentanyl) injected intravenously into a rat in a single bolus dose of 50 micrograms per kilogram body weight. The distribution and elimination half-lives are shown as 7.9 and 44.6 minutes, respectively. The horizontal line drawn at 1 nanogram (billionths of a gram) per milliliter plasma concentration is the level needed for analgesic effect. Thus, analgesia would be lost about 130 minutes after drug injection. [Data from C. C. Hug, Jr., and M. R. Murphy, "Tissue Redistribution of Fentanyl and Termination of Its Effects in Rats," *Anesthesiology* 55 (1981): 369–375.]

Figure 2.13 shows that the peak levels of pain relief produced by the drug fentanyl (a narcotic analgesic) are reached within seconds after intravenous injection. Fentanyl is highly lipid soluble and is rapidly redistributed to muscle and fat, reducing blood concentrations of the drug in the process. The elimination half-life is about 45 minutes.

TABLE 2.2   Half-life calculations.

Number of half-lives	Amount of drug in the body	
	Percent eliminated	Percent remaining
0	0	100
1	50	50
2	75	25
3	87.5	12.5
4	93.8	6.2
5	96.9	3.1
6	98.4	1.6

As shown in Table 2.2, it takes four half-lives for 90 percent of a drug to be eliminated by the body (3 hours) and six half-lives for 98 percent to be eliminated (4.5 hours). At that point, the patient is, for most practical purposes, drug-free. It is important to remember that even though the analgesia became minimal after 2 hours, the drug persists at low levels in a patient's body for up to 4.5 hours. The so-called drug hangover is a result of such a prolonged elimination half-life. Whenever it is appropriate throughout the text, drug half-lives will be cited to describe the duration of action of psychoactive drugs in the body. Some drug half-lives can be measured by days; thus, recovery from the drug may take a week or more. Diazepam (Valium) is an example of a drug that can have a half-life lasting several days, especially in the elderly. This is discussed further in Chapter 4.

Drug Half-Life, Accumulation, and Steady State

Not only is the biological half-life of a drug the time required for the drug concentration in blood to fall by one-half, but it is also the determinant of the length of time necessary to reach a steady state of concentration.[3] If one administers a second full dose of drug before the body has eliminated the first dose, the total amount of drug in the body and the peak level of the drug in blood will be greater than the total amount and peak level produced by the first dose. For example, if 100 milligrams of a drug with a 4-hour half-life were administered at 12 o'clock noon, 50 milligrams of drug would remain in the body at 4 P.M. If an additional 100 milligrams of drug were then taken at 4 o'clock, 75 milligrams of drug would remain in the body at 8 o'clock

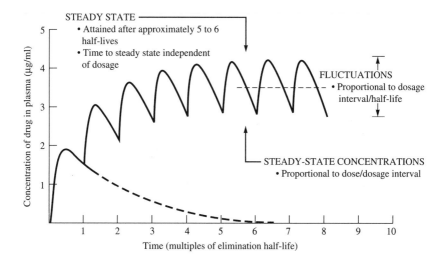

FIGURE 2.14   Plasma drug concentrations during repeated oral administration of a drug at intervals equal to its elimination half-life. The dashed line illustrates the elimination curve if only a single dose is given. Since only 50 percent of each dose is eliminated before the next dose is given, the drug accumulates, reaching steady-state concentration in 5 to 6 half-lives. The sinusoidal curve shows the maximal and minimal drug concentrations at the beginning and end of each dosage interval, respectively. The dotted line illustrates the average concentration achieved at steady state.

(25 milligrams of the first dose and 50 milligrams of the second). If this administration schedule were continued, the amount of drug in the body would continue to increase until a plateau, or steady state, concentration was reached (Figure 2.14).

In general, the time to reach steady-state concentration is about six times the drug's elimination half-life and is independent of the actual dosage of the drug. The reason for this is as follows. In one half-life, a drug reaches 50 percent of the concentration that will eventually be achieved. As shown above, after two half-lives, the drug achieves 75 percent concentration; at three half-lives, the drug achieves the initial 50 percent (of the third dose), the next 25 percent (from the second dose), plus half of the remaining 25 percent (from the first dose). At 98.4 percent (the concentration achieved after six half-lives), the drug concentration is essentially at steady state; this is the rationale behind our general rule. The *steady-state concentration* (the level of drug achieved in blood with repeated, regular-interval dosing) is achieved when the amount administered per unit time equals the amount eliminated per unit time. The interdependent variables that determine the

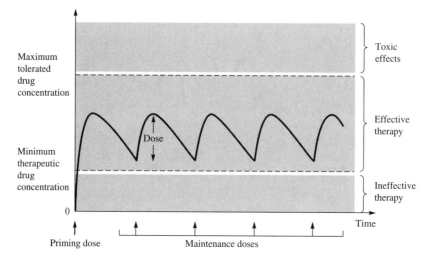

FIGURE 2.15   The blood concentration of a drug is plotted in arbitrary units against time on the abscissa. The dashed lines are placed at the blood concentrations that bracket the minimal therapeutic drug concentration and the maximal tolerated drug concentration. After the initial *priming dose,* the peak concentration rises into the effective therapeutic, but not toxic, range of blood concentrations. The administration of *maintenance doses* of the appropriate dose and frequency keeps the blood concentration out of the ineffective zone and below the level associated with toxic effects. [From C. M. Smith and A. M. Reynard, *Textbook of Pharmacology* (Philadelphia: Saunders, 1992), p. 70.]

ultimate concentration (or steady-state blood level of drug) are the dose (which determines the blood level but not the time to steady state), the dose interval, the half-life of the drug, and other, more complex factors that can affect drug elimination.

In summary, steady, regular-interval dosing leads to a predictable accumulation, with a steady-state concentration reached after about six half-lives; the magnitude of the concentration is proportional to dose and dosage interval. Clinically, these factors guide drug therapy when blood levels of drug are monitored and correlated with therapeutic results (Figure 2.15).

In law enforcement, these facts about drug half-lives are used to estimate the blood level of alcohol at a specific, earlier time when the only available fact is the blood level of alcohol at a known time after an event (such as an automobile accident).

Therapeutic Drug Monitoring

Therapeutic drug monitoring (TDM) can make a critical difference in therapeutic applications. Indeed, in psychopharmacology, TDM can dramatically improve the prognosis of psychiatric disorders, making previously difficult-to-treat disorders much more treatable.[4]

The basic principle underlying TDM is that a threshold plasma concentration of a drug is needed at the receptor site in order to initiate and maintain a pharmacological response. Critically important is that plasma concentrations of psychoactive drugs correlate well with tissue or receptor concentrations. Therefore, TDM is an indirect, although usually quite accurate, measurement of drug concentration at the receptor site in the tissue of interest (here, the CNS). To make the correlation between TDM, dosage, and therapeutic response, large-scale clinical trials are performed, and blood samples are drawn at multiple time periods during both acute and chronic (long-term) therapy. Statistical correlation is made between the level of drug in plasma and the degree of therapeutic response. A dosage regimen can then be designed to achieve this plasma level of drug.

Limiting factors to TDM include the following: imprecision in detecting and quantifying improvement in psychiatric illness, difficulty in detecting early signs of toxicity, and delays in the onset of therapeutic response.

The goals of TDM are many. One goal is to assess whether a patient is taking medication as prescribed; if plasma levels of the drug are below the therapeutic level (because the patient has not been taking the required medication), therapeutic results will be poor. Another goal is to avoid toxicity: If plasma levels of the drug are above the therapeutic level, the dosage can be lowered, effectiveness maintained, and toxicity minimized. A third goal is to enhance therapeutic response by focusing not on the amount of drug taken but on the measured amount of drug in plasma. Other goals include possible reductions in the cost of therapy (since a patient's illness is better controlled) and the substantiation of the need for unusually high doses in patients who require higher-than-normal intake of prescribed medication.

Drug Tolerance and Dependence

Drug tolerance may be defined as a state of progressively decreasing responsiveness to a drug. A person who develops tolerance requires a larger dose of the drug to achieve the effect originally obtained by a smaller dose.

At least three mechanisms are involved in developing drug tolerance: Two are pharmacological mechanisms, and one is a behavioral mechanism. *Metabolic tolerance* is the first of the two classically described types of pharmacological tolerance. Here, the presence of drugs in blood perfusing the liver induces the synthesis of hepatic drug-metabolizing enzymes that are involved in the metabolism of drugs and other chemicals by the liver. Because of this enzyme induction, drugs are metabolized at a faster rate, and so more drug must be given to maintain the same level of drug in the body. A second type of pharmacological tolerance is *cellular-adaptive* (or *pharmacodynamic*) *tolerance*. Here receptors in the brain adapt to the continued presence of the drug. Neurons adapt either by increasing the number of receptors (thereby requiring more drug to occupy them) or by reducing their sensitivity to the drug (a process called "down regulation"). With pharmacodynamic tolerance, higher levels of drug in plasma are necessary to maintain the same biological effect. This effect is seen in people who develop problems with narcotics, barbiturates, and alcohol (although in the latter two, enzyme induction is also involved).

More recently identified is the role of *behavioral conditioning processes* in the development of tolerance. Indeed, simple exposure of drugs to receptors does not account for the substantial degree of tolerance that many people acquire to opioids, barbiturates, ethyl alcohol, and other drugs. Here, tolerance can be demonstrated when a drug is administered in the context of usual predrug cues, but not in the context of alternative cues.[5] Poulos and Cappell propose a model of *homeostatic theory of drug tolerance*.[6] They found that, with morphine analgesia, testing in an environment in which tolerance had developed effected the manifestation of tolerance, and an environmental cue could maintain the tolerance. This "contingent tolerance" is pervasive and represents a general process underlying the development of all forms of systemic tolerance.

> The environmental cues routinely paired with drug administration will become conditioned stimuli that elicit a conditioned response that is opposite in direction to, or compensation for, the direct effects of the drug. Over conditioning trials, the compensatory conditioned response grows in magnitude and counteracts the direct drug effects, that is, tolerance develops.[7]

An example of enzyme-induction tolerance is presented in Table 2.3. In the experiment, rabbits were pretreated with three daily doses of pentobarbital (a short-acting barbiturate) and then given a single challenging dose of pentobarbital. The length of time that the rabbits slept and the amount of pentobarbital in the animals' bloodstreams at

TABLE 2.3 Effect of pentobarbital pretreatment on the duration of pentobarbital action.

Pretreatment	Sleeping time (min)	Plasma level of pentobarbital on awakening (μg/ml)	Pentobarbital half-life in plasma (min)
None	67 ± 4	9.9 ± 1.4	79 ± 3
Pentobarbital	30 ± 7	7.9 ± 0.6	26 ± 2

Source: H. Remmer, "Drugs as Activators of Drug Enzymes," in B. B. Brodie and E. G. Erdos, eds., Metabolic Factors Controlling Duration of Drug Action (Proceedings of the First International Pharmacological Meeting), vol. 6 (New York: Macmillan, 1962), p. 235.
Note: Rabbits were pretreated with three daily doses of pentobarbital (60 mg/kg) subcutaneously, then given a single challenging dose of 60 mg/kg intravenously.

the time of awakening were measured and compared with the sleeping time and the blood levels of pentobarbital in rabbits that were not pretreated but were given an identical dose of the drug. Although the pretreated animals slept less than half as long as the control rabbits, their blood levels of the drug on awakening were approximately the same. Pretreatment had raised the animals' tolerance for the drug not by affecting the "sleep center" in the brain, but by inducing metabolizing enzymes in the liver, which caused the drug to be metabolized and excreted more rapidly.

Physical dependence is an entirely different phenomenon, even though it is associated with drug tolerance in most cases. A person who is physically dependent on a drug needs it to function normally. The state of physical dependence is revealed by withdrawing the drug and noting the occurrence of withdrawal symptoms (*abstinence syndrome*) some time after the drug has been withheld. The symptoms of withdrawal can be terminated by readministering the drug.

PHARMACODYNAMICS: DRUG–RECEPTOR INTERACTIONS

Before producing any pharmacological effect, a drug must physically interact with one or more constituents of a cell. The cell component that is directly involved in the initial action of a drug is called the receptor. One of the basic concepts in pharmacology is that drug

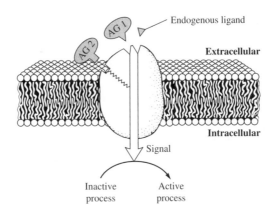

FIGURE 2.16   Diagrammatic representation of classical receptors located on a membrane-spanning protein. A type I agonist (AG 1) fits the receptor site for an endogenous ligand. A type II agonist (AG 2) binds to an adjacent site, thereby influencing (amplifying) signal transmission. Signal transmission activates intracellular processes that are inactive without receptor activation.

molecules must attach to specific receptors either on a cell membrane or within a cell, and such occupation (of a receptor) by a drug must lead to a change in the functional properties of that cell, thus producing a pharmacological response. As described below, drug occupation of a receptor either activates (an *agonist* action) or inactivates (an *antagonist* action) that receptor. Ultimately, this drug–receptor interaction produces a cascade of cellular events involving changes in subcellular components of the target cell, resulting in clinically relevant therapeutic effects and side effects.[8,9]

Figure 2.16 illustrates several important points about drug–receptor interactions.[9] First, receptors are usually located on the surface of membrane-spanning proteins. These proteins, in turn, have one or more types of binding sites, usually for one endogenous transmitter chemical ("ligand"); these sites can be differentiated pharmacologically.

Second, attachment (reversible binding) of the endogenous ligand specific for that receptor activates the receptor, usually by changing the structure of the protein. This change allows a signal to be transmitted through the membrane to the intracellular side of the cell membrane.

Third, the intensity of the resulting transmembrane signal is determined either by the percentage of the available receptors that are occupied by the endogenous ligand (or exogenous agonist drug) or by the rate of reversible binding by either the ligand or the drug.

Fourth, a drug can either enhance or diminish the generation, transmission, or receipt of the transmembrane signal by binding to the receptor for the endogenous ligand. Binding accompanied by drug-induced mimicry of ligand action is an agonist (or stimulant) action. Drug occupation of a receptor that is not accompanied by ligand-like activation blocks the access of the ligand to the receptor and is an antagonist (or inhibitory) action. Agonists and antagonists can bind either to the ligand binding site (to activate or block transduction), to other sites that influence signal transmission within the membrane, or to intracellular signal reception points (Figure 2.16).

Drug–Receptor Affinity

A characteristic of the drug receptor is its high (but not absolute) degree of specificity (or *affinity*) for a particular drug molecule. What may appear to be a slight or insignificant variation in the chemical structure of a drug may greatly alter the intensity of a cell's response to it. For example, amphetamine and methamphetamine are both power-ful stimulants of the central nervous system (CNS). Although their chemical composition is extremely similar, methamphetamine is much more potent and produces much greater behavioral stimulation at the same dosage. Both drugs probably affect the same receptors in the brain, but methamphetamine exerts a much more powerful action on them.

The drug molecule with the "best fit" to the receptor will elicit the greatest response from the cell. Thus, methamphetamine might fit the receptor better than amphetamine does. It is currently thought that the cellular response that follows the attachment of a drug to its receptor is followed by a change in the conformation of the cell membrane that ultimately alters brain or body function.

Selectivity or specificity of drug action is not due to the selective distribution of drug molecules; rather, it is a function of the selective localization of drug receptors, the specificity of drugs that bind to particular receptors, the strength of the drug's attachment, and the consequences of the interaction between drugs and their receptors.

Current drug research is attempting to characterize in molecular terms (and in more and more detail) the primary sites and mecha-nisms of drug action. A drug with a seemingly wide variety of actions can frequently be shown to act quite specifically on a particular type of cell or tissue component (such as an enzyme, a specific neurotrans-mitter, a DNA molecule, and so on). For example, aspirin exerts a wide variety of effects (analgesic, anti-inflammatory, and fever reducing), most of which can be explained in terms of inhibition of the action of one or more of the enzymes that are involved in the inflammatory process. Similarly, the benzodiazepine tranquilizers may exert their sedative, antianxiety, and antiepileptic actions by interacting with specific receptor sites in the brain, thereby potentiating the action of an inhibitory neurotransmitter (gamma-aminobutyric acid) (Chapter 4). One goal of this text will be to demonstrate, whenever possible, those single actions that may account for the wide variety of effects that a drug or specific class of drugs produces.

That drugs act on specific molecular receptors has three important implications. First, a drug is potentially capable of altering the rate at which any bodily (or brain) function proceeds. Second, a drug does not create effects but merely modulates ongoing functions. Third, a drug cannot impart new functions to a cell.

The affinity of a drug for its receptor (that is, its ability to bind to a receptor), its intrinsic activity (agonist versus antagonist), and its potency are intimately related to the drug's chemical structure. Indeed, in this text, chemical structures are illustrated only to demonstrate that small structural changes can result in profound differences in action. This presumably follows from the supposition that small structural changes can significantly alter the fit of a drug for its receptor, significantly affecting the drug-induced conformational changes that occur in the three-dimensional structure of a receptor.

It should be noted that receptors themselves are subject to many regulatory, intrinsic, homeostatic controls, and their sensitivity (and even their absolute numbers) can be modulated (increased or decreased). Such mechanisms appear to be involved in the mechanisms of pharmacodynamic tolerance, genetic variability, and so on.

Dose–Response Relationship

One way of quantifying drug–receptor interactions (that is, the formation of reversible drug–receptor complexes) is to use what are known as *dose–response curves*. In Figure 2.17, two types of dose–response curves are illustrated. In graph A, the dose is plotted against the percentage of persons who exhibit a characteristic effect. In graph B, the dose is plotted against the intensity, or the magnitude, of the response in a single person. These curves indicate that a dose exists that is low enough to produce little or no effect; at the opposite extreme, a dose exists beyond which no greater response can be elicited.

All dose–response curves demonstrate important characteristics, three of which are *potency* (the absolute amount of drug necessary to

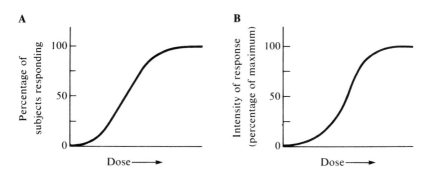

FIGURE 2.17 Two types of dose–response curves. **(A)** Curve obtained by plotting the dose of drug against the percentage of subjects showing a given response at any given dose. **(B)** Curve obtained by plotting the dose of drug against the intensity of response observed in any single individual at a given dose. The intensity of response is plotted as a percentage of the maximum obtainable response.

produce a defined effect), *efficacy* (the maximum effect obtainable), and the *dose* required to produce the maximum effect (Figure 2.17B). Finally, one can use dose–response curves to estimate variability of response and drug safety. The latter two factors are discussed in the next section.

The location of the dose–response curve along the horizontal axis reflects the potency of the drug. If two drugs produce sedation, but one exerts this action at half the dose level of the other, the first drug is considered to be twice as potent as the second drug. Potency, however, is a relatively unimportant characteristic of a drug, because it makes little difference whether the effective dose of a drug is 0.1 gram or 10 grams as long as the drug is administered in an appropriate dose with no undue toxicity. Thus, a more potent drug is not necessarily a better one. High potency, in fact, is usually a disadvantage, because an extremely potent drug may be much more toxic (or dangerous) and require much more careful administration to reach a given therapeutic or behavioral endpoint.

Slope refers to the more or less linear, central portion of the dose–response curve. A steep slope on a dose–response curve implies that there is only a small difference between the dose that produces a desired effect and the dose that causes toxicity. The steeper the slope, the smaller the increase in dose that is required to go from a minimum response to a maximum effect.

The peak of the dose–response curve indicates the maximum effect, or efficacy, that can be produced by a drug, regardless of further

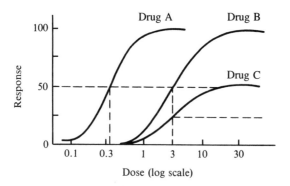

FIGURE 2.18 Dose–response curves for three drugs. See text for discussion.

increases in dose. Not all psychoactive drugs can exert the same level of effect. For example, caffeine, even in massive doses, cannot exert the same intensity of CNS stimulation that amphetamine can. Similarly, aspirin can never achieve the maximum analgesic effect that morphine does. Thus, the maximum effect is an inherent property of a drug and is one measure of a drug's efficacy. Most psychoactive drugs, however, are not used to the point of their maximum effect, because side effects limit the upper range of dosage. Thus, the usefulness of a compound is correspondingly limited, even though the drug may be inherently capable of producing a greater effect.

To review these concepts, evaluate the three curves in Figure 2.18. Drugs A and B exhibit the same maximum response, and drug C has significantly less efficacy (less intrinsic activity). Drug B is about 10 times less potent than drug A, while drug C is equally as potent as drug B. Drug C has a flatter slope than either drug A or drug B. Thus, drug C may be easier to administer despite its lower intrinsic activity. Note that these curves do not predict safety, side effects, toxicity, or therapeutic superiority.

DRUG SAFETY AND EFFECTIVENESS

Variability in Drug Responsiveness

Variability is another factor to be considered when evaluating drug responses. The dose of a drug that will produce a specific response will vary considerably among subjects. Figure 2.19 illustrates a Gaussian (bell-shaped) distribution of drug variability in a population of animals. Although the average dose required to elicit a given response in this population of animals can be calculated easily (illustrated by the dotted line), some animals respond at doses that are very much lower than the average and others only respond at doses that are very much higher. Thus it is extremely important that the dose of all drugs be individualized. Generalizations about "average doses" are risky at best. Because of the Gaussian distribution, however, we can estimate the dose of a drug that will produce the desired effect in 50 percent of the subjects. This dose is called the ED_{50} for the drug (the effective dose for 50 percent of the subjects). Similarly, we can estimate an LD_{50} (lethal dose for 50 percent of the subjects). The LD_{50} is calculated in exactly the same way as the ED_{50} except that the dose of the drug is plotted against the number of animals that die after being administered various doses of the compound. Both the ED_{50} and the LD_{50} must be determined to prevent accidental drug-induced deaths in humans. Both the ED_{50} and the LD_{50} are usually determined in laboratory mice, and the ratio of the LD_{50} to the ED_{50} is used as an index of the relative safety of the drug, called the *therapeutic index*.

To illustrate, two dose–response curves are shown in Figure 2.20. The curve at the left illustrates the dose of drug necessary to induce sleep in a population of mice, and the one at the right illustrates the dose of drug necessary to kill a similar population. In this example, the LD_{50}:ED50 ratio is seen to be 100:10, or 10. This may seem like a

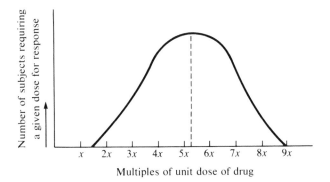

FIGURE 2.19   Biological variation in susceptibility to drugs. This curve is a Gaussian distribution, with the dose of drug plotted against the number of subjects requiring a given dose for a given response to occur. Note that, for a given response, some animals will require only a small amount of the drug while others will require much more than what is considered normal.

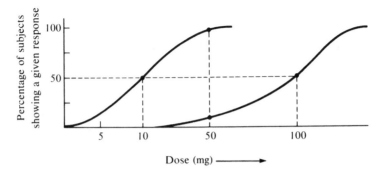

FIGURE 2.20 Two dose–response curves. *Left,* the dose of drug required to induce a given response. *Right,* the lethal dose of the compound.

rather large margin, but note that, at a dose of 50 milligrams, 95 percent of the mice sleep while 5 percent of the mice die. This overlap demonstrates both the difficulty in assessing the relative safety of drugs for use in large populations and the biological variation in individual responses to drugs. With this particular compound, a dose cannot be administered that guarantees that 100 percent of the mice will sleep and none will die. Thus, a more useful indication of the margin of safety is a ratio of the lethal dose for 1 percent of the population to the effective dose for 99 percent of the population ($LD_1:ED_{99}$). A sedative drug with an $LD_1:ED_{99}$ of 1 would be a safer compound than the drug illustrated in Figure 2.20.

Note that such indices, which are obtained from laboratory animals, are of limited usefulness, because they do not reflect the occasional unexpected response that can seriously harm a patient. Variability, either among different persons or in the same person on different occasions, results from (1) differing concentrations of the drug at its site of action, (2) differing physiological responses to the same drug concentrations, and (3) unusual, idiosyncratic (genetically determined) or allergic (immunologically sensitized) responses that are wholly unanticipated.

Variations of the first kind result from differences in how a dose of drug affects people (pharmacokinetic variation) due to differences in drug absorption, distribution, metabolism, and excretion. Variations of the second kind result from variations in response to a similar concentration of a drug at the receptor (pharmacodynamic variation). For example, receptors could be either desensitized or hypersensitive to the drug. Age, genetic factors, drug interactions, and certain disease states all contribute to variability in how sensitive receptors are to a drug.

These causes of variability will be discussed as we consider individual drugs.

Drug variability is intimately associated with drug toxicity. Therefore, the side effects that are invariably associated with a drug, as well as its more serious toxicities (including those that can be fatal), must always be considered.

Drug Interactions

It is widely appreciated that the effects of one drug can be modified by the concurrent administration of another drug. This is particularly important in psychopharmacology.[10] For example, alcohol taken after a sleeping pill or a tranquilizer has been ingested increases sedation and the loss of coordination. This action may have little consequence if the doses of each drug are low (one or two tablets and one or two drinks), but higher doses of either or both drugs can be dangerous both to the user and to others. Even though a person may normally be able to ingest a limited amount of alcohol and still drive a car without significant loss of control or coordination, the concurrent ingestion of a tranquilizer may profoundly impair his or her driving performance, endangering the driver, the passengers, and other motorists. Numerous other examples could be given, and one must always be aware of the danger of significant interactions that can occur when two or more drugs are taken at the same time.

We have already discussed two of the primary factors that contribute to drug interactions: protein binding of drugs and cross-tolerance caused by drug-metabolizing enzymes. Both processes are relatively nonspecific and can result in clinically important interactions of two or more drugs. For example, with protein binding, if a second drug competes for the same binding site and displaces a drug that has already bound to a protein, more of the previously bound drug will be freed to pass out of the bloodstream and, therefore, be available to the receptor. Thus, a more intense effect may be produced as the second drug (the displacing drug) increases the effects or the toxicity of the first drug (the displaced drug).

As can be seen, a wide variety of factors influence a drug's action in the body, making the use of more than one drug at a time risky, whether the drugs are used separately or mixed in one concoction. Mixtures often complicate therapy, because in many cases it has not been established whether more than one drug is needed; furthermore, if toxic effects do occur, it can be difficult to determine which drug is responsible.

Drug Toxicity

All drugs can produce harmful effects as well as beneficial ones. The nature of these unwanted effects falls into two categories:[11] (1) effects that are related to the principal pharmacological action of a drug and (2) effects that are unrelated to this action.

It is important to categorize harmful effects of drugs in terms of their severity and to distinguish between those effects that cause a temporary inconvenience or discomfort and those that can lead to permanent disability or death. Many unwanted effects in the first category can be readily predicted from knowledge about the mode of action of a drug.

Virtually all drugs exert effects on several different body functions, despite the fact that one is usually interested in obtaining a single, or perhaps a small number of, the drug's many possible effects. The desired effect is usually considered the *main effect,* while the unwanted effects are labeled *side effects.* To achieve the main effect, the side effects must be tolerated; this is possible if the side effects are minor, but if they are more serious, they may be a limiting factor in the use of the drug.

The distinction between main effects and side effects is relative and depends on the purpose of the drug. One person's side effect may be another person's main effect. For example, in one patient morphine's pain-relieving properties may be sought, while the intestinal constipation that morphine induces becomes an undesirable side effect that must be tolerated. For a second patient, however, morphine may be used to treat diarrhea, in which case the constipation induced is the main effect and any relief of pain becomes a side effect.

In addition to side effects that are merely irritating, some drugs may cause reactions that are very serious. Such side effects include serious allergies, blood disorders, liver or kidney toxicity, or abnormalities in fetal development. Fortunately, the incidence of these serious toxic effects is quite low.

Allergies to drugs may take many forms, from mild skin rashes to fatal shock. Allergies differ from normal side effects, which can often be eliminated or at least made tolerable by a simple reduction in dosage. However, a reduction in the dose of a drug may have no effect on a drug allergy, because exposure to any amount of the drug can be hazardous and possibly catastrophic for the patient.

Organ damage to the liver and kidneys results from their role in concentrating, metabolizing, and excreting toxic drugs. One example of drug-induced liver damage is that caused by alcohol. Similarly, a class of major tranquilizers, the phenothiazines (for example, chlorpromazine [Thorazine]), may induce jaundice by increasing the viscosity of bile in the liver.

The thalidomide tragedy dramatically illustrated how the side effects of drugs can harm fetal development. The seriousness of the problem of drug action on the fetus and the wide range of possible consequences was noted as early as 1968:

> It is clear that the risks of chemical teratogenesis . . . are accentuated during the first trimester of pregnancy. Until much more information becomes available, the very diversity of known teratogens and mutagens (drugs that alter the structure of chromosomes in the cell) should dictate caution. . . . A woman who is known to be pregnant should not be exposed to drugs at all during the first trimester unless the need is pressing. At least until experimental or statistical investigations show them to be harmless, caffeine, nicotine, and alcohol, to which people are so frequently exposed, should be regarded as possibly hazardous to the fetus during the first three months of pregnancy.[12]

Finally, the toxicity to fetuses of socially abused drugs should be mentioned. The considerable data compiled since 1968 quite clearly show the adverse effects of nicotine and ethyl alcohol on the fetus. More recently, the effects of cocaine abuse on the fetus have received much attention. Indeed, these drugs are thought to be responsible for a majority of preventable fetal toxicities and are three of the major health hazards in the country today.

Placebo Effects

The term *placebo* refers to a pharmacologically inert substance that elicits a significant therapeutic response. Placebos work best on symptoms or diseases that vary (wax and wane) over time; perhaps the most prominent examples are major depression and chronic pain.[13–16] Because the placebo action is independent of any chemical property of the drug, it arises largely because of what the patient expects or desires. A placebo response may result from a person's mental set or from the entire environmental setting in which the drug is taken. In certain predisposed persons, a placebo may produce extremely strong reactions with far-reaching consequences. Indeed, placebos can therapeutically empower patients to stimulate their psychophysiological self-regulation abilities. Possible mechanisms for the placebo effect include conditioning, expectancy, and self-liberation of endogenous neurotransmitters, including endorphins and adrenalin-like catecholamines (discussed later in this text).

Remarkably, placebos have been shown to evoke patterns of altered behavior that are similar to and as long-lasting as those observed when a pharmacologically active drug is ingested. Thus, in analyzing the pharmacology of a psychoactive agent, we must pay particular attention to the mental set of expectations, the social setting, and the predisposition of the subjects taking the placebo if we are to describe the pharmacological effects of a drug accurately.

The placebo effect is important in understanding the often neglected psychological aspects of therapy. Responses that closely mimic those produced by pharmacologically active drugs can be learned without drugs or placebos. For instance, meditation techniques can produce states that closely resemble those produced by drugs, especially altered states of consciousness. Meditation may be used to alter activity in certain centers of the brain in much the same way that a drug would. Certainly, the placebo effect is a powerful element in drug-induced responses.

Development of New Drugs

To complete our discussion of the effects of drugs in the body, let us mention the processes by which new drugs are developed and evaluated before they are released for public use.

The earliest medicinal products were usually natural in origin: crude powders of leaves or roots, or extracts from a variety of plants or animals. One of the great advances of the twentieth century was the development of organic chemistry, which made it practical to synthesize new drug molecules that offer more promise than many products obtained from natural sources. Although new drugs are occasionally discovered by accident, they usually result from systematic and tedious laboratory investigation and careful scientific observation.

The development and marketing of new drugs in the United States is rigidly controlled by the federal government through the Food and Drug Administration (FDA). Before a drug is marketed for general clinical use, it is subjected to thorough laboratory and clinical pharmacological studies that demonstrate its usefulness and safety. Before studies in humans are permitted, the pharmacological effects of a new drug on animals must be extensively analyzed. These studies establish the range of effective doses, the doses at which side effects occur, and the lethal doses in various animals. The studies on the safety and toxicity of a drug are evaluated after administration of single doses as well as during long-term use. From all these studies, a risk-to-benefit ratio is determined. Because of differences among species of animals, these studies must usually be carried out on at least three different species. In this preliminary testing on animals, neither the mechanism of a drug's action nor the range of its possible clinical usefulness needs to be completely described, but the absorption, distribution, metabolism, and excretion of the drug are carefully documented.

After it has been found safe to use in animals, a compound may be taken into an initial clinical trial (phase 1), which is usually conducted on normal volunteer subjects, as well as on patients; this phase is aimed at establishing the drug's safety, dose range, and possible problems requiring further study (Figure 2.21). If phase 1 studies indicate safety, the drug may be subjected to a thorough clinical pharmacological evaluation (phase 2). These studies are closely controlled to eliminate such variables as placebo response and investigator bias. Statistical validation is of paramount importance. Finally, if a drug still looks promising, it will enter phase 3 of the human studies—a period of extended clinical evaluation. During this phase, the compound is made available to investigators throughout the country for use in a variety of clinical situations. This procedure is followed to elicit information about the drug's safety, efficacy, side effects, dosage, variability of response, and so on.

If a drug passes all these trials, it may receive conditional approval by the FDA (phase 4) for broad use by physicians and medical centers who agree to a procedure of organized reporting of therapeutic results, limitations, and problems.

Currently it costs a pharmaceutical manufacturer more than $30 million to take a new compound through laboratory and clinical testing to the marketing stage. Although this attention to detail may seem excessive, it works to the benefit of the public. Most drugs that are currently on the legitimate market have reasonable risk-to-benefit ratios. Although none of the drugs available are completely without risk, most are relatively safe.

Study Questions

1. Distinguish between *pharmacokinetics* and *pharmacodynamics*.
2. Why must a psychoactive drug be altered metabolically in the body before it can be excreted?
3. Discuss the advantages and disadvantages of the various methods of administering drugs.

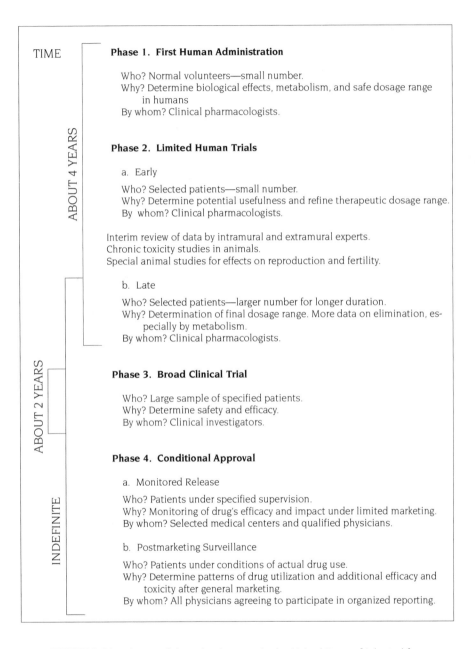

FIGURE 2.21 Phases of drug development in the United States. [Adapted from E. M. Ross and A. G. Gilman, "Pharmacodynamics: Mechanism of Drug Action and the Relationship between Drug Concentration and Effect," in A. G. Gilman, L. S. Goodman, T. W. Rall, and F. Murad, eds., *Goodman and Gilman's The Pharmacological Basis of Therapeutics,* 7th ed. (New York: Macmillan, 1985), p. 59.]

4. List the various membrane barriers that may affect drug distribution.
5. Discuss the placental barrier as it affects the distribution of psychoactive drugs.
6. If a drug has an elimination half-life of 6 hours, how long will it take for the drug to be eliminated from the body after a person has taken a single dose?
7. What is drug *tolerance* and why does it occur? Discuss three mechanisms underlying the development of tolerance.
8. Distinguish between *agonist* and *antagonist* as they relate to drug–receptor interactions.
9. Discuss the factors that influence the time course of drug action in the body.
10. Discuss how two drugs might interact with each other in the body.
11. Discuss the term *therapeutic drug monitoring*, what it implies, and how it applies to the therapeutic use of drugs.

Notes

1. L. Z. Benet, J. R. Mitchell, and L. B. Sheiner, "Pharmacokinetics: The Dynamics of Drug Absorption, Distribution and Elimination," in A. G. Gilman, T. W. Rall, A. S. Nies, and P. Taylor, eds., *Goodman and Gilman's The Pharmacological Basis of Therapeutics*, 8th ed. (New York: Pergamon, 1990), pp. 3–32.
2. M. W. B. Bradbury, "The Structure and Function of the Blood–Brain Barrier," *Federation Proceedings* 43 (1984): 186–190.
3. C. M. Smith and A. M. Reynard, *Textbook of Pharmacology* (Philadelphia: Saunders, 1992), pp. 67–71.
4. S. H. Preskorn, M. J. Burke, and G. A. Fast, "Therapeutic Drug Monitoring: Principles and Practice," in D. L. Dunner, ed., *The Psychiatric Clinics of North America* 16 (1993): 611–641.
5. S. Siegel, "Drug Anticipation and the Treatment of Dependence," in B. A. Ray, ed., *Learning Factors in Substance Abuse*, NIDA Research Monograph 84 (1988): 1–24.
6. C. X. Poulos and H. Cappell, "Homeostatic Theory of Drug Tolerance: A General Model of Physiological Adaptation," *Psychological Reviews* 98 (1991): 390–408.
7. S. T. Tiffany and P. M. Maude-Griffin, "Tolerance to Morphine in the Rat: Associative and Nonassociative Effects," *Behavioral Neuroscience* 102 (1988): 534–543.
8. E. M. Ross, "Pharmacodynamics: Mechanisms of Drug Action and the Relationship between Drug Concentration and Effect," in A. G. Gilman, T. W. Rall, A. S. Nies, and P. Taylor, eds., *Goodman and Gilman's The Pharmacological Basis of Therapeutics*, 8th ed. (New York: Pergamon, 1990), p. 33.

9. L. B. Wingard, T. M. Brody, J. Larner, and A. Schwartz, *Human Pharmacology: Molecular to Clinical* (St. Louis: Mosby Year Book, 1991), pp. 10–17.

10. A. M. Callahan, M. Fava, and J. F. Rosenbaum, "Drug Interactions in Psychopharmacology," in D. L. Dunner, ed., *The Psychiatric Clinics of North America* 16 (1993): 647–671.

11. H. P. Rang and M. M. Dale, *Pharmacology* (Edinburgh: Churchill Livingstone, 1987), p. 692.

12. A. Goldstein, L. Aronow, and S. M. Kalman, *Principles of Drug Action* (New York: Harper & Row, 1968), p. 733.

13. R. Rothschild and F. M. Quitkin, "Review of the Use of Pattern Analysis to Differentiate True Drug and Placebo Responses," *Psychotherapy and Psychosomatics* 58 (1992): 170–177.

14. E. D. Peselow, M. P. Sanfilipo, C. Difiglia, and R. R. Fieve, "Melancholic/Endogenous Depression and Response to Somatic Treatment and Placebo," *American Journal of Psychiatry* 149 (1992): 1324–1334.

15. C. Peck and G. Coleman, "Implications of Placebo Theory for Clinical Research and Practice in Pain Management," *Theoretical Medicine* 12 (1991): 247–270.

16. L. White, B. Tursky, and G. E. Schwartz, eds., *Placebo: Theory, Research, and Mechanisms* (New York: Guilford, 1985).

CHAPTER 3

CENTRAL NERVOUS SYSTEM DEPRESSANTS: CONCEPTS AND TRADITIONAL AGENTS

The central nervous system (CNS) depressants are a group of drugs with diverse chemical structures. Nonetheless, all can induce behavioral depression such as relief from anxiety, release from inhibitions, sedation, sleep, unconsciousness, general anesthesia, and coma (Figure 3.1). These drugs are divided into five categories: (1) the barbiturates, (2) the nonbarbiturate hypnotics, (3) the general anesthetics, (4) ethyl alcohol, and (5) the benzodiazepines. The first three are covered in this chapter, as are the inhalants of abuse. The benzodiazepines are discussed separately because of their popularity, mechanism of action, and wide clinical use and abuse (Chapter 4). Similarly, the unique, nonmedical use of alcohol in our culture justifies a separate discussion (Chapter 5).

GENERAL CONCEPTS

The terms *sedative, tranquilizer, anxiolytic,* and *hypnotic* can be applied to any CNS depressant, because each may diminish environmental awareness, spontaneity, and physical activity; higher doses produce drowsiness and lethargy; and even higher doses produce sleep. Individual compounds differ little from one another in their pharmacokinetics, clinical uses, and abilities to induce various stages of depression, but they do differ in their individual potencies and chemical makeup, which cause them to be handled differently by the body.

51

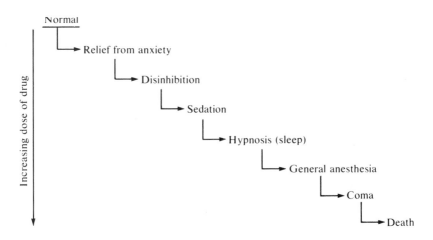

FIGURE 3.1   Continuum of behavioral sedation. How increasing doses of sedative-hypnotic drugs affect behavior.

In past years, low doses of these drugs were used clinically to calm anxious patients. This role in daytime sedation is now largely restricted to the benzodiazepines, which are inherently less dangerous. Today, the use of barbiturate and nonbarbiturate sedatives has decreased, being largely restricted to use in anesthesia and as antiepileptic agents. Even for these uses, newer agents are largely supplanting the barbiturates.

Five Principles of CNS Depressants

Five general principles apply fairly uniformly to all the CNS depressants (the traditional agents as well as alcohol and the benzodiazepines).

First, *the effects of CNS depressants are additive with one another and with the mental set of the user.* For example, alcohol will exaggerate the depression induced by barbiturates, and barbiturates will intensify the impairment of driving ability in a person who has been drinking alcohol. Similarly, a person who is depressed or physically tired may be profoundly affected by a dose of depressant drug that would only slightly affect someone who feels normal or excited.

The depressant effects of sedative drugs are also frequently supra-additive. Thus, the depression that is observed in a person who has taken more than one drug is greater than would be predicted if the person had taken only one. Such intense depression is often unpredictable and unexpected, and it can lead to dangerous or even fatal consequences. Depressant drugs should not be used in combination without the advice and guidance of a physician, especially if one of the drugs is ethyl alcohol (Chapter 5).

Second, *nonspecific antagonism occurs between the CNS depressants and the behavioral stimulants.* When a person is profoundly depressed by a sedative drug, the administration of a stimulant will not specifically block the action of the depressant and return the patient to normal, although the stimulant may arouse the patient temporarily. In fact, the stimulant may do more harm than good, because when it wears off, the patient will become even more depressed.

Clinically, we have long needed a specific antagonist to CNS depressants—a drug that actually displaces the depressant from its receptors in the brain, thus immediately terminating the action of the depressant. Such a drug would be lifesaving, especially in treating persons who have attempted suicide by ingesting lethal amounts of CNS depressants. The first great step in this area occurred in 1992 when the specific benzodiazepine antagonist, flumazenil (Chapter 4), became available for clinical use. Specific antagonists for the barbiturates and alcohol, however, have not been discovered.

Third, *older concepts of pharmacology held that general depressants exerted a depressant action on all neurons in the brain* (thus the phrase "nonselective depressant"). The drunkenness or "disinhibition" was thought to follow from an early depression of inhibitory synapses that occurred at lower doses than those required to depress excitatory neurotransmission. This, however, creates a theoretical correlation between behavioral and neuronal processes of disinhibition—a correlation that does not exist. More specific neuronal effects that are as yet unidentified are probably involved.

Fourth, in general, *the behavioral depression induced by a single dose of depressant drug seldom presents a problem.* As the drug is metabolized and excreted, the person slowly reverts from a drug-depressed state to a normal one. However, if large doses of depressants are repeatedly administered over a prolonged period of time, the depression induced is followed by a period of rebound hyperexcitability, which may be quite severe. For this reason, these agents can induce physiological dependence.

Fifth, *the use of any CNS depressant carries the risk of inducing psychological dependence and tolerance.* The former probably follows from the drug's positive reinforcement effects (Chapter 15). Tolerance occurs as a result of the induction of drug-metabolizing enzymes in the liver and to the adaptation of cells in the brain. In addition, a remarkable degree of cross-tolerance may occur, in which tolerance to one drug results in a lessened response to another drug. Cross-dependence, too, may be exhibited, in which one drug can prevent the withdrawal symptoms that are associated with physical dependence on a different drug.

Essentially any CNS depressant can substitute for any other CNS depressant, regardless of its chemical structure. This fact can be applied in clinical use, as in the use of the benzodiazepines to help ameliorate the symptoms that accompany withdrawal from alcohol.

Historical Background

> From time immemorial, human beings have sought ways and means both of achieving release from subjectively distressing and disabling anxiety, and of inducing sleep to counteract debilitating insomnia.[1]

Alcohol is certainly the oldest of the sedative-hypnotic agents; it is ingested to ease anxiety, tension, and agitation, and to lull the imbiber into a soporific state. The *opium alkaloids* (such as heroin) have similarly been used historically to induce a somnolent stupor for relief from anxiety. The addiction potential of the opioids, as well as their lethal potential, have limited their (usually illicit) use as antianxiety agents to relatively small groups of individuals.

In the latter part of the nineteenth century *bromide* and *chloral hydrate* became available as safer, more reliable alternatives to alcohol and opium when used as sedative agents. Then, in 1912, *phenobarbital* was introduced into medicine as a sedative drug, inaugurating an ongoing search for even safer sedative-anxiolytic agents. Between 1912 and about 1950, approximately 50 other barbiturates were marketed.

In the early 1950s, *meprobamate* (Equanil) was introduced as the first "modern day" tranquilizer. Then, in 1960, *chlordiazepoxide* (Librium) became the first available benzodiazepine tranquilizer. As opposed to the older agents, the benzodiazepines exert effects on a specific neurotransmitter receptor (discussed in Chapter 5), effects that are independent of the nonspecific neuronal depression that is observed at higher doses. Recognizing the limitations to the use of the benzodiazepines, scientists have been searching for potentially superior agents. The search has culminated in the mid-1990s introduction of two chemically unique anxiolytic agents: buspirone and zolpidem. Indeed, the search continues for agents that are as clinically useful as benzodiazepines but have fewer adverse effects and a lower risk of dependency and withdrawal.

Sites and Mechanisms of Action

The barbiturates, the nonbarbiturate sedative-hypnotics, ethyl alcohol, and the general anesthetics all reversibly depress the activity of all excitable tissues of the body, including that of the CNS, which is exquisitely sensitive.[2] At low and normal doses of these compounds, the poly-synaptic, diffuse brain stem pathways are the first to be depressed.[3] Such brain stem depression accounts for the deep coma and death that can follow barbiturate overdosage. Newer agents exert minimal effects on these polysynaptic brain stem pathways.

This concept of polysynaptic brain stem depression by the sedative-hypnotic agents, however, fails to explain why these neurons are depressed. Although there is no single, unifying answer, we will nevertheless attempt an explanation, beginning in this chapter and continuing in the next.

To begin, we will discuss the GABA receptor (see Appendix III); more specifically, we will look at a specific subtype of GABA receptor, the GABA$_A$ receptor, as a site of depressant drug action. The GABA$_A$ receptor is a membrane-spanning ion channel (Figure 3.2), which is common through the CNS, being particularly prominent in the amygdala and the midbrain. When the neurotransmitter GABA is released

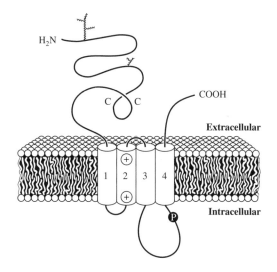

FIGURE 3.2   Model for the GABA$_A$ receptor subunits. This diagram of a GABA$_A$ receptor subunit shows four membrane-spanning regions. The figure depicts the amino acid backbone of a receptor subunit (dark line) with both the amino (H$_2$N) and carboxy (COOH) termini in the extracellular space. On the amino terminal portion of the molecule are sites for glycosylation (branches). A disulfide bridge between paired cysteine (C) residues produces an extracellular loop in the molecule. The hydrophobic regions of the protein span the membrane four times (cylinders). At the extracellular and intracellular sides of the protein are collections of positively charged amino acids (+), which provide sites for interaction with chloride ions as they traverse the channel. On the intracellular loop between the third and fourth transmembrane-spanning regions of the beta- and gamma-2-subunits is a consensus site for phosphorylation (P) by cAMP-dependent protein kinase. [Zorumski and Isenberg,[4] p. 167.]

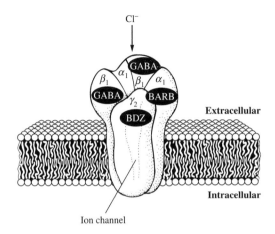

Ion channel

FIGURE 3.3   Schematic model of the gamma-aminobutyric acid– (GABA–) chloride ionophore. GABA binding to its receptor (GABA) activates and opens the chloride channel, thus increasing the inward flux of chloride ions. Benzodiazepines bind to specific receptors (BDZ) and increase the effect of GABA on the chloride channel. Barbiturates bind to their receptors (BARB) and prolong the GABA-induced opening of the chloride channel. In high doses, barbiturates may directly open the chloride channel. [Zorumski and Isenberg,[4] p. 168.]

from presynaptic terminals, it binds to this receptor, inducing a conformational change which, in turn, opens an ionic channel that allows negatively charged chloride ions to pass into the neuron. This hyperpolarizes the nerve membrane, making the neuron less excitable by other transmitters (Appendix III). Located on the outer surface of the $GABA_A$ receptor are specific binding sites for both the benzodiazepines and the barbiturates (Figure 3.3). Drugs of either class, when bound, affect the structure of the ion channel, making it easier to open or prolonging its opening; this action enhances or potentiates the inhibitory neurotransmitter effect of GABA.

Barbiturates do not bind to the same site on the $GABA_A$ receptor as the benzodiazepines do. As a consequence of binding, barbiturates increase the affinity of GABA for its receptor and prolong the length of time that chloride channels remain open fourfold to fivefold.[4,5] In high doses, barbiturates open chloride channels in the absence of GABA,[6] at least partially accounting for their high-dose hypnotic and anesthetic effects. The effects of *benzodiazepines* on $GABA_A$ receptors are discussed at length in Chapter 4.

Uses

Use of both the barbiturates and the nonbarbiturate sedatives has declined rapidly in recent years for several reasons.

1. They lack selective CNS action.
2. They are inherently less safe than the benzodiazepines.
3. They have a high potential for inducing tolerance and dependence.
4. They interact dangerously with many other drugs.

Despite these disadvantages, the barbiturates continue to be used clinically as anticonvulsants and as intravenous anesthetics. On rare occasions, barbiturates are also used in psychiatry to sedate (for example, the "amytal interview") and in medicine to help protect the brain after severe head injury (by reducing neuronal activity, blood flow to the brain, and intracranial pressure). Some of the older chloral hydrate derivatives are still used as bedtime sedatives for the elderly. Most other sedatives are of such long duration of action that their use for the elderly is restricted. The decreased availability of barbiturates has tended to limit their recreational use and abuse, although these have not totally disappeared.

Drug-Induced "Brain Syndrome"

Certain psychiatric and neurological disorders, such as the dementias, produce characteristic behavioral, intellectual, and cognitive patterns. Sedative-hypnotic drugs can induce a state that closely resembles dementia. One way to diagnose drug-induced dementia (an "organic brain syndrome") is to perform a mini mental status examination that evaluates 12 areas of mental functioning (Table 3.1).

Different psychiatric disorders cause patients to manifest different deficits in this examination. Schizophrenics, for example, have an intact sensorium and adequate memory and behavior; are cooperative; and may speak with a normal stream of talk. Their mental status examination is characterized by disturbed thought processes with an absence of logic and frequent misperceptions of reality. (The pathological processes involved in patients who suffer from schizophrenia are discussed in Chapter 11).

In instances where a person's neurons are reversibly depressed by alcohol, nonselective depressants, or benzodiazepine tranquilizers, or

TABLE 3.1 Mental status examination: Twelve areas of mental functioning.

1. General appearance
2. Sensorium
   a. Orientation to time, place, and person
   b. Clear vs. clouded thinking
3. Behavior and mannerisms
4. Stream of talk
5. Cooperativeness
6. Mood (inner feelings)
7. Affect (surface expression of feelings)
8. Perception
   a. Illusions (misperception of reality)
   b. Hallucinations (not present in reality)
9. Thought processes: logical vs. strange or bizarre
10. Mental content (fund of knowledge)
11. Intellectual function (ability to reason and interpret)
12. Insight and judgment

when a patient's neurons are irreversibly destroyed (as in dementia), 5 of the 12 functions of the mental status examination are particularly altered (sensorium, affect, mental content, intellectual function, and insight and judgment). The person's sensorium becomes clouded, which causes disorientation in time and place; memory becomes impaired, which is evidenced by forgetfulness and loss of short-term memory; the intellect becomes depressed, and judgment is altered. The person's affect becomes shallow and labile; that is, he or she becomes extremely vulnerable to external stimuli and may be sullen and moody at one moment and exhibit mock anger at the next. When such a mental status is seen, it is diagnosed as a "brain syndrome" caused by depressed nerve cell function.

Certain persons (such as the elderly) who already have some natural loss of nerve cell function are more likely to be adversely affected by these drugs, experiencing increased disorientation and further clouding of consciousness. Frequently these persons exhibit a state of drug-induced "paradoxical excitement," which is characterized by a labile personality with marked anger, delusions, hallucinations, and confabulations. Treating such a drug-induced disorder requires that administration of the sedative drug be stopped.

FOUR AGENTS OF CENTRAL NERVOUS SYSTEM DEPRESSION

Barbiturates

The barbiturates were the mainstays in treating anxiety and insomnia for almost 50 years, from 1912 to about 1960. During this period, they were associated with thousands of suicides, deaths from accidental ingestion, wide dependency and abuse, and many serious interactions with other drugs and alcohol. They remain, however, the classic prototype of sedative-hypnotic drugs against which newer drugs are compared.

Pharmacokinetics

Barbiturates are classified according to their pharmacokinetics. As shown in Table 3.2, their half-lives can be quite short (a 3-minute redistribution half-life for thiopental), longer (a 24- to 48-hour elimination half-life for amobarbital, pentobarbital, and secobarbital), or very long (an 80- to 100-hour elimination half-life for phenobarbital). The reader may recall from Chapter 2 that the hypnotic action of ultra-short-acting barbiturates (such as thiopental) is terminated by redistribution, while the action of other barbiturates is determined by metabolism and excretion.

Taken orally, barbiturates are rapidly and completely absorbed and are well distributed to most body tissues. The ultra-short-acting barbiturates are exceedingly lipid soluble, cross the blood–brain barrier rapidly, and induce sleep within seconds. Because the longer-acting barbiturates are more water soluble, they are slower to penetrate the CNS. Sleep induction with these compounds, therefore, is delayed, and redistribution plays less of a role in the termination of clinical effect. Thus, drug-induced "hangover" is prominent (especially since the plasma half-lives of most of these drugs vary from 10 to 48 hours).

Urinalysis is used to screen for the presence of barbiturates as well as other psychoactive drugs of abuse. Depending on the specific barbiturate, tests will be positive as short as 30 hours or as long as several weeks after the drug is ingested. When urinalysis is positive for barbiturates, more specific confirmation is needed to determine the exact drug that was taken.

TABLE 3.2 Structures, half-lives, and uses of some barbiturates.

General formula

Drug name		R_1	R_2	R_3	Half-life		Uses		
Trade	Generic				Distribution (min)	Elimination (hr)	Insomnia	Anesthesia	Epilepsy
Amytal	Amobarbital	Ethyl	Isopentyl	H		10–40	X		
Alurate	Aprobarbital	Allyl	Isopentyl	H		12–34	X		
Butisol	Butabarbital	Ethyl	sec-Butyl	H		34–42	X		
Mebaral	Mephobarbital	Ethyl	Phenyl	CH_3		50–120			X
Brevital	Methohexital	Allyl	1-methyl, 2-Pentynyl	CH_3		1–2		X	
Nembutal	Pentobarbital	Ethyl	Methyl butyl	H		15–50	X		
Luminal	Phenobarbital	Ethyl	Phenyl	H		24–120	X		X
Seconal	Secobarbital	Allyl	Methyl butyl	H		15–40	X		
Lotusate	Talbutal	Allyl	sec-Butyl	H			X		
Surital	Thiamylal	Allyl	Methyl butyl	H				X	
Pentothal	Thiopental	Ethyl	Methyl butyl	H	3	3–6		X	

ᵃO= except in thiamylal and thiopental, where it is replaced by S=.

Pharmacological Effects

> The barbiturates possess a low degree of selectivity and therapeutic index. Thus, it is not possible to achieve a desired effect without evidence of general depression of the CNS. Pain perception and reaction are relatively unimpaired until the moment of unconsciousness, and in small doses the barbiturates increase the reaction to painful stimuli. Hence they cannot be relied upon to produce sedation or sleep in the presence of even moderate pain. In some individuals and in some circumstances, such as the presence of pain, barbiturates cause overt excitement instead of sedation.[3]

This state of overt excitement is caused by the drug-induced brain syndrome. The degree of excitement depends on the person and the circumstances under which the drugs were taken. Physical aggression can be seen during the period of intoxication, especially in individuals experiencing pain or in patients with paranoia or paranoid ideation.

Sleep patterns are markedly affected by the barbiturates. The initial brain wave (EEG) alterations induced by the barbiturates resemble a high-voltage, low-frequency pattern that is characteristic of slow-wave sleep. Rapid eye movement (REM) sleep is markedly suppressed. Because dreaming occurs during REM sleep and is largely absent during slow-wave sleep, barbiturate-induced sleep differs electrographically from normal sleep. The absence of REM sleep (with loss of dreaming) may be harmful and even precipitate psychotic episodes. Also, during drug withdrawal, dreaming becomes vivid and excessive. Such rebound increase in dreaming during withdrawal, termed "REM rebound," is one example of a withdrawal effect following prolonged periods of barbiturate ingestion. Indeed, the vivid nature of the dreams can lead to insomnia, often clinically relieved by restarting the drug and thus negating the attempt at withdrawal.

Drowsiness ("hangover") and more subtle alterations of judgment, motor skill, and behavior may persist for hours or days until the barbiturate is completely metabolized and eliminated.

Sedative doses of barbiturates have minimal effect on respiration, but overdoses can result in death. Barbiturates appear to have no significant effects on the cardiovascular system, the gastrointestinal tract, the kidneys, or other organs until toxic doses are reached. In the liver, barbiturates stimulate the synthesis of enzymes that metabolize these as well as other drugs, an effect that produces significant tolerance to such drugs.

Psychological Effects

Many of the behavioral effects caused by barbiturates are similar to those caused by alcohol-induced inebriation and may even be indistinguishable from them. A person may respond to low doses either with relief from anxiety (the expected effect) or with withdrawal, emotional depression, or aggressive and violent behavior. Higher doses (or low doses combined with another depressant) lead to more general behavioral depression and sleep.

The person's mental set and his or her physical or social setting can determine whether relief from anxiety, mental depression, aggression, or other unexpected or unpredictable responses are experienced.

Another important behavioral effect is the ataxia (staggering) and loss of motor coordination that may accompany a person's use of barbiturates or other depressant drugs. For instance, driving skills will be severely impaired, and this effect is a predictable and inseparable consequence. As noted, the effects of barbiturates are additive with the effects produced by other depressants (including alcohol) that may be present.

Adverse Reactions

Side Effects and Toxicity Drowsiness is one of the primary effects induced by barbiturates; obviously, such drowsiness is often the effect a person seeks.

Barbiturates significantly impair motor and intellectual performance and judgment:

> A person need not be rendered staggering drunk before his motor performance and, probably more important, his judgment are significantly impaired. The most common offending agent in this regard is alcohol. . . . At this time it should be emphasized that all sedatives are equivalent to alcohol in their effects; that all are additive in their effects with alcohol; and that their effects persist longer than might be predicted.[7]

There are no specific antidotes to the serious effects of barbiturate overdosage. Treatment of overdosage is aimed at supporting the respiratory and cardiovascular system until the drug is metabolized and eliminated.

Tolerance The barbiturates can induce tolerance by the two mechanisms discussed earlier: (1) the induction of metabolizing enzymes in the liver and (2) the adaptation of neurons in the brain to the presence of the drug. However, a person who takes barbiturates does not develop tolerance to all of their effects. Tolerance develops primarily to the sedative effects and much less so to the depressant effects on respiration. Thus, the margin of safety for the person who uses the drug decreases. Accidental poisonings have been attributed to this effect on respiration.

Physical Dependence   Barbiturates induce physical dependence; however, the dose required to produce this dependence is considerably higher than the usual clinical dose. For example, while 100 milligrams of pentobarbital (Nembutal) may induce sleep, serious physical dependence does not develop until daily dosages of 800 milligrams or more are used. Indeed, only after such large doses does removal of the drug lead to serious withdrawal symptoms. This is not to say that normal doses of barbiturates cannot produce some degree of physical dependence, but any withdrawal symptoms are usually not serious or life threatening. REM rebound is common and is accompanied by increased dreaming, which can progress to sleep deprivation, vivid dreams, and nightmares. Withdrawal from high doses of barbiturates may result in hallucinations, restlessness, disorientation, and even life-threatening convulsions.

Psychological Dependence   Psychological dependence refers to a compulsion to use a drug for a pleasurable effect. This phenomenon usually results from an effect of the drug on reward centers in the brain (Chapter 15). All CNS depressants, especially alcohol, are subject to such effect and are known to be abused compulsively. Because they can relieve anxiety, induce sedation, and produce a state of euphoria, these drugs may be used to achieve a variety of psychological states in a variety of abuse situations.

Effects in Pregnancy   Barbiturates, like all psychoactive drugs, are freely distributed to the fetus. Because the newborn has limited metabolizing and excreting systems, it may be depressed for a significant period of time after delivery if the mother had been ingesting barbiturates. Should the drug ingestion have been quite continuous before delivery, withdrawal signs may be seen in the newborn. Thus, barbiturates and other sedatives are generally contraindicated during pregnancy. One exception involves the administration of an ultra-short-acting barbiturate to induce anesthesia for an emergency cesarean section. In this situation, neonatal depression is minimal and no signs of withdrawal are observed.

Administering sedatives must be closely monitored throughout the entire pregnancy. Data on barbiturates are limited but suggestive of developmental abnormalities. However, mothers with epilepsy must take antiepileptic medications (including barbiturates) to prevent seizures. Although some congenital problems have been reported in the offspring of epileptic mothers, the benefit to pregnant epileptic mothers of continuing medication during pregnancy outweighs the rare occurrence of congenital abnormalities. Otherwise, unless medically indicated, barbiturates and other sedatives are contraindicated during pregnancy.

Traditional Nonbarbiturate Hypnotics

In the early 1950s, three nonbarbiturate sedatives, glutethimide (Doriden), ethchlorvynol (Placidyl), and methyprylon (Noludar), were introduced to produce sedation, anxiolytic effects, and sleep. However, their chemical structures are similar to those of the barbiturates, and they offered few advantages—their toxicity and abuse potential were as great as those of barbiturates. Today, they are generally considered obsolete, although they are still occasionally encountered both as drugs in therapeutic use and as drugs of abuse.

Methaqualone (Quaalude) was a fourth nonbarbiturate depressant that had little to justify its widespread use. During the late 1970s and early 1980s, the illicit use of methaqualone rose dramatically, and it trailed only marijuana and alcohol in its level of abuse. Such attention was due to an undeserved reputation as an aphrodisiac. Extensive illicit use and numerous deaths led to its removal from sale in 1984. Methaqualone was pharmacologically similar to the barbiturates and, as a sedative drug, was actually an anaphrodisiac. Methaqualone, far from being a "love drug," was merely one of several nonselective depressants that were thought to affect the user favorably when they were taken in the right setting and with a particular set of expectations.[8]

Meprobamate (Equanil, Miltown), now largely of historical interest, was introduced as an antianxiety agent in 1955 as another alternative to the barbiturates for daytime sedation and anxiolysis. Around it developed the term *tranquilizer,* in a marketing attempt to distinguish it from the barbiturates, a distinction that was not borne out in reality. Meprobamate produces long-lasting daytime sedation, mild euphoria, and relief from anxiety. Its relative lack of potency and efficacy implied a large placebo component to its therapeutic effects. Unfortunately, meprobamate is teratogenic and thus contraindicated during pregnancy.

Meprobamate can produce tolerance, physical dependence, and psychological dependence. Because it is not as potent a respiratory depressant as the barbiturates, its margin of safety may be greater. Attempted suicides from overdosage are rarely successful. Despite a continuing reduction in clinical use, abuse and dependency continue and are difficult to treat.[9]

Chloral hydrate is yet another drug of largely historical interest, having been available clinically since the late 1800s. It is rapidly metabolized to trichlorethanol (a derivative of ethyl alcohol), which is a nonselective CNS depressant and the active form of chloral hydrate. It has been noted that REM sleep is not greatly depressed by chloral hydrate, and REM rebound is minimal upon discontinuation. Chloral hydrate appears to be a relatively safe and effective sedative-hypnotic, with a plasma half-life of about 4 to 8 hours. Hangover is less likely to occur than with compounds having longer half-lives. Its liability in producing tolerance and dependence is similar to that of the barbiturates. Occasionally chloral hydrate is utilized as a bedtime sedative in elderly patients. One interesting aside is that chloral hydrate in combination with alcohol leads to a loss of consciousness. This mixture is often called a "Mickey Finn."

General Anesthetics

General anesthetic agents are reversible CNS depressants that produce a loss of sensation accompanied by unconsciousness. General anesthesia is therefore the most severe state of intentional drug-induced CNS depression. The agents that are used as general anesthetics are of two types: (1) those that are administered by inhalation through the lungs and (2) those that are injected.

The inhalation anesthetics in current use include one gas (nitrous oxide) and four volatile liquids (isoflurane, halothane, desflurane, and enflurane), whose vapors are delivered into the patient's lungs by means of an anesthesia machine. These drugs produce a generalized, graded, dose-related depression of all functions of the CNS: an initial period of sedation followed by the onset of sleep. As anesthesia deepens, the patient's reflexes become progressively depressed and analgesia is induced. At that point, a patient is said to be anesthetized. Deepening of anesthesia results in loss of reflexes, depression of both respiration and brain excitability, amnesia, and analgesia.

TABLE 3.3 Sites and mechanisms of action of general anesthetics.

I. Neuronal systems selectively influenced by general anesthetics (by function)
  A. Consciousness
    1. Cerebral cortex
    2. Reticular and other ascending activating systems
    3. EEGs reveal at least two classes of anesthetics: one exemplified by halothane (chloroform and trichloroethylene), and another that includes nitrous oxide, diethyl ether, and cyclopropane
  B. Memory/amnesia
    1. Cerebral cortex, hippocampus, amygdala
  C. Analgesia/pain perception
    1. Descending pain modulating systems, midbrain periaqueductal gray matter, spinal cord dorsal horn gray matter (endorphin release after nitrous oxide, ethanol)

II. Neuronal systems functionally impaired by higher concentrations of most general anesthetics
  A. Respiration
    1. Respiratory centers; carotid chemoreceptors by halothane, enflurane
  B. Blood pressure
    1. Hypothalamic center control of cardiovascular system by way of autonomic outflow
  C. Skeletal muscle movement and tone
    1. Cerebellum, midbrain, basal ganglia, cerebral cortical systems involved in initiation of movement, spinal cord

III. Synaptic processes potentially affected by general anesthetics
  A. Transmitter synthesis
  B. Transmitter release—halothane (cerebral cortex)
  C. Transmitter metabolism
  D. Postsynaptic effects
    1. Augmentation of inhibition
    2. Augmented or prolonged presynaptic inhibition (benzodiazepines, barbiturates, ethanol, ether)

Of the injectable anesthetics, thiopental and methohexital (ultrashort-acting barbiturates) are the most widely used. Propofol (Diprovan) and etomidate (Amidate) are also used in special situations. The mechanism of action of the latter two anesthetics is probably the same as that of the barbiturates, that is, nonselective CNS depression produced secondary both to GABA$_A$-receptor occupancy as well as to depression of synaptic transmission in polysynaptic pathways.

Prominent scientists have studied the possible mechanisms of action of the inhaled general anesthetics for over 100 years.[10] The mechanisms proposed have been so diverse that one recent textbook of pharmacology devotes 7 pages to this puzzle;[11] a summary is presented in

TABLE 3.3 Sites and mechanisms of general anesthetics (*continued*)

      3. Augmented endorphin release (nitrous oxide and possibly ether, but not halothane)

      4. Augmented GABA-induced inhibition

  E. Depression of transmitter-induced postsynaptic excitation (all inhalation anesthetics in high concentrations as well as barbiturates, ethanol)

  F. Alteration of neurotransmitter receptor proteins (demonstrated to date with an acetylcholine receptor); anesthetics cause desensitization of the receptor and accelerated closing of the ion channels associated with the receptor (other receptor systems and proteins are likely to be affected by anesthetics)

IV. Direct effects on neurons

  A. Depression of membrane excitability, decrease in sodium conductance, possibly the consequence of increased membrane thickness/volume, increased fluidity of membranes

      1. Hyperpolarization of small fibers in the cerebral cortex

      2. Intracellular components: mitochondria oxidative systems depressed (hypoxia produces unconsciousness, hypoxia and anesthetics are additive or synergistic in actions); calcium-mediated mitochondrial functions are depressed by anesthetics

      3. General anesthetics are localized selectively to lipids and hydrophobic regions of proteins; anesthetic potencies are correlated with lipid solubility as well as hyperpolarization of small fibers

V. Outline of differential actions of various general anesthetics

  A. Markedly different chemical structures and physical properties, some actions appear to be *receptor-mediated*, whereas for others the receptors not readily identified

  B. Different EEGs with different agents

  C. Different margins of safety and spectra of neural actions

  D. Differential sensitivities of various synaptic and neural systems to different agents

  E. Differential genetically determined sensitivities among agents

  F. Genetic influences occur as demonstrated in mice, *Drosophila*, and nematodes

From Smith and Reynard,[11] p. 189.

Table 3.3. Despite all these theories, we are still unsure whether general anesthesia is a "physical" phenomenon (discussed next) or a specific, rapidly reversible "receptor interaction" involving GABA[12] or other receptors.[13]

To me, the most plausible explanation for the action of anesthetics involves alteration in the physicochemical processes of nerve membranes. This follows from the linear correlation (Figure 3.4) between the potency of various drugs as general anesthetic agents and their solubility in lipid. By dissolving in the nerve membranes, the structure of the lipid matrix of the membranes becomes distorted, thereby perturbing the function of the ion channels and the membrane proteins.

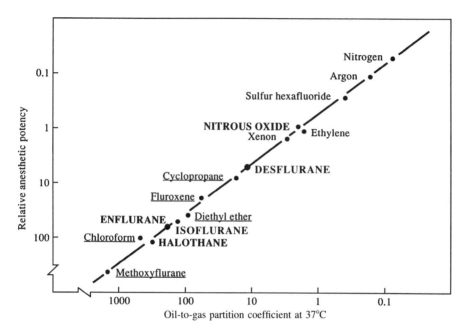

FIGURE 3.4   Correlation of anesthetic potency with the oil-to-gas partition coefficient. The correlation is shown for a number of general anesthetic agents and for other inert gases that are not usually used for anesthesia. Note the log scales and the excellent correlation over a very wide range of fat solubilities and potencies. Agents that are used today in anesthesia are shown in boldface capital letters. Agents that were formerly used as anesthetics are underscored.

Indeed, Diliger and coworkers recently demonstrated anesthetic-induced disruption of ion flows through acetylcholine channels, an action exerted either directly on the channel protein itself or at the interface between the protein and the lipid membrane.[14] By depressing transmembrane ion flow, nerve function is depressed and a state of clinical anesthesia is produced. When administration of the anesthesia is discontinued, the anesthetic is absorbed back into the bloodstream and exhaled through the lungs, and normal membrane structure and function return.

Occasionally certain anesthetic agents are misused. Nitrous oxide, a gas of low anesthetic potency, is an example. At a 50 percent concentration in oxygen, nitrous oxide induces a state of behavioral disinhibition, analgesia, and mild euphoria. Since at least 50 percent of the inhaled gas mixture must consist of nitrous oxide to achieve these effects, extreme caution must be exercised in order to prevent hypoxia. This necessitates administration through an anesthesia machine or similar device. If the nitrous oxide were mixed only with room air, hypoxia would result, which would produce irreversible brain damage. This danger also exists with other forms of inhalant abuse, as discussed below.

Inhalants of Abuse

Besides nitrous oxide, other inhaled substances are involved in the problems of "inhalant abuse" and "recreational anesthesia." Here classification is difficult, because (while some inhalants are anesthetic) they have little in common pharmacologically; the commonality is the mode of administration.

Abused inhalants are a group of volatile or gaseous substances used for altering mental status that are rarely, if ever, administered by routes other than inhalation.[15] The inhaled substances involved include the following:

1. anesthetics (especially nitrous oxide and halothane)

2. industrial or household solvents, including paint thinners or solvents, degreasers, and solvents in glues

3. art and office supply solvents, including typewriter correction fluid and marker pen solvents

4. gases used in household or commercial products, including butane lighters, aerosol cream dispensers, and propane tanks

5. household aerosol propellants, including paint, hair spray, and fabric protector sprays

6. aliphatic nitrites and organic solvents, including amyl nitrite capsules

The aliphatic nitrites are most commonly found as amyl nitrite (in ampules for patients with heart disease) and as butyl nitrites (in "room deodorizers"). Some of the substances found in these different products are listed in Table 3.4. When inhaled, these substances dilate blood vessels, causing reduced blood pressure, cerebral ischemia, dizziness, and a flushed feeling.

Inhalants are usually abused in conjunction with sexual activity for a claimed ability to enhance orgasms.[15] Inhalant abusers are usually from one of three classes:

1. young males between the ages of 14 and 20 years

2. inhalant-dependent adults

3. polydrug users

TABLE 3.5 Chemicals commonly found in inhalants.

	Inhalant	Chemical
ADHESIVES	Airplane glue	Toluene, ethyl acetate
	Other glues	Hexane, toluene, methyl chloride, acetone, methyl ethyl ketone, methyl butyl ketone
	Special cements	Trichloroethylene, tetrachloroethylene
AEROSOLS	Spray paint	Butane, propane (U.S.), fluorocarbons, toluene, hydrocarbons, "Texas shoe shine" (a spray containing toluene)
	Hair spray	Butane, propane (U.S.), CFCs
	Deodorant, air freshener	Butane, propane (U.S.), CFCs
	Analgesic spray	Chlorofluorocarbons (CFCs)
	Asthma spray	Chlorofluorocarbons (CFCs)
	Fabric spray	Butane, trichloroethane
	PC cleaner	Dimethyl ether, hydrofluorocarbons
ANESTHETICS	Gas	Nitrous oxide
	Liquid	Halothane, enflurane
	Local	Ethyl chloride
CLEANING AGENTS	Dry cleaning	Tetrachloroethylene, trichloroethane
	Spot remover	Xylene, petroleum distillates, chlorohydrocarbons
	Degreaser	Tetrachloroethylene, trichloroethane, trichloroethylene
SOLVENTS AND GASES	Nail polish remover	Acetone, ethyl acetate
	Paint remover	Toluene, methylene chloride, methanol acetone, ethyl acetate
	Paint thinner	Petroleum distillates, esters, acetone
	Correction fluid and thinner	Trichloroethylene, trichloroethane
	Fuel gas	Butane, isopropane
	Lighter	Butane, isopropane
	Fire extinguisher	Bromochlorodifluoromethane
FOOD PRODUCTS	Whipped cream	Nitrous oxide
	Whippets	Nitrous oxide
"ROOM ODORIZERS"	Locker Room, Rush, poppers	Isoamyl, isobutyl, isopropyl or butyl nitrite (now illegal), cyclohexyl

From Sharp,[15] pp. 4–5.

The majority of deaths involving use of these inhalants occurs in male teenagers; most of the remainder are adults in their twenties. About 90 percent of all inhalant-caused deaths occur in males.[16] A relatively high percentage (about 20 percent) of youths have experience with inhalant abuse by the end of the eighth grade. Today most fatalities seem to follow inhalation of lighter fluid products containing butane or propane.

These volatile substances appear to act as general anesthetics, producing the continuum of sedation (Figure 3.1) that leads from euphoria to alcohol-like intoxication, to disinhibition and loss of consciousness. Serious problems, however, arise from several sources.

1. The volatile substances are often put into a plastic bag or on rags that are placed over the user's face and head. Spraying the gas directly into the mouth is also commonplace. Suffocation is a constant hazard, especially when bags or rags are used.

2. Hypoxia leading to anoxia (lack of oxygen) follows the replacement of room air with the vapors, and with the lack of oxygen in a bag placed over the face.

3. Respiration and the cardiovascular system are not properly monitored (as an anesthesiologist would do during a surgery).

4. The hypoxia, together with the direct cardiotoxic effects of these volatile substances, leads to ischemia of heart tissue, life-threatening cardiac arrhythmias, and cardiac collapse.

5. Some agents cause peripheral nerve damage; others are toxic to the liver or kidneys.

The reader interested in a detailed review of this topic is referred to the recent symposium listed in references 15 and 17.

Study Questions

1. List the various classes of nonselective CNS depressants, and give examples of each class.
2. Describe the gradation of action that occurs in a person as a result of taking progressively increasing doses of a nonselective CNS depressant.
3 Describe what is meant by "supra-additive CNS depression."
4. Describe the two types of drug tolerance that can develop as a result of repeated use of barbiturates.
5. Describe the mechanism of action of nonselective CNS depressants.

6. What is meant by "drug-induced, reversible brain syndrome"?
7. What mechanisms are responsible for the differing durations of action of various barbiturates?
8. Describe the effects of barbiturates on sleep patterns both acutely and during drug withdrawal.
9. Compare the effects of barbiturates and chloral hydrate on the elderly.
10. Compare the mechanism of action of barbiturates with that of an inhaled general anesthetic.
11. Summarize some of the problems associated with the abuse of inhalants.

Notes

1. P. G. Janicak, J. M. Davis, S. H. Preskorn, and F. J. Ayd, Jr., *Principles and Practice of Psychopharmacotherapy* (Baltimore: Williams & Wilkins, 1993), p. 405.
2. T. W. Rall, "Hypnotics and Sedatives: Ethanol," in A. G. Gilman, T. W. Rall, A. S. Nies, and P. Taylor, eds., *Goodman and Gilman's The Pharmacological Basis of Therapeutics,* 8th ed. (New York: Pergamon, 1990), p. 345.
3. T. W. Rall, "Hypnotics and Sedatives: Ethanol," in A. G. Gilman, T. W. Rall, A. S. Nies, and P. Taylor, eds., *Goodman and Gilman's The Pharmacological Basis of Therapeutics,* 8th ed. (New York: Pergamon, 1990), pp. 358–360.
4. C. F. Zorumski and K. E. Isenberg, "Insights into the Structure and Function of GABA-Benzodiazepine Receptors: Ion Channels and Psychiatry," *American Journal of Psychiatry* 148 (1991): 162–173.
5. R. W. Olsen, "GABA–Drug Interactions," *Progress in Drug Research* 31 (1987): 224–238.
6. R. E. Twyman, C. J. Rogers, and R. L. MacDonald, "Pentobarbital and Picrotoxin Have Reciprocal Actions on Single GABA$_A$ Receptor Channels," *Neuroscience Letter* 96 (1989): 89–95.
7. H. Meyers, E. Jawetz, and A. Goldfien, *Review of Medical Pharmacology,* 3rd ed. (Los Altos, Ca.: Lange Medical Publications, 1972), p. 219.
8. C. V. Wetli, "Changing Patterns of Methaqualone Abuse," *Journal of the American Medical Association* 249 (1983): 621.
9. J. D. Roache and R. R. Griffiths, "Lorazepam and Meprobamate Dose Effects in Humans: Behavioral Effects and Abuse Liability," *Journal of Pharmacology and Experimental Therapeutics* 243 (1987): 978.
10. J. H. Tinker, "Voices from the Past: From Ice Crystals to Fruit Flies in the Quest for a Molecular Mechanism of Anesthetic Action," *Anesthesia and Analgesia* 77 (1993): 1–3.
11. C. M. Smith and A. M. Reynard, *Textbook of Pharmacology* (Philadelphia: Saunders, 1992), pp. 188–194.
12. D. L. Tanelian, P. Kosek, I. Mody, and M. B. MacIver, "The Role of the GABA$_A$ Receptor/Chloride Channel Complex in Anesthesia," *Anesthesiology* 78 (1993): 757–776.

13. R. Allada and H. A. Nash, "*Drosophila melanogaster* as a Model for Study of General Anesthesia: The Quantitative Response to Clinical Anesthetics and Alkanes," *Anesthesia and Analgesia* 77 (1993): 19–26.

14. J. P. Diliger, A. M. Vidal, H. I. Mody, and Y. Liu, "Evidence for Direct Actions of General Anesthetics on an Ion Channel Protein," *Anesthesiology* 81 (1994): 431–442.

15. C. W. Sharp, "Introduction to Inhalant Abuse," in C. W. Sharp, P. Beauvais, and R. Spence, eds., *Inhalant Abuse: A Volatile Research Agenda*, NIDA Research Monograph 129 (Rockville, Md.: U.S. Department of Health and Human Services, 1992), pp. 1–10.

16. J. Ramsey, H. R. Anderson, K. Bloor, and R. J. Flanagan, "An Introduction to the Practice, Prevalence and Chemical Toxicology of Volatile Substance Abuse," *Human Toxicology* 8 (1989): 261–269.

17. J. C. Garriott, "Death among Inhalant Abusers," in C. W. Sharp, P. Beauvais, and R. Spence, eds., *Inhalant Abuse: A Volatile Research Agenda*, NIDA Research Monograph 129 (Rockville, Md.: U.S. Department of Health and Human Services, 1992), pp. 181–191.

CHAPTER 4

CENTRAL NERVOUS SYSTEM DEPRESSANTS: BENZODIAZEPINES, "SECOND GENERATION" ANXIOLYTICS, AND ANTIEPILEPTIC DRUGS

Anxiety can be described as apprehension, tension, or uneasiness related to anticipated danger. It may be a response to external stimuli, or it may be devoid of any apparent precipitating stimulus.[1] Anxiety is also a fundamental emotion, and it is a normal response to an experience that mimics a past experience that posed a significant problem.

Anxiety is a complex of subjective feelings and characteristic behavior, consisting of tension, fear, worry, helplessness, apprehension, and difficulties with thought, concentration, or sleep. The behavioral signs may include headaches, nausea, diarrhea, rapid heart rate, rapid breathing, tremors, muscle tension, restlessness, and fatigue. Certainly these feelings, behaviors, and symptoms are normal, appropriate, and necessary responses for survival in a hostile world (serving as the cognitive and emotional concomitant of a behavioral alarm system). However, anxiety can be harmful when carried to extremes, whether it is psychologically induced in response to the environment or neurochemically induced as a result of dysfunction. The distinction here may be vital, because individuals suffering from the dysfunctional form may require more prolonged pharmacological therapy.

It is important to recognize the variety of anxiety disorders. Accurate diagnosis is vital because both pharmacological and non-pharmacological treatment varies for each (Chapter 16). The disorders include the following:

1. generalized anxiety disorder
2. stress-related anxiety
3. panic disorder
4. phobias
5. anxiety secondary to medical illness (e.g., hyperthyroidism, Cushing's disease, and coronary artery disease)
6. anxiety accompanying another, primary mental disorder (e.g., schizophrenia, drug abuse, dementia, depression, post-traumatic stress disorder, obsessive-compulsive disorder)
7. drug-induced anxiety (e.g., from cocaine, caffeine, asthma medications, nasal decongestants, and withdrawal from alcohol or sedatives)

In the following discussion, we describe the use of drugs in treating these disorders, especially generalized anxiety disorder and phobias.

The distinction between "normal" and "pathological" anxiety is difficult. Thus, anxiolytics are often tried (rightly or wrongly) to alleviate the distress. Because of the uncertainty of diagnosis and the wide prevalence of anxiety in our society, the benzodiazepines have become one of the most widely prescribed classes of drugs.

> Given the high population prevalence and significant levels of morbidity associated with anxiety, it is not surprising that anti-anxiety drugs are among the most widely used of all medications. Anti-anxiety agents are the fourth most frequently prescribed class of medication, with over 55 million prescriptions written for benzo-diazepines alone in 1989.[2]

The benzodiazepines and related drugs can relieve anxiety in many of the listed syndromes; they are perhaps most useful in managing stress-related anxiety. However, as we shall see, their therapeutic use in most instances is best restricted to relatively short periods of time, perhaps 1 to 6 weeks, and only for conditions where such short-term therapy is beneficial. Such conditions include acute situational grief, acute incapacitating stress reactions, and insomnia caused by anxiety over short-lived external events.

These drugs are generally not utilized for chronic anxiety disorders, depression, situations requiring fine motor skills or mental alertness, situations where alcohol or other CNS depressants will be used, the elderly, or individuals prone to drug misuse. There are, as always, exceptions to these restrictions. A newer, nonbenzodiazepine, second-generation anxiolytic (buspirone) may have less abuse potential. Also, as stated by Unlenhuth and associates, "Many patients continue to derive benefit from long-term treatment with benzodiazepines. . . . Attitudes strongly against the use of these drugs may be depriving many anxious patients of appropriate treatment."[3] Perhaps these patients represent those with a neurochemical basis of anxiety, and continued treatment may be indicated, at least in the absence of signs of dependence or abuse. Such sustained treatment, however, is likely to remain controversial.

BENZODIAZEPINES

With the continuing decline in the use of barbiturates, the benzo-diazepines have been the drugs of choice for the short-term pharmaco-logical treatment of stress-related anxiety and insomnia. The history of the benzodiazepines can be divided into three phases (the third is discussed on page 89).[4] The first phase began with the introduction of chlordiazepoxide (Librium) in 1960 and lasted until 1977. During this period there was an exponential increase in the clinical use (and therapeutic misuse) of benzodiazepines, and a dozen competing benzodiazepines were introduced. Slowly we began to understand their limitations, side effects, toxicities, and potential for abuse.

The second phase in benzodiazepine history began in 1977, when it was established that diazepam (Valium) binds specifically and with high affinity to a distinct population of receptors in the brain. Since 1977 the clinical use of benzodiazepines has not significantly increased, but our understanding of their mechanism of action and, indeed, our understanding of the neurochemistry of anxiety, fear, and panic disorders has increased dramatically.

The Benzodiazepine-GABA Receptor

In Chapter 3 we introduced the $GABA_A$ receptor as a site of barbiturate action. It is now clear that most, if not all, of the actions of the benzo-diazepines are also mediated through specific binding to $GABA_A$ recep-tors. Even the affinity of the various types of benzodiazepines for these receptors correlates closely with their individual pharmacological potencies.

GABA depresses neuronal excitability by selectively increasing the transmembrane conductance of chloride ions; that is, GABA opens chloride channels in the nerve membrane of $GABA_A$ receptors. The benzodiazepine binding site on this receptor is distinct from the barbiturate binding site, and yet it is located next to the site where GABA binds (Figure 4.1), both of which are located on the same protein subunit.[4,5] Benzodiazepine binding serves to potentiate and facilitate GABA-induced increases in chloride conductance, which, in turn, inhibits synaptic action.

Two further points complicate this concept of benzodiazepine receptors. First, there are at least two types of benzodiazepine receptors, $GABA_A$ and $GABA_B$. The former act to increase chloride ion conductance (inducing fast-acting inhibitory postsynaptic potentials [IPSPs]; see Appendix II). The $GABA_A$ receptor is also the site of action of barbiturates and benzodiazepines. $GABA_B$ receptors were not discovered until the early 1980s; only now, with the discovery of specific $GABA_B$-receptor blockers, is their function becoming better known.*

Second, the actual role of $GABA_A$ receptors and anxiolysis is not straightforward; the relationship might, in fact, be expressed through GABA-induced modification of other neurotransmitters. The importance of this second point will become clearer when we discuss two new drugs, zolpidem and buspirone.

A recently introduced benzodiazepine antagonist (flumazenil, Romazicon) can occupy the benzodiazepine binding site on the $GABA_A$ receptor. Such binding distorts the GABA binding site, thus reducing membrane binding of GABA and preventing the chloride channels from opening (see Figure 4.1). Flumazenil is used clinically to displace benzodiazepines from the $GABA_A$ receptors, thus terminating the depressant effects of overdosage. In this situation, acute anxiety reactions can be precipitated if the individual has developed benzodiazepine dependency.

---

*$GABA_B$ receptors operate as neuromodulators. They are located on the presynaptic nerve terminals of other neurons that secrete such neurotransmitters as GABA, glutamate, dopamine, norepinephrine, serotonin, substance P, and others. These $GABA_B$ receptors are coupled to potassium ion channels via intracellular G-proteins (see Appendix III), and they mediate late IPSPs. A $GABA_B$ receptor agonist (like GABA itself) would inhibit the release of a number of neurotransmitters and neuropeptides. Baclofen is the only currently available selective $GABA_B$ receptor agonist; it is a clinically useful muscle relaxant and antispastic drug. The effects of $GABA_B$ receptor antagonists are discussed later in this chapter.

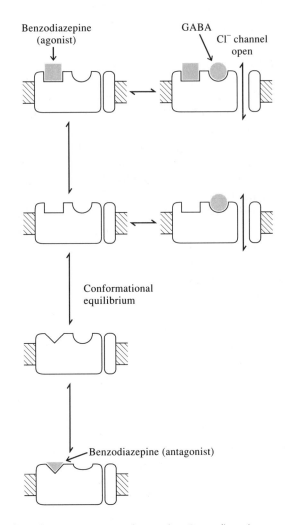

FIGURE 4.1   Benzodiazepine-GABA receptor interaction. Benzodiazepine agonists (e.g., diazepam) and antagonists (e.g., flumazenil) are believed to bind to a site on the GABA receptor that is distinct from the GABA binding site. A conformational equilibrium exists between states in which the benzodiazepine receptor exists in its *agonist binding* conformation (*top*) and in its *antagonist binding* conformation (*bottom*). In the latter state, the GABA receptor has a much reduced affinity for GABA, so the chloride channel remains closed. [Modified from H. P. Rang and M. M. Dale,[5] fig. 25.6.]

The existence of both a specific, endogenous benzodiazepine agonist and a specific, endogenous antagonist has been postulated but not proven. This is certainly an intriguing postulate, since it suggests that benzodiazepine receptors exist for reasons other than the possible future ingested of drugs! Several substances (including naturally occurring benzodiazepines) have been proposed as endogenous anxiolytics, and several substances have been proposed as endogenous "anxiogenic" (anxiety-inducing) compounds.[2,5]

Pharmacokinetics

Approximately 12 benzodiazepine derivatives are commercially available. They are marketed for use as sedatives, anxiolytics, muscle relaxants, intravenous anesthetics, and anticonvulsants. They differ from each other mainly in such pharmacokinetic measures as lipid solubility, rate of metabolism to pharmacologically active intermediates, and plasma half-lives of both the parent drug and any active metabolites.

The basic structure of the benzodiazepines is shown in Figure 4.2, along with a list of currently available derivatives. Note that all these drugs share the same basic structure, differing only in their substituent groups.

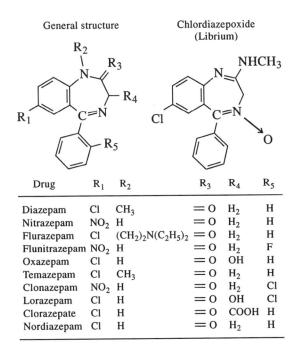

Drug	R_1	R_2	R_3	R_4	R_5
Diazepam	Cl	CH_3	$=O$	H_2	H
Nitrazepam	NO_2	H	$=O$	H_2	H
Flurazepam	Cl	$(CH_2)_2N(C_2H_5)_2$	$=O$	H_2	H
Flunitrazepam	NO_2	H	$=O$	H_2	F
Oxazepam	Cl	H	$=O$	OH	H
Temazepam	Cl	CH_3	$=O$	H_2	H
Clonazepam	NO_2	H	$=O$	H_2	Cl
Lorazepam	Cl	H	$=O$	OH	Cl
Clorazepate	Cl	H	$=O$	COOH	H
Nordiazepam	Cl	H	$=O$	H_2	H

FIGURE 4.2   Structures of some benzodiazepines.

TABLE 4.1 Benzodiazepines.

Drug name		Dosage form		Active metabolite	Active compounds in blood	Mean elimination half-life in hours (range)
Trade	Generic	Oral	Parent-eral			
LONG-ACTING AGENTS						
Valium	Diazepam	X	X	Yes	Diazepam	24 (20–50)
					Nordiazepam	60 (50–100)
Librium	Chlordiazepoxide	X		Yes	Chlor-diazepoxide	10 (8–24)
					Nordiazepam	60 (50–100)
Dalmane	Flurazepam	X		Yes	Desalkyl-flurazepam	80 (70–160)
Paxipam	Halazepam	X		Yes	Halazepam	14 (10–20)
					Nordiazepam	60 (50–100)
Centrax	Prazepam	X		Yes	Nordiazepam	60 (50–100)
Tranxene	Chlorazepate	X		Yes	Nordiazepam	60 (50–100)
INTERMEDIATE-ACTING AGENTS						
Ativan	Lorazepam	X	X	No	Lorazepam	15 (10–24)
Klonopin	Clonazepam	X		No	Clonazepam	30 (18–50)
Dormalin	Quazepam	X		Yes	Quazepam	35 (25–50)
					Desalkyl-flurazepam	80 (70–160)
ProSom	Estazolam	X		Yes	Hydroxy-estazolam	18 (13–35)
SHORT-ACTING AGENTS						
Versed	Midazolam		X	No	Midazolam	2.5 (1.5–4.5)
Serax	Oxazepam	X		No	Oxazepam	8 (5–15)
Restoril	Temazepam	X		No	Temazepam	12 (8–35)
Halcion	Triazolam	X		No	Triazolam	2.5 (1.5–5)
Xanax	Alprazolam	X		No	Alprazolam	12 (11–18)

Absorption and Distribution

Benzodiazepines are well absorbed when they are taken orally; peak plasma concentrations are achieved in about one hour. Some (e.g., oxazepam and lorazepam) are absorbed more slowly, while others (e.g., triazolam) are absorbed more rapidly.

About 15 benzodiazepines are commercially available in the United States (Table 4.1). Of these, 14 are available in a dosage form for oral ingestion, 2 of these are also available for parenteral use (diazepam and lorazepam), and 1 is available only in parenteral formulation (midazolam).

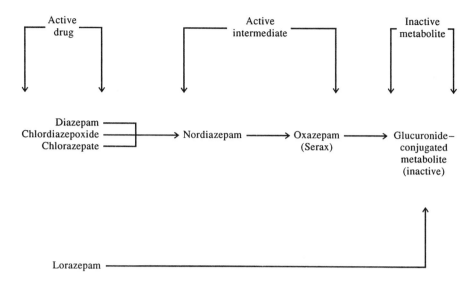

FIGURE 4.3   Metabolism of benzodiazepines. The intermediate metabolite nor-diazepam is formed from many agents. Oxazepam (Serax) is commercially available and is also an active intermediate in the metabolism of nordiazepam to its inactive products.

Metabolism and Excretion

In Chapter 2 we stated that most psychoactive drugs must be metabo-lized to pharmacologically inactive, water-soluble products, which are then excreted in urine. While this holds true for several benzo-diazepines, some of them are first biotransformed to intermediate products that are pharmacologically active; these, in turn, must be detoxified by further metabolism before they can be excreted (Figure 4.3). As we can see from Table 4.1 and Figure 4.3, several long-acting compounds are biotransformed into long-lasting pharmacologically active metabolites, such as nordiazepam, the half-life of which is about 60 hours. Figure 4.4 demonstrates the buildup and slow metabolism of active metabolite in a human volunteer who was given diazepam daily for 14 days. The short-acting benzodiazepines are metabolized directly into inactive products.

The elderly have a severely reduced ability to metabolize long-acting benzodiazepines and their active metabolites. In this popula-tion, the elimination half-life (for both the parent drug and the active metabolite) is often more than 10 days. Since it takes about six half-lives to rid the body completely of a drug (Chapter 2, Table 2.2), it would take an elderly patient as long as 60 days to become completely drug-free after even a single dose of diazepam. Because these drugs

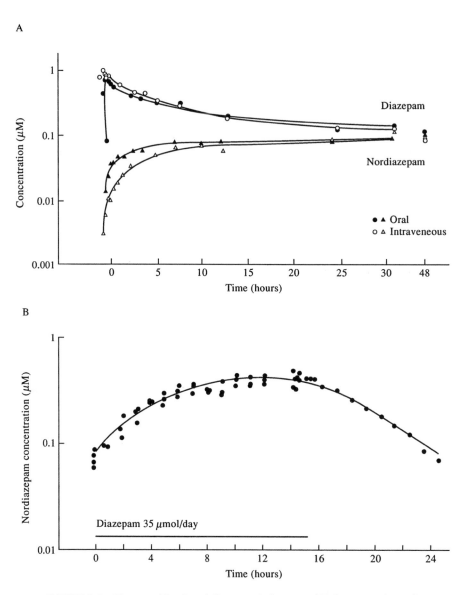

FIGURE 4.4   Pharmacokinetics of diazepam in humans. (**A**) Concentrations of diazepam and its active metabolite, nordiazepam, following a single oral or intravenous dose. Note the negligible disappearance of both substances after the first 20 hours. (**B**) Accumulation of nordiazepam during two weeks of daily administration of diazepam followed by a slow decline (half-life about 3 days) after cessation of diazepam administration. [From H. P. Rang and M. M. Dale,[5] fig. 25.8, p. 636.]

can induce a "brain syndrome," elderly patients can become pro-foundly and persistently drug-demented as a result. In general, no long-acting benzodiazepine should be administered to an elderly patient. As stated by Rang and Dale:

> At the age of 91, the grandmother of one of the authors was growing increasingly forgetful and mildly dotty, having been taking nitraz-epam for insomnia regularly for years. To the author's lasting shame, it took a canny general practitioner to diagnose the problem. Cancellation of the nitrazepam prescription produced a dramatic improvement.[6]

It must be added that my 85-year-old grandmother experienced the identical problem with diazepam. Two months after discontinuation of the drug, her dementia disappeared and she remained lucid until her death 10 years later.

Because of the long elimination times, a person who has been using one of these drugs for prolonged periods may maintain detectable urinary concentrations of the drug for many days to several weeks after discontinuing its use.

Pharmacodynamics

The clinical and behavioral effects of the benzodiazepines all occur as a result of facilitation of GABA-induced neuronal inhibition at the various locations of $GABA_A$ receptors throughout the CNS. Low doses alleviate anxiety, agitation, and fear by their actions on receptors located in the hippocampus and the amygdala. The mental confusion and amnesia seem to be associated with effects on GABA neurons located in the cerebral cortex and the hippocampus. The sedative-hypnotic effects appear to arise from effects on receptors located in the cerebral cortex. The mild muscle-relaxant effects of the benzodiazepines are probably caused both by their anxiolytic actions and to some action on GABA receptors located in the spinal cord, cerebellum, and brain stem. The antiepileptic actions seem to follow from actions on GABA receptors located in the cerebellum and the hippocampus. The abuse potential and psychological dependency may follow from actions on GABA receptors that modulate the discharge of other neurons involved in the behavior-reinforcing systems within the brain (see Chapter 15).

Benzodiazepines probably bind to some degree to both $GABA_A$ and $GABA_B$ receptors, although $GABA_A$ binding dominates. Given that there may be a great number of subgroups of $GABA_A$ receptors, binding differences might account for slight differences in the spectrum of action of these agents. For example, alprazolam may be less sedating than diazepam (and may even be antidepressant); clonazepam and alprazolam may be of more use in treating panic attacks than are other benzodiazepines; diazepam may be more efficacious for relieving muscle spasm; and clonazepam may be of particular value as an anticonvulsant. Much remains to be done in classifying the actions of the benzodiazepines.

Higher doses of benzodiazepines cause a syndrome of sedation and hypnosis characteristic of the barbiturates. Tolerance appears to build to the sedative effects but less to the antianxiety effects.[7]

Uses

The major indication for benzodiazepine therapy is anxiety that is so debilitating that the patient's life-style, work, and interpersonal - relationships are severely hampered. However, the absolute necessity for concurrent psychological support and counseling cannot be over-emphasized (Chapter 16).

Benzodiazepines have been called *minor tranquilizers* to differentiate them from *major tranquilizers,* the antipsychotic compounds (discussed in Chapter 11). Benzodiazepines do not substitute for antipsychotic agents and are not effective in treating psychotic depression. However, some benzodiazepines (especially alprazolam) are useful in patients who are suffering from depression accompanied by severe anxiety.

Panic attacks and phobias are now being treated with the benzodiazepine alprazolam.[8-10] Here, however, the efficacy of benzodiazepines, especially in comparison to antidepressants such as imipramine (Chapter 8), is still uncertain. The uncertainty probably results from the concept that panic and phobic disorders are chronic, recurring conditions, with frequent relapses after short-term therapy. Controlled trials of pharmacotherapy in this area are just being conducted. Chapter 16 discusses therapy of panic attacks and phobias in more detail.

Because benzodiazepines can substitute for alcohol, they are widely used both in treating acute alcohol withdrawal and in long-term therapy to reduce the rate of relapse to previous drinking habits.[11]

All benzodiazepines exert antiepileptic actions because they raise the hippocampal threshold for generating seizures.

Side Effects and Toxicity

Common acute side effects in benzodiazepine therapy are dose-related extensions of the intended actions. These include sedation, drowsiness, ataxia, lethargy, mental confusion, disorientation, slurred speech, amnesia, and induction or extension of the symptoms of dementia. At higher doses, impairments of mental and psychomotor function dominate.

Respiration is not seriously depressed, even at high doses. Indeed, attempted suicides by overdose are rarely successful unless the benzodiazepine is taken along with another CNS depressant, such as alcohol. Indeed, this combination can cause a most serious (and potentially fatal) drug interaction.

Sleep patterns can be altered markedly. When short-acting agents are taken at bedtime, both early-morning wakening and rebound insomnia for the next night are common. When long-acting agents are taken at bedtime, daytime sedation can be a problem.

An additive impairment of motor abilities—especially a person's ability to drive an automobile—is common. This impairment is compounded by the drug-induced suppression of one's ability to assess his or her own level of physical and mental impairment.

The cognitive deficits associated with benzodiazepine use are significant. As $GABA_A$ agonists, these drugs are exceedingly effective amnestic agents—a desirable effect when used in anesthesia but a potentially serious side effect when the retention of mental capacity is important. Benzodiazepines also significantly interfere with learning behaviors. The potential usefulness of GABA antagonists as cognitive enhancers is discussed below.

Possible side effects associated with long-term, chronic use of benzodiazepines include the dementing effects of the drugs. Memory, thinking, and cognition are severely affected and can appear as dementia in the elderly. Because of the long half-lives of benzodiazepines, a prolonged period of drug abstinence is required in order to determine accurately a patient's normal mental capacity.

Tolerance and Dependence

When benzodiazepines are taken for long periods of time, a pattern of dependence develops. Even in therapeutic dosages, long-term, daily use of the drugs followed by discontinuation can cause a predictable abstinence (withdrawal) syndrome.[12,13] Early withdrawal signs include a return of the symptoms for which the drug originally was given, possibly in a more intense form.[14,15] Next, rebound increases in insomnia, restlessness, agitation, irritability, and muscle tension gradually appear as the blood level of the drug falls. The shorter acting the drug, the quicker the onset of these withdrawal symptoms. In rare instances hallucinations, psychoses, and seizures can occur. Most of these withdrawal symptoms subside within 1 to 4 weeks, depending on the half-life of the drug being used. When the patient has developed a dependence on a drug of short duration, treatment involves gradual tapering of the dose and substitution of a long-acting benzodiazepine. With benzodiazepine withdrawal, there is an unmasking of the formerly drug-occupied benzodiazepine receptors as well as an increased number of receptors formed in response to chronic exposure to the drug.[13]

Tolerance can develop, which can necessitate small increases in dose. This tolerance, however, is not nearly as marked as that which occurs following long-term use of the barbiturates. The mechanism of tolerance involves receptor adaptation ("down regulation" of both the binding activity and the function of benzodiazepine-GABA$_A$ receptors);[13] it is not caused by metabolic pharmacokinetic changes, because benzodiazepines do not induce the production of hepatic drug-metabolizing enzymes.[16]

Fetal Effects

Benzodiazepines administered during the first trimester of pregnancy have been reported to cause fetal abnormalities, although it was unclear whether the mothers had taken other drugs. Other data dispute this relationship.[17] It does appear, however, that a fetus can develop benzodiazepine dependence, and withdrawal may occur in the newborn. Unless it is absolutely necessary (as in an epileptic mother who takes a benzodiazepine as an anticonvulsant), benzodiazepines should be avoided during pregnancy.

Finally, benzodiazepines can be detected in breast milk. Maternal intake and infant behavior should be carefully monitored if the mother plans to breast-feed the baby.

Nonmedical Use and Abuse

Benzodiazepines were introduced during the 1960s, and their popularity peaked during the mid-1970s, when 100 million prescriptions for these drugs were written each year. Having recognized the overuse, physicians wrote only 65 million prescriptions in 1981. In 1990, however, 88 million prescriptions were written.[18] This level of use probably does not represent gross misuse. Rather, it may represent legitimate use for the treatment of short-term anxiety and for nonanxiety-related conditions, such as the treatment of epilepsy and panic. More women still use benzodiazepines than do men, but such a distribution appears to be appropriate, because men are both more reluctant to seek medical care and more likely to use alcohol to relieve anxiety.[1]

Benzodiazepine abuse is always a prominent topic in conferences on prescription drug abuse,[19] despite the fact that

> benzodiazepines rarely are primary drugs of abuse—people rarely use them alone to produce intoxication. Most people who are not anxious do not like the effects of benzodiazepines. Some abusers of other sedatives, including alcoholics, find the effects of benzodiazepines desirable, but very rarely as primary intoxicants.[16]

The nonmedical use of benzodiazepines peaked between 1975 and 1977 and has been modestly declining ever since. The only apparent abuse of benzodiazepines now involves polydrug abusers rather than persons who use one drug alone in an abusive pattern. As part of a polydrug pattern, benzodiazepines (especially diazepam and alprazolam) may be taken for a euphoriant effect or to enhance the euphoriant effect of narcotics.[20] In patients who take methadone as part of the treatment protocol for opioid dependency (Chapter 10), benzodiazepines can reduce the anxiety that is often present. Indeed, clonazepam (Klonopin), nicknamed "super Valium," has become a common drug of abuse among methadone-maintenance patients.[19] Many alcohol and cocaine abusers take benzodiazepines, presumably for their reinforcing and anxiolytic properties and to self-medicate symptoms of cocaine toxicity.

GABA_A- and GABA_B-Receptor Antagonists

GABA Antagonists and Cognition

Benzodiazepines are cognitive inhibitors possibly because they ultimately inhibit cholinergic neurons in the basal forebrain (by increasing GABA function). Therefore, benzodiazepine antagonists might enhance cognition by their ability to selectively disinhibit these same cholinergic neurons.[21] Miller and coworkers[22] recently demonstrated that an experimental $GABA_A$ antagonist enhanced learning acquisition in animal models by secondarily enhancing cortical and hippocampal cholinergic function. The mechanism appeared to involve binding of the antagonist at a site on the $GABA_A$ receptor that is different from that to which the benzodiazepines bind. The drug did not induce either anxiety or seizures, as might be predicted if the brain contains an endogenous GABA agonist that acts to prevent these conditions.

Bittiger and coworkers[23] recently reviewed the pharmacology of a series of selective antagonists of $GABA_B$ receptors and the potential therapeutic applications resulting from such blockade. These agents (one being phaclifen) not only block the muscle-relaxant effects of the $GABA_B$-receptor agonist baclofen but also increase the release of neurotransmitters in the cerebral cortex.

Potential therapeutic applications of $GABA_B$-receptor antagonists include use as cognitive enhancers, as antidepressants, and as anticonvulsants in the treatment of absence (petit mal) epilepsy. Improvement in memory and cognitive processes were studied by Mondadori, Preiswerk, and Jaekel,[24] who attribute such improvement to increased transmitter release, reduction of late IPSPs, and increased neuronal excitability. Pratt and Bowery[25] note that the antidepressant desipramine (Chapter 8) altered $GABA_B$ receptors in a manner consistent with its antidepressant action. Thus, $GABA_B$-receptor antagonists might promote antidepressant activity. Finally, $GABA_B$ antagonists suppress the typical EEG pattern characteristic of absence epilepsy.

Flumazenil: A $GABA_A$ Antagonist

Flumazenil (Romazicon) is a benzodiazepine derivative that binds with high affinity to benzodiazepine receptors on the $GABA_A$ complex (see Figure 4.1) but exhibits no intrinsic activity after binding. As a consequence, it competitively blocks the binding of pharmacologically active benzodiazepines.[26] Flumazenil thus effectively reverses the antianxiety and sedative effects of the benzodiazepines.

Flumazenil is metabolized quite rapidly in the liver and has a short half-life (about 50 to 70 minutes). Because this half-life is much shorter than that of most benzodiazepines, the benzodiazepine effects can reappear as flumazenil is lost, thus necessitating reinjection. Flumazenil has become a routinely used antidote for both diagnostic and therapeutic use in coma where benzodiazepine ingestion is suspected; flumazenil reverses benzodiazepine overdosage. There is also indication that flumazenil may be useful in the differential diagnosis of some cognitive disorders and in the diagnosis of panic disorder.[27]

"SECOND GENERATION" ANXIOLYTICS

Today we are in the third phase of benzodiazepine history as we begin to appreciate the variety of anxiety and other psychological disorders; this understanding is leading to more sophisticated treatment paradigms (Chapter 16). In addition, there is the belief that "second generation" anxiolytics, acting on a totally different set of receptors than do the benzodiazepines, may prove to be pharmacologically superior to the benzodiazepines.

Zolpidem

Zolpidem (Ambien) is a newly available nonbenzodiazepine that has been approved for the short-term treatment of insomnia.[28] Although chemically unrelated to the benzodiazepines, it binds to a specific subtype (type 1) of the $GABA_A$ receptor.[29,30] Zolpidem is therefore classified as a specific agonist of benzodiazepine type 1 receptors. As such, it displays some, but not all, of the actions of all other benzodiazepine agonists, which, as stated earlier, bind nonspecifically to all $GABA_A$ receptors.

Pharmacokinetics

Zolpidem is rapidly and completely absorbed from the gastrointestinal tract after oral administration. Peak plasma levels are reached in about 1 hour. Following metabolism in the liver, the end products are excreted by the kidneys. The metabolic half-life is about 2.5 hours (longer in the elderly). Because of this short half-life, the drug is usually compared to triazolam (Halcion).

Pharmacodynamics

At doses of 5 to 10 milligrams, zolpidem produces sedation and promotes a physiological pattern of sleep in the absence of anxiolytic, anticonvulsant, or muscle-relaxant effects. It is claimed that, at these doses, memory is less affected than after comparable doses of triazolam, even in the elderly.[31] Dependency, rebound insomnia, and withdrawal signs have not yet been reported.

Adverse Effects

Dose-related adverse effects include drowsiness, dizziness, and nausea. In the elderly taking 20 milligrams or more, confusion, falls, memory loss, and psychotic reactions have been reported. A high-dose incidence of nausea and vomiting may tend to limit overdosage, such as in suicide attempts. Overdoses to 400 milligrams (20 times the high-dose therapeutic amount) have not been fatal. Flumazenil appears to effectively antagonize the effects of zolpidem. In conclusion,

> zolpidem is an effective non-benzodiazepine hypnotic that binds to benzodiazepine receptors in the brain. Its minimal effect on the stages of sleep is an advantage over benzodiazepine hypnotics. Whether zolpidem is less likely than benzodiazepines to have residual effects the next day, induce tolerance, or be abused remains to be determined.[28]

Buspirone

Buspirone (BuSpar) is an anxiolytic drug that differs from the benzodiazepines both structurally and pharmacologically. It is not only an effective therapy for certain anxious patients but also a useful tool for investigating the neurochemistry of anxiety. Buspirone relieves anxiety in a unique fashion:

1. Its anxiolysis occurs without significant sedation, drowsiness, or hypnotic action, even in overdosage.

2. Amnesia, mental confusion, and psychomotor impairment are minimal or absent.

3. It does not potentiate the CNS depressant effects of alcohol, benzodiazepines, or other CNS sedatives (i.e., synergism does not occur).

4. It does not substitute for benzodiazepines in treating anxiety or benzodiazepine withdrawal.

5. It does not exhibit cross tolerance or cross dependence with benzodiazepines.

6. It exhibits little potential for addiction or abuse.

7. It exhibits an antidepressant effect in addition to its anxiolytic effect, making it potentially useful in depressive disorders with accompanying anxiety (Chapter 8).

8. Its effect has a gradual onset rather than the immediate onset of the action of the benzodiazepines.

9. It is ineffective as a hypnotic to promote the onset of sleep.

Mechanism of Action

To this point, we have correlated anxiolytic action with drug binding to $GABA_A$ receptors. Buspirone is unique as an anxiolytic in that it selectively binds to a subgroup of serotonin (5-hydroxytryptamine, or 5-HT) receptors. Because this subclass is called the 1-A group, the receptors are called $5\text{-}HT_{1A}$. After binding, buspirone exerts a weak stimulant action; the drug is therefore termed a "weak agonist" of $5\text{-}HT_{1A}$ receptors. Such binding relates to anxiolytic action since electrical lesions of these seritonergic neurons are accompanied by a loss of anxiolytic action.[32] Furthermore, this selective receptor binding is confined to areas of the brain thought to be involved in mechanisms of anxiety (hippocampus, neocortex, and dorsal raphe).*

Clinical Uses

Buspirone is considered a drug of first choice for the pharmacological treatment of generalized anxiety disorders, chronic anxiety, and anxiety in the elderly. It is also prescribed for many patients of all ages who suffer from mixed symptoms of anxiety and depression.[34] Buspirone seems to be of little value in treating panic disorder.

> Buspirone seems to be most helpful in anxious patients who do not demand immediate gratification or the immediate response they associate with the benzodiazepine response. Slower and more gradual onset of anxiety relief is balanced by the increased safety andlack of dependency-producing aspects of buspirone.[34]

To see clinical effects takes several weeks of continuous, three-times-per-day treatment. Patients who have previously been taking benzodiazepines do poorly on buspirone. This has led to an impression in some clinicians that buspirone, despite lower toxicity, possesses lower efficacy. This reminds me of tricyclic antidepressants (Chapter 8), the efficacy of which was also questioned during their first 20

---

*As summarized by Yocca:

Buspirone . . . binds selectively to presynaptic (dorsal raphe) and postsynaptic (hippocampus, cortex) $5\text{-}HT_{1A}$ receptor binding sites. . . . Azopirones in general display partial agonist activity at postsynaptic $5\text{-}HT_{1A}$ receptors linked negatively to adenyl cyclase and appear to demonstrate a similar profile in hippocampal CA_1 pyramidal neurons sensitive to the effects of 5-HT. Through their actionat presynaptic $5\text{-}HT_{1A}$ receptors, these agents . . . dose-dependently inhibit cortical and hippocampal 5-HT synthesis while inhibiting the firing of 5-HT-containing dorsal raphe neurons. . . . These interactions initiate long-term changes in central 5-HT neurotransmission.[33]

years. Only time and experience will prove this second-generation anxiolytic drug will be a viable or nonviable alternative to the benzodiazepines.

ANTIEPILEPTIC DRUGS USED IN TREATING PSYCHOLOGICAL DISORDERS

Seizures are manifestations of electrical disturbances in the brain. The term *epilepsy* refers to CNS disorders characterized by relatively brief, chronically recurring seizures that have a rapid onset. Epileptic seizures are often associated with focal (or localized) lesions within the brain. In laboratory animals, epileptic seizures can be induced by a variety of techniques, including "kindling" (repeated low-voltage electrical stimulation to increase the sensitivity of neurons in the limbic system).

Interestingly, Post and Weiss[35] associate kindling not only with antiepileptic drug action but also with the treatment of bipolar disorders. Historically, a few individuals have advocated the use of antiepileptic drugs in treating "disturbed nonepileptic psychiatric patients."[36] For example, phenytoin has been used to treat uncontrolled bouts of mania, panic, and aggression. Since phenytoin acts by "stabilizing" neuronal membranes and increasing the activity of GABAergic neurons, it limits seizures by limiting the spread of abnormal electrical activity. The same mechanism suggests the efficacy of phenytoin in nonepileptic, psychological disorders. More recently, newer antiepileptic drugs (such as carbamazepine, valproic acid, and clonazepam) have been studied for treating psychological disorders.

The fact that both the barbiturates and the benzodiazepines are not only anxiolytic but also antiepileptic encourages the notion that epilepsy and mania can be treated with similar drugs. For reference, Table 4.2 lists the antiepileptic drugs that are available and the year in which each one was introduced.

Relationships between Structure and Activity

Most antiepileptic drugs belong to one of a relatively small number of chemical classes, some of which we have already discussed. The barbiturates (e.g., phenobarbital), the oldest of these drugs, and the hydantoins (such as phenytoin) had been the most widely used

TABLE 4.2 Antiepileptic drugs available in the United States.

Year introduced	Generic name	Trade name
1912	Phenobarbital	Luminal
1935	Mephobarbital	Mebaral
1938	Phenytoin	Dilantin
1946	Trimethadione	Tridione
1947	Mephenytoin	Mesantoin
1949	Paramethadione	Paradione
1951	Phenacemide	Phenurone
1952	Metharbital	Gemonil
1953	Phensuximide	Milontin
1954	Primidone	Mysoline
1957	Methsuximide	Celontin
1957	Ethotoin	Peganone
1960	Ethosuximide	Zarontin
1968	Diazepam	Valium
1974	Carbamazepine	Tegretol
1975	Clonazepam	Klonopin
1978	Valproic acid	Depakene
1981	Clorazepate	Tranxene
1981	Lorazepam	Ativan
1993	Felbamate	Felbatol
1994	Gabapentin	Neuronin

Source: Modified from R. M. Julien, "Antiepileptic Drugs," in N. T. Smith and A. N. Corbascio, eds., *Drug Interactions in Anesthesia*, 2nd ed. (Philadelphia: Lea & Febiger, 1986), p. 246.

antiepileptic compounds. More recently several benzodiazepines have been found to be exceedingly useful.

Older drugs used to treat epilepsy that are structurally similar to either the barbiturates or the hydantoins include the *succinimides,* the *oxazoladines,* and *primidone* (Figure 4.5). These drugs are not used to treat nonepileptic, psychological disorders and will not be further discussed here. Finally, two structurally dissimilar agents introduced in the late 1970s are effective in treating both epilepsy and nonepileptic psychological disorders: *carbamazepine* (Tegretol) and *valproic acid* (Depakene). Carbamazepine structurally resembles both phenytoin and imipramine. Valproic acid exerts specific actions at GABA synapses.

Recently, *felbamate* and *gabapentin* were introduced as effective new antiepileptic drugs. Felbamate structurally resembles meproba-

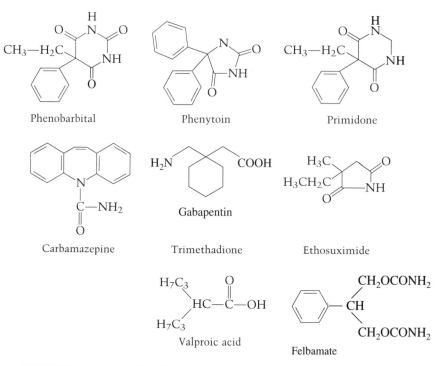

FIGURE 4.5   Representative drugs used to treat epilepsy.

mate (Chapter 3), demonstrating that one drug can be effective in treating both neurological and psychological disorders.[37] To date, nonepileptic, psychological uses of felbamate have not been reported, although the structural resemblance to meprobamate implies anxiolytic effect. At first thought to be free of serious side effects, felbamate's use was suspended in late 1994 because of serious hematological reactions. Felbamate is currently used only when it is obviously necessary and irreplaceable as an antiepileptic.

Gabapentin, a structural analogue of GABA, was synthesized as a GABA-mimetic drug that crosses the blood-brain barrier. It is an effective adjunct antiepileptic drug when used with other drugs for certain types of seizures.[38] Recently, in a case report, gabapentin was effective in treating an anxiety disorder (phobia) and pain (reflex sympathetic dystrophy) in a female patient.[39] Gabapentin binds to neocortex and hippocampus, but its receptors and biochemical function are unknown.

Barbiturates

Phenobarbital (Chapter 3), introduced in 1912, was the first widely effective antiepileptic drug. It replaced the more toxic agent bromide that had been used for many years. Two other barbiturates are also used occasionally for treating epilepsy: mephobarbital (Mebaral) and metharbital (Gemonil).

Because of their relative lack of toxicity, these drugs are still used occasionally even though more effective, more specific, and less sedating antiepileptic agents are now the drugs of first choice. Because of their long duration of action, the barbiturates can be administered only once each day. Epileptic children given barbiturates can display adverse neuropsychological reactions (behavioral hyperactivity and interference with learning ability).

Primidone (Mysoline) is an antiepileptic agent that is structurally very similar to phenobarbital (see Figure 4.5). Primidone is metabolized to phenobarbital, which might well be the major active form of the drug.

Hydantoins

Phenytoin (Dilantin), which was introduced in 1938, remains a commonly used anticonvulsant. At an effective dose level, phenytoin produces less sedation than do barbiturates. Phenytoin appears to act by limiting the involvement of neurons in the spread of seizure activity. The drug is slowly but completely absorbed when taken orally and has a half-life of about 24 hours. Thus, daytime sedation can be minimized if the patient takes the full daily dose at bedtime. Although phenytoin has been tried in the treatment of mania, results have generally been disappointing.

Benzodiazepines

All benzodiazepines possess antiepileptic and anxiolytic properties. Two of them, clonazepam (Klonopin) and clorazepate (Tranxene), are promoted by their manufacturers for treating seizures, especially for patients who suffer from certain types of seizures that are difficult to treat (such as petit mal variant, myoclonic, and akinetic seizures). Because these drugs are frequently used to treat chronic seizures in children, drug-induced personality changes and learning disabilities must be carefully monitored.

Diazepam (Valium) and midazolam (Versed), available in parenteral formulation, are administered intravenously to rapidly control episodes of status epilepticus (an emergency situation that is characterized by rapidly recurring, intense seizures).

In nonepileptic applications, alprazolam (Xanax, see Table 4.1) is used to treat panic disorder accompanied by depression;[40,41] lorazepam and clonazepam have been widely studied for psychiatric applications including the treatment of acute mania and other agitated psychotic conditions, usually in combination with other mood stabilizers (Chapter 9). Indeed, clonazepam has been referred to as a "behavioral suppressor" rather than as a "mood stabilizer."[42]

Carbamazepine

Carbamazepine (Tegretol) is structurally related both to the tricyclic antidepressant imipramine (Chapter 8) and to the anticonvulsant phenytoin. As an antiepileptic drug, it is administered either alone or with other antiepileptic drugs to treat generalized major motor seizures and complex partial seizures. For children, it is often preferred to phenobarbital. Carbamazepine is also effective in treating psychomotor types of epilepsy (a type of seizure that does not respond to phenytoin). Possibly because of its structural resemblance to imipramine, its sedative effect is much less intense than that of the other antiepileptic agents. The primary limitations of carbamazepine include rare but potentially serious alterations in the cellular composition of blood (reduced numbers of white blood cells), presumably secondary to its effects on bone marrow.

For nonepileptic, psychiatric use, carbamazepine is being increasingly used to prevent recurrences in bipolar disorder; it is slightly less effective than lithium for acute mania but slightly more effective for maintenance and prophylactic treatment.[43-45] This use is discussed at length in Chapter 9.

Valproic Acid

Valproic acid (Depakene, Depakote, valproate) is a simple organic compound (see Figure 4.5) that suppresses a wide variety of seizures. It is quite effective in treating both petit mal and generalized major motor seizures in children. Like the benzodiazepines, valproic acid augments the postsynaptic action of GABA. Valproic acid is rapidly absorbed, but because it has a short half-life (about 6 to 12 hours), it must be administered several times a day. About 75 percent of epileptic patients receiving valproic acid respond favorably to it. Serious side effects from valproic acid are rare but do include liver failure in children.

With both antiepileptic action and GABAergic actions, it is not surprising that valproic acid has been tried in nonepileptic situations as a "mood stabilizer." Administered as maintenance therapy for bipolar disorder (Chapter 9), valproic acid is effective in treating the acute manic phase.[46-48] "Currently, valproic acid is the best-studied of the mood stabilizers and is emerging as a highly effective alternate treatment to lithium for acute mania."[49]

Study Questions

1. Describe the progression in understanding the mode of action of the benzodiazepines.
2. Describe evidence for and against the existence of a "natural anxiolytic" in the brain.
3. Describe the structure and function of the benzodiazepine receptor.
4. How might you describe anxiety or panic in terms of receptors or neurochemicals?
5. List some of the clinical uses of benzodiazepines.
6. List three processes that might prolong the half-life of a benzodiazepine.
7. Why should the elderly avoid using long-acting benzodiazepines?
8. Describe the most significant drug interaction that involves benzodiazepines.
9. Discuss benzodiazepine withdrawal and its treatment.
10. What is flumazenil and for what purpose can it be used?
11. How can GABA-receptor antagonists be used clinically and why?
12. Compare and contrast the mechanisms of action and uses of the benzodiazepines and buspirone.
13. Name the three newest antiepileptic drugs. For what use other than seizures can two of these drugs be used?

Notes

1. American Medical Association, "Drugs Used for Anxiety and Sleep Disorders," in *Drug Evaluations Annual 1994* (Milwaukee, Wis.: American Medical Association, 1993), p. 219.
2, A. Breier and S. M. Paul, "The GABA-A/Benzodiazepine Receptor: Implications for the Molecular Basis of Anxiety," *Journal of Psychiatric Research* 24, Suppl. 2 (1990): 91–104.
3. H. Unlenhuth, H. DeWit, M. B. Balter, C. E. Johanson, and G. D. Mellinger, "Risks and Benefits of Long-term Benzodiazepine Use," *Journal of Clinical Psychopharmacology* 8 (1988): 161–167.

4. D. W. Hommer, P. Skolnick, and S. M. Paul, "The Benzodiazepine/GABA Receptor Complex and Anxiety," in H. Y. Meltzer, ed., *Pharmacology: The Third Generation of Progress* (New York: Raven, 1987), pp. 977–983.

5. H. P. Rang and M. M. Dale, *Pharmacology,* 2nd ed. (Edinburgh: Churchill Livingstone, 1991), pp. 634–635.

6. Ibid., p. 637.

7. G. J. DiGregorio, "Antianxiety Drugs," in J. R. DiPalma and G. J. DiGregorio, eds., *Basic Pharmacology in Medicine,* 3rd ed. (New York: McGraw-Hill, 1990), pp. 222–229.

8. E. Schweizer, K. Rickels, S. Weiss, and S. Zavodnick, "Maintenance Drug Treatment of Panic Disorder: 1. Results of a Prospective, Placebo-Controlled Comparison of Alprazolam and Imipramine," *Archives of General Psychiatry* 50 (1993): 51–60.

9. K. Rickels, E. Schweizer, S. Weiss, and S. Zavodnick, "Maintenance Drug Treatment for Panic Disorder: 2. Short- and Long-Term Outcome after Drug Taper," *Archives of General Psychiatry* 50 (1993): 61–68.

10. D. J. Greenblatt, J. S. Harmatz, and R. I. Shader, "Plasma Alprazolam Concentrations: Relation to Efficacy and Side Effects in the Treatment of Panic Disorder," *Archives of General Psychiatry* 50 (1993): 715–722.

11. R. Saitz, M. F. Mayo-Smith, M. S. Roberts, H. A. Redmond, D. R. Bernard, and D. R. Calkins, "Individualized Treatment for Alcohol Withdrawal: A Randomized Double-blind Controlled Trial," *Journal of the American Medical Association* 272 (August 17, 1994): 519–523.

12. R. L. DuPont, "A Practical Approach to Benzodiazepine Discontinuation," *Journal of Psychiatric Research* 24, Suppl. 2 (1990): 81–90.

13. D. J. Greenblatt, L. G. Miller, and R. L. Shader, "Benzodiazepine Discontinuation Syndromes," *Journal of Psychiatric Research* 24, Suppl. 2 (1990): 73–80.

14. C. Salzman, "The APA Task Force Report on Benzodiazepine Dependence, Toxicity, and Abuse," *American Journal of Psychiatry* 148 (1991): 151–152.

15. American Psychiatric Association, *Benzodiazepine Dependence, Toxicity and Abuse: A Task Force Report of the American Psychiatric Association* (Washington, D.C.: American Psychiatric Association, 1990).

16. American Psychiatric Association, "Clinical Pharmacology of Benzodiazepines," in *Benzodiazepine Dependence, Toxicity, and Abuse: A Task Force Report of the American Psychiatric Association* (Washington D.C.: American Psychiatric Association, 1990), pp. 3–6.

17. L. S. Cohen, V. C. Heller, and J. F. Rosenbaum, "Treatment Guidelines for Psychiatric Drug Use in Pregnancy," *Psychosomatics* 30 (1989): 25–33.

18. C. Winick, "Epidemiology of Alcohol and Drug Abuse," in J. H. Lowinson, P. Ruiz, R. B. Millman, and J. G. Langrod, eds., *Substance Abuse: A Comprehensive Textbook,* 2nd ed. (Baltimore: Williams & Wilkins, 1992), pp. 15–29.

19. D. R. Wesson, D. E. Smith, and R. B. Seymour, "Sedative-Hypnotics and Tricyclics," in J. H. Lowinson, P. Ruiz, R. B. Millman, and J. G. Langrod, eds., *Substance Abuse: A Comprehensive Textbook,* 2nd ed. (Baltimore: Williams & Wilkins, 1992), pp. 271–279.

20. American Psychiatric Association, "Abuse Liability of Benzodiazepines," in *Benzodiazepine Dependence, Toxicity, and Abuse: A Task Force Report of the American Psychiatric Association* (Washington, D.C.: American Psychiatric Association, 1990), pp. 49–53.

21. M. Sarter, J. P. Bruno, and P. Dudchenko, "Activating the Damaged Basal Forebrain Cholinergic System: Tonic Stimulation versus Signal Amplification," *Psychopharmacology* 101 (1990): 1–17.

22. J. A. Miller, M. W. Dudley, J. H. Kehne, S. M. Sorensen, and J. M. Kane, "MDL 26,479: A Potential Cognition Enhancer with Benzodiazepine Inverse Agonist-Like Properties," *British Journal of Pharmacology* 107 (1992): 78–86.

23. H. Bittiger, W. Froestl, S. J. Mickel, and H.-R. Olpe, "GABA$_B$ Receptor Antagonists: From Synthesis to Therapeutic Applications," *Trends in Pharmacological Sciences* 14 (1993): 391–394.

24. C. Mondadori, J. Jaekel, and G. Preiswerk, "CGP 36742: The First Orally Active GABA$_B$ Blocker Improves the Cognitive Performance of Mice, Rats, and Rhesus Monkeys," *Behavioral and Neural Biology* 60 (1993): 62–68.

25. G. D. Pratt and N. G. Bowery, "Repeated Administration of Desipramine and a GABA-B Receptor Antagonist, CGP 36742, Discretely Up-regulates GABA-B Receptor Binding Sites in Rat Frontal Cortex," *British Journal of Pharmacology* 110 (1993): 724–735.

26. A. Nilsson, "Autonomic and Hormonal Responses after the Use of Midazolam and Flumazenil," *Acta Anaesthesiologica Scandinavica,* Suppl. 92 (1990): 51–54.

27. D. J. Nutt, P. Glue, C. Lawson, and S. Wilson, "Flumazenil Provocation of Panic Attacks. Evidence for Altered Benzodiazepine Receptor Sensitivity in Panic Disorder," *Archives of General Psychiatry* 47 (1990): 917–925.

28. "Zolpidem for Insomnia," *The Medical Letter on Drugs and Therapeutics* 35, no. 895 (30 April 1993): 35–36.

29. I. Berlin, D. Warot, T. Hergueta, P. Molinier, C. Bagot, and A. J. Puech, "Comparison of the Effects of Zolpidem and Triazolam on Memory Functions, Psychomotor Performances, and Postural Sway in Healthy Subjects," *Journal of Clinical Psychiatry* 13 (1993): 100–106.

30. D. Ruana, J. Benavides, A. Machado, and J. Vitorica, "Regional Differences in the Enhancement by GABA of [3H]Zolpidem Binding to Omega-1 Sites in Rat Brain Membranes and Sections," *Brain Research* 600 (1993): 134–140.

31. M. Roger, P. Attali, and J. P. Coquelin, "Multicenter, Double-blind, Controlled Comparison of Zolpidem and Triazolam in Elderly Patients with Insomnia," *Clinical Therapeutics* 15 (1993): 127–136.

32. D. P. Taylor and S. L. Mood, "Buspirone and Related Compounds as Alternative Anxiolytics," *Neuropeptides* 19, suppl. (1991): 15–19.

33. F. D. Yocca, "Neurochemistry and Neurophysiology of Buspirone and Gepirone: Interactions at Presynaptic and Postsynaptic 5-HT$_{1A}$ Receptors," *Journal of Clinical Psychopharmacology* 10, Suppl. 3 (1990): 6S–12S.

34. K. Rickels, "Buspirone in Clinical Practice," *Journal of Clinical Psychiatry* 51, suppl. (1990): 51–54.

35. R. M. Post and S. R. B. Weiss, "Sensitization, Kindling, and Anticonvulsants in Mania," *Journal of Clinical Psychiatry* 50, Suppl. 12 (1989): 23–30.

36. T. W. Rall and L. S. Schleifer, "Drugs Effective in the Therapy of the Epilepsies," in A. G. Gilman, L. S. Goodman, and A. Gilman, eds., *Goodman and Gilman's The Pharmacological Basis of Therapeutics*, 6th ed. (New York: MacMillan, 1980), p. 455.

37. K. J. Palmer and D. McTavish, "Felbamate: A Review of Its Pharmacodynamic and Pharmacokinetic Properties, and Therapeutic Efficacy in Epilepsy," *Drugs* 46 (1993): 1041–1065.

38. R. H. Mattson, editor, "Managing Epilepsy: The Role of Gabapentin," *Neurology* 44, No. 6, Suppl. 5 (1994).

39. G. A. Mellick and M. L. Seng, "The Use of Gabapentin in the Treatment of Reflex Sympathetic Dystrophy and a Phobic Disorder," *American Journal of Pain Management* 5 (1995): 7–9.

40. P. G. Janicak, J. M. Davis, S. H. Preskorn, and F. J. Ayd, *Principles and Practice of Psychopharmacotherapy* (Baltimore: Williams & Wilkins, 1993), pp. 239–240.

41. G. L. Klerman, N. Argyle, and J. A. Deltito, "The Effects of Alprazolam, Imipramine, and Placebo on the Depressive Symptoms Associated with Panic Disorder," *Journal of Clinical Psychopharmacology*, in press.

42. Janicak, Davis, Preskorn, and Ayd, *Principles and Practice of Psychopharmacotherapy*, p. 358.

43. Ibid., p. 369.

44. J. G. Small and others, "Carbamazepine Compared with Lithium in the Treatment of Mania," *Archives of General Psychiatry* 48 (1991): 915–921.

45. N. Coxhead, T. Silverstone, and J. Cookson, "Carbamazepine versus Lithium in the Prophylaxis of Bipolar Affective Disorder," *Acta Psychiatrica Scandinavia* 85 (1992): 114–118.

46. P. G. Janicak, R. Newman, and J. M. Davis, "Advances in the Treatment of Mania and Related Disorders: A Reappraisal," *Psychiatric Annals* 22 (1992): 92–103.

47. H. G. Pope, S. L. McElroy, P. E. Keck, and J. L. Hudson, "A Placebo-Controlled Study of Valproate in Mania," *Archives of General Psychiatry* 48 (1991): 62–68.

48. T. W. Freeman, J. L. Clothier, P. Pazzaglia, M. C. Lesem, and A. C. Swann, "A Double-Blind Comparison of Valproate and Lithium in the Treatment of Acute Mania," *American Journal of Psychiatry* 149 (1992): 108–111.

49. Janicak, Davis, Preskorn, and Ayd, *Principles and Practice of Psychopharmacotherapy*, p. 382.

CHAPTER 5

CENTRAL NERVOUS SYSTEM DEPRESSANTS: ALCOHOL

When we use the term *alcohol* we mean ethyl alcohol (ethanol)—a psychoactive drug that is similar in most respects to the sedative-hypnotic compounds; the main difference from the other depressants is that it is used primarily for recreational rather than medical purposes. Because it is the second most widely used psychoactive substance in the world (after caffeine), alcohol has created special problems for both individual users and society in general.

Pharmacology of Alcohol

Pharmacokinetics

Absorption   Alcohol is a simple molecule containing two carbon atoms; a hydroxyl (OH) group is attached to one of those carbons (Figure 5.1). Alcohol is soluble in both water and fat, and it diffuses easily through biological membranes. Thus, it is rapidly and completely absorbed from the entire gastrointestinal tract, most being absorbed from the upper intestine (because of its large surface area).

The rate of absorption can be modified in various ways. In a person with an empty stomach, approximately 20 percent of a single dose of alcohol is absorbed directly from the stomach, usually quite rapidly. The remaining 80 percent is absorbed rapidly and completely from the upper intestine; the only limiting factor is the time it takes to empty the stomach. If a person drinks alcohol on a full stomach, gastric emptying is delayed, and the rapid absorption that usually occurs in the upper intestine is slowed. Thus, blood levels of alcohol increase much

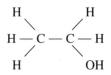

FIGURE 5.1 Structure of ethanol (CH_3CH_2OH).

faster in a person who has fasted than in someone who has just eaten a large meal. In either case, however, the alcohol is completely absorbed eventually.

Distribution After absorption, alcohol is evenly distributed throughout all body fluids and tissues. The blood–brain barrier is freely permeable to alcohol. When alcohol appears in the blood and reaches a person's brain, 90 percent of it crosses the blood–brain barrier almost immediately. This high rate of entry implies that there is little hindrance to the penetration of alcohol into the brain and that equilibrium of the levels of alcohol in brain and plasma is rapid.

Alcohol is also freely distributed from a pregnant woman's blood to the fetus. It crosses both the placenta and the infant's blood–brain barrier rapidly and easily. Fetal alcohol levels become the same as those of the drinking mother. Alcohol can be detected on a baby's breath at birth, in amniotic fluid during pregnancy, and in the baby's blood. Research on the impact of maternal alcohol consumption on human infants has demonstrated the occurrence of *fetal alcohol syndrome,* which consists of serious birth defects in 30 to 50 percent of all babies born to alcoholic mothers. The fetal alcohol syndrome can result when alcohol is ingested by a pregnant woman at critical times during embryonic development.[1] This syndrome is discussed more completely later in this chapter.

Metabolism and Excretion Approximately 95 percent of the alcohol that a person ingests is enzymatically metabolized by alcohol dehydrogenase. The other 5 percent is excreted unchanged, mainly through the lungs.* Most metabolism of alcohol (about 85 percent) is

---

*Small amounts of alcohol are excreted from the body through the lungs. Most of us are familiar with the "alcohol breath" that results from exhalation of alcohol. This feature forms the basis for breath analysis tests, because alcohol equilibrates rapidly across the membranes of the lungs. Indeed, in the breathalyzer test, a ratio of 1:2100 exists between alcohol in exhaled air and in venous blood. The blood alcohol concentration is easily extrapolated from the alcohol concentration in the expired air.

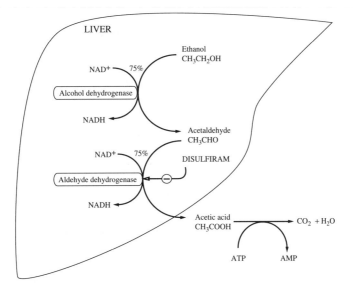

FIGURE 5.2   Metabolism of ethanol.

carried out by alcohol dehydrogenase enzyme, which is located in the liver. A small but significant amount of alcohol metabolism (up to 15 percent) is carried out by gastric alcohol dehydrogenase, which is located in the lining of the stomach.[2] This gastric enzyme metabolizes significant amounts of alcohol as the alcohol is absorbed across the stomach wall into the bloodstream (so-called first-pass metabolism). Indeed, gastric metabolism significantly decreases the amount of alcohol that must be absorbed, which attenuates its systemic toxicity. Frezza and coworkers[3] reported that when women and men consume comparable amounts of alcohol (after correction for differences in body weight), women have higher blood ethanol concentrations than do men. Indeed, women have about 50 percent less first-pass metabolism of alcohol than do men because women, whether alcoholic or nonalcoholic, have a lower level of gastric alcohol dehydrogenase. These factors may contribute to the enhanced vulnerability of some women to both acute intoxication and to the chronic complications of alcoholism.

Once alcohol is absorbed, the metabolism of alcohol in the liver occurs in two steps (Figure 5.2).[2] The first step is initiated by alcohol dehydrogenase, which converts alcohol to acetaldehyde. In the second step, the enzyme aldehyde dehydrogenase helps convert acetaldehyde to acetic acid, which is ultimately broken down into carbon dioxide and water, thus releasing energy (calories). Other than providing calories, alcohol has no nutritional value.

The rate of metabolism of alcohol in the liver is unusual because it is independent of the concentration of alcohol in the blood and is linear with time (in biochemical terms, this is called "zero order" metabolism). Virtually all other drugs are metabolized by "first order" metabolism, which means that the amount of drug metabolized per unit time depends on the amount (or concentration) of drug in blood.

In an adult, approximately 10 milliliters (one-third ounce) of 100 percent ethanol is metabolized per hour regardless of the blood alcohol concentration. In other words, it would take an adult 1 hour to metabolize the amount of alcohol that is contained in a 1-ounce glass of 80-proof whiskey (about 40 percent ethanol), a 4-ounce glass of wine, or a 12-ounce bottle of beer. Thus, consumption of 4 ounces of wine, 12 ounces of beer, or 1 ounce of whiskey per hour would keep the blood levels of alcohol in a person fairly constant. If a person ingests more alcohol in any given hour than is metabolized, his or her blood concentrations will increase. Consequently, there is a limit to the amount of alcohol that a person can consume in an hour without becoming drunk.

Factors that may alter this predictable rate of metabolism of alcohol are usually not clinically significant. With long-term use, however, alcohol can induce drug-metabolizing enzymes in the liver, thereby increasing the liver's rate of metabolizing alcohol (and so inducing tolerance) as well as its rate of metabolizing other compounds that are similar to alcohol (cross tolerance).

Mention should be made here of disulfiram (Antabuse), a drug frequently used to treat chronic alcoholism. Disulfiram inhibits aldehyde dehydrogenase, the enzyme responsible for metabolizing acetaldehyde into acetic acid (see Figure 5.2). As a result, acetaldehyde accumulates in the body, making the patient extremely uncomfortable, with headache, nausea, vomiting, drowsiness, hangover, and so on. Disulfiram makes alcoholics feel so dreadful when they drink that they are discouraged from drinking.

> Disulfiram is not a cure for alcoholism; it merely affords a volunteer a crutch by which the sincere desire to stop drinking can be fortified. The rationale for its use is that the patients know that if they are to avoid the devastating experience of the "acetaldehyde syndrome" they cannot drink for at least 3–4 days after taking disulfiram.[4]

Pharmacodynamics

Identifying the mechanism of action of alcohol has been and continues to be difficult because of alcohol's variety of behavioral and neuro-chemical actions. Indeed, a "unitary hypothesis," where one single neurochemical effect can explain all of alcohol's actions, may not be possible at all.

For almost 90 years, it was presumed that alcohol (as a small, organic, relatively low-potency drug) acted as the general anesthetics were presumed to act—exerting a general depressant action on nerve membranes and synapses. Being both water soluble (hydrophilic) and lipid soluble (lipophilic, or hydrophobic), ethanol interacts with and dissolves into both water and lipid. This property led to a unitary hypothesis of action: that the drug dissolves in cell membranes, dis-torting, disorganizing, or swelling the lipid bilayer of the membrane. This dissolving has the result of nonspecifically and indirectly altering membrane processes, such as electrical transmission, transmembrane ion currents, and release of synaptic transmitter chemicals. The neu-ronal membrane in essence becomes more "fluid," and its functions are disrupted. A process of fluidization would amplify neuronal dis-ruption because of the swelling and distortion of lipid membranes in areas surrounding ion channels and synaptic receptors. This would account for the nonspecific neuronal and synaptic depression that alcohol produces.[5] Various terms placed on this concept include "membrane fluidization," "membrane hypothesis," and "membrane lipid perturbation hypothesis."

Although this membrane hypothesis may correlate with and explain the high-dose or anesthetic properties of alcohol, it poorly explains the low-dose effects on behavioral reinforcement, anxiolysis, incoordination, cognition, and memory. It also does not explain the tolerance and dependence that can develop to alcohol.

A critical question is whether specific receptors are altered by alcohol. Tabakoff and Hoffman[6] and Samson and Harris[7] review the actions of alcohol on GABA, dopamine, enkephalin, NMDA-glutamate, and serotonin neurotransmission. The latter authors state:

> Neurotransmission at two types of excitatory receptor, nicotinic acetylcholine and serotonin, is enhanced by acute ethanol exposure. Most other excitatory receptors are inhibited by alcohol, while in-hibitory systems are augmented. . . . Our current understanding of al-cohol's action is most advanced for the $GABA_A$ receptor. Both behav-ioral and neurochemical studies provide evidence of enhancement of GABA receptor activity by alcohol.[7]

This action on GABA_A differs from that of the barbiturates and benzodiazepines; alcohol binds to a different site on the receptor. A particular subunit of the GABA receptor (the gamma-2L subunit) is required for alcohol's enhancing action; this subunit is not necessary for the action of other GABA agonists.[8] Action on this subunit seems to be coupled to phosphorylation (by a protein kinase), which leads to changes in channel function. A chronic adaptive effect seems to involve changes in intracellular mRNA, suggesting that chronic alcohol can affect gene expression.[9–11] As a result of this GABA agonist action, other transmitter systems are affected. Three are of importance here: the cholinergic (acetylcholine), the NMDA, and the dopamine.

Alcohol inhibits the release of acetylcholine in the central nervous system (CNS), which is an anticholinergic effect. Since the anticholinergic drug scopolamine (Chapter 12) is an exceedingly effective amnesic, and since cholinergic mechanisms are involved in learning and memory, this anticholinergic action likely contributes to alcohol's impairment of cognition.

Alcohol also inhibits N-methyl-D-aspartate (NMDA) receptors for the excitatory neurotransmitter glutamate, and this action may be in-

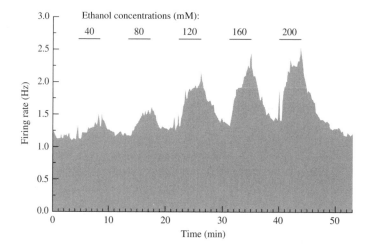

FIGURE 5.3 This ratemeter record of the firing rate of a single putative dopamine-containing ventral tegmental area (VTA) neuron in a brain slice preparation illustrates the effect of ethanol on spontaneous neuronal activity. Horizontal bars indicate duration of ethanol superfusion. The firing rate was averaged over 12-second intervals, and the height of each vertical bar indicates the mean firing rate in that interval. Concentrations of from 40 to 200 mM ethanol produced a concentration-dependent increase in firing rate. [From Harris, Brodie, and Dunwiddie (1992).[12]]

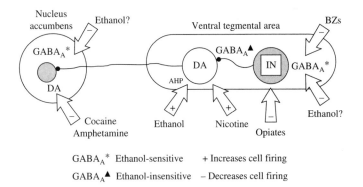

FIGURE 5.4 Putative substrates of pharmacological reinforcement. This illustrates schematically some of the ways in which drugs of abuse might interact with the ventral tegmental area/nucleus accumbens system. Cocaine and amphetamine are likely to act by potentiating dopamine (abbreviated DA) effects in nucleus accumbens, which would have a primarily depressant effect on cell firing, whereas nicotine appears to have a direct excitatory effect upon DA neurons (DA) in the ventral tegmental area. Opiates, benzodiazepines (BZs), and ethanol may all act to inhibit the firing of inhibitory interneurons (IN) via effects on opiate receptors or an ethanol-sensitive GABA$_A$ receptor, respectively, and these interneurons could then inhibit the DA cells via ethanol-insensitive GABA$_A$ receptors. Alternatively, ethanol might have a direct excitatory effect upon the DA cells via a mechanism that does not involve a GABAergic receptor. [From Harris, Brodie, and Dunwiddie (1992).[12]

volved in both the learning impairment and the antiepileptic effects of the drug, both in acute intoxication and after chronic use. Binding to NMDA receptors also alters ion channel fluxes and is linked to inhibition of intracellular nucleotides that modulate neuron function.[6]

Finally, the GABA agonist action of ethanol has been linked to the positive reinforcing effects of the drug.[7,12] Indeed, the abuse potential of alcohol follows from an ultimate action to augment dopamine neurotransmitter systems, particularly the dopaminergic projection from the ventral tegmental area (VTA) to the nucleus accumbens and to the frontal cortex (Chapter 15). As Figure 5.3 demonstrates, alcohol increases the discharge rate of neurons in the ventral tegmental area. Harris, Brodie, and Dunwiddie postulate that "the excitatory effects of ethanol on dopamine neurons in the VTA might come about as a result of an inhibition of inhibitory interneurons mediated via GABA$_A$ receptors."[12]

The same authors also state that ethanol may act directly on dopamine neurons to increase their firing, not indirectly via the interneurons. These possible effects of ethanol are summarized in Figure 5.4.

Pharmacological Effects

The graded, reversible depression of CNS function is the primary pharmacological effect of alcohol. Respiration, though transiently stimulated at low doses, becomes progressively depressed and, at very high blood concentrations of alcohol, is the cause of death. Alcohol is also anticonvulsant, although it is not clinically used for this purpose. On the other hand, when one stops drinking alcohol, withdrawal is accompanied by a prolonged period of hyperexcitability, and seizures can occur, with the seizure activity peaking approximately 8 to 12 hours after the last drink.

The effects of alcohol are additive with those of other sedative-hypnotic compounds, resulting in more sedation and greater impairment of driving ability. Other sedatives (especially the benzodiazepines) and marijuana are the drugs that are most frequently combined with alcohol, and they increase its deleterious effects on a person's motor and intellectual skills as well as on one's state of alertness.

The combination of alcohol and sedatives may produce supra-additive effects that can result in fatal depression of cardiac and respiratory functions. Thus, these combinations can be hazardous and occasionally fatal.

Alcohol also affects the circulation and the heart. Alcohol dilates the blood vessels in the skin, producing a warm flush and a decrease in body temperature. Thus, it is pointless and possibly dangerous to drink alcohol to keep warm when one is exposed to cold weather. Long-term use of alcohol is also associated with diseases of the heart muscle, which can result in heart failure. Several reports have noted that low doses of alcohol consumed daily (up to 2.5 ounces) may reduce the risk of coronary artery disease. This protective effect occurs because of an alcohol-induced increase in high-density lipoprotein in blood with a corresponding decrease in low-density lipoprotein. (The higher the concentration of high-density lipoprotein and the lower the concentration of low-density lipoprotein, the lower the incidence of coronary heart disease.) Unfortunately, the cardioprotective effect of low doses of alcohol is lost on persons who also smoke cigarettes.

Alcohol exerts a diuretic effect on the body by increasing the excretion of fluids as a result of its effects on renal function, by decreasing the secretion of an antidiuretic hormone, and by the diuretic action produced simply by ingesting large quantities of fluid. Alcohol, however, does not appear to harm either the structure or the function of the kidney.

Alcohol (like all depressant drugs) is not an aphrodisiac. In fact, the behavioral disinhibition induced by low doses of alcohol may appear to cause some loss of restraint, but alcohol depresses body function and actually interferes with sexual performance. As Shakespeare wrote in *Macbeth,* "It [alcohol] provokes the desire, but it takes away the performance."

Psychological Effects

The short-term psychological and behavioral effects of alcohol are primarily restricted to the CNS. Figure 5.5 correlates the effects of alcohol with levels of the drug measured in the blood. The behavioral reaction to disinhibition, which occurs at low doses, is unpredictable. It is largely determined by the person, his or her mental expectations, and the environment. In one setting a person may become relaxed and euphoric; in another he or she may become withdrawn or violent. Mental expectations and the physical setting become progressively less important at increasing doses, because the sedative effects increase and behavioral activity decreases.

At low doses, a person may still function (although with less coordination) and attempt to drive or otherwise endanger himself and others. Memory, concentration, and insight are progressively dulled

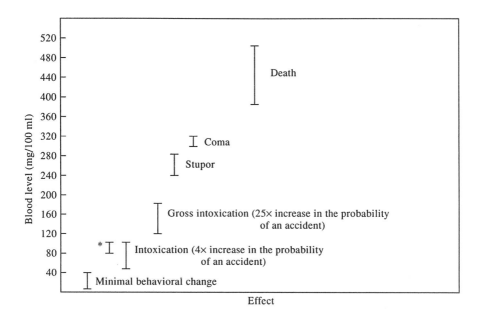

FIGURE 5.5   Correlation of the blood level of ethanol with degrees of intoxication. The legal level of intoxication (*) varies by state; the range of values is shown.

and then lost. As the dose increases, the drinker becomes progressively incapacitated.

Alcohol intoxication, with its resulting disinhibition, plays a major role in a large percentage of violent crimes, including rape, sexual assault, and certain kinds of deviant behaviors.[13] More than 50 percent of crimes and highway accidents are alcohol related, a number that has changed little in 20 years.[14] Over 10 million individuals in the United States suffer the consequences of alcohol abuse, which include arrests, traffic accidents, occupational injuries, violence, and health and occupational losses. This number does not include the 10 million individuals considered to be alcohol dependent (with their own suffering of negative consequences). Thus, about 10 percent of our society are personally afflicted with (or suffer the consequences of) another's alcohol use.

Long-term effects of alcohol may involve many different organs of a person's body, depending on whether the drinking is moderate or heavy. Long-term ingestion of moderate amounts of alcohol seems to produce few physiological, psychological, or behavioral changes in a person. But long-term ingestion of larger amounts of alcohol leads to a variety of serious neurological, mental, and physical disorders. These disorders are described in the section on alcoholism.

As stated previously, alcohol is quite caloric but has little nutritional value. Thus, a person may survive for years on a diet of alcohol and not much else, but he or she will slowly develop vitamin deficiencies and nutritional diseases, which may result in physical deterioration. Indeed, alcohol abuse has been suggested as the most common cause of vitamin and trace element deficiencies in adults.[15]

Tolerance and Dependence

The patterns and mechanisms for the development of tolerance, physical dependence, and psychological dependence on alcohol are similar to those for all the depressant compounds. The extent of tolerance depends on the amount, pattern, and extent of alcohol ingestion. Persons who ingest alcohol only intermittently on sprees or more regularly but in moderation develop little or no tolerance; persons who regularly ingest large amounts of alcohol develop marked tolerance. The tolerance that does develop is of three types:

1. metabolic tolerance, where the liver increases its amount of drug-metabolizing enzyme (This type accounts for at most 25 percent of the tolerance that develops to alcohol.)

2. tissue, or functional, tolerance, where neurons in the brain adapt to the amount of drug present (Individuals who develop this type of tolerance characteristically display blood alcohol levels about twice those of a nontolerant individual at a similar level of behavioral intoxication.)

3. associative, contingent, or homeostatic tolerance[16] (A variety of environmental manipulations can counter the effects of ethanol, and these counterresponses are a possible mechanism of tolerance.)

The relationship of tolerance to the development of excessive drinking has yet to be determined.[7] No evidence has been demonstrated that any degree of tolerance to the positive reinforcing effects of ethanol develops. Tolerance develops only to the motor-disrupting, the hypothermic, the sedative, the anxiolytic, and the anticonvulsant effects.

When physical dependence develops from chronic ingestion of alcohol, withdrawal of the drug results, within several hours, in a period of rebound hyperexcitability that may eventually lead to convulsions and even death. Concomitant with this hyperexcitability is a period of tremulousness, with hallucinations, psychomotor agitation, confusion and disorientation, sleep disorders, and a variety of associated discomforts—a syndrome that is sometimes referred to as *delirium tremens* (DTs) or *rum fits* (discussed more fully in the section on alcoholism).

Side Effects and Toxicity

Many of the side effects and toxicities associated with alcohol have already been mentioned, but let us summarize and expand on them here. In acute use, a reversible drug-induced brain syndrome is induced. This syndrome is manifested as a clouded sensorium with disorientation, impaired insight and judgment, amnesia ("blackouts"), and diminished intellectual capabilities. The person's affect may be labile, with emotional outbursts precipitated by otherwise innocuous events. With high doses of alcohol, delusions, hallucinations, and confabulations may occur. In social functioning, these alterations result in unpredictable states of disinhibition (drunkenness), alterations in driving performance, and uncoordinated motor behavior.

Liver damage is the most serious physiological long-term consequence of excessive alcohol consumption. Irreversible changes in both the structure and the function of the liver are common. The significance of alcohol-induced liver dysfunction is illustrated by the fact that 75 percent of all deaths attributed to alcoholism are caused by cirrhosis of the liver,[17] and cirrhosis is the seventh most common cause of death in the United States.[15] Cirrhosis appears to result from alcohol-induced interference with normal body immune functions. Indeed, cirrhosis is a clear indication of the immunosuppressive effect of alcohol.[18]

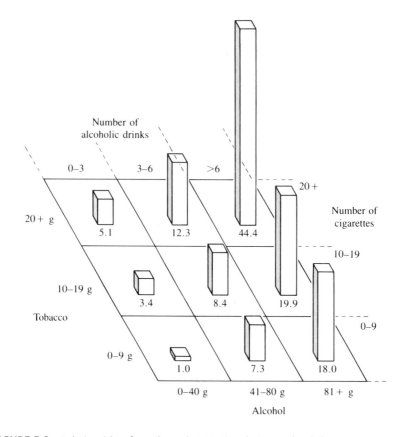

FIGURE 5.6 Relative risks of esophageal cancer in relation to the daily consumption of alcohol and tobacco. The risk is 44.4 times greater for persons who consume 20 grams or more of tobacco and 80 grams or more of alcohol per day (upper right block) than for persons who consume little or none of either drug (lower left block). One ounce of ethyl alcohol is approximately 23.4 grams; thus 40 grams is 1.7 ounces, or approximately equivalent to three drinks. [From *Third Special Report to the U.S. Congress on Alcohol and Health.*[21] Data from A. J. Tuyns, G. Pequignot, and O. M. Jenson, "Le cancer de l'oesophage en Ille et Vilaine en fonction des niveaux de consommation d'alcool et de tabac: Des risques qui se multiplient," *Bulletin du Cancer* 65, no. 1 (1977): 45–60.]

In addition, long-term alcohol ingestion may irreversibly destroy nerve cells, producing a permanent brain syndrome with dementia (Korsakoff's syndrome). The digestive system may also be affected. Pancreatitis (inflammation of the pancreas) and chronic gastritis (inflammation of the stomach), with the development of peptic ulcers, may occur.

A great deal of epidemiological evidence now shows that chronic excessive alcohol consumption is a major risk factor for cancer in humans. Although ethanol alone may not be carcinogenic, heavy drinking increases a person's risk of developing cancer of the tongue, mouth, throat, voice box, and liver.[19] This cancer-potentiating effect can be explained by the role of alcohol in modifying the action of other cancer-causing agents. Indeed, alcohol clearly exerts a synergistic action with tobacco. For example, the risk of head and neck cancers for heavy drinkers who smoke is 6 to 15 times greater than for those who abstain from both. The risk of throat cancer is 44 times greater for heavy users of both alcohol and tobacco than for nonusers (Figure 5.6). Thus, alcohol may promote tumor growth—an effect that may follow from its immunosuppressive action and the resultant reduction in body defense mechanisms against tumor cells.[18]

During the mid-1980s, data appeared that linked a minimal-to-moderate alcohol intake in women with increases in the incidence of breast cancer. More recent data dispute this claim,[20] leading to the current impression that no strong correlation exists.

Teratogenic Effects

Alcohol is a clearly delineated teratogen. A fetal alcohol syndrome occurs in the offspring of mothers having high blood levels of alcohol during critical stages of fetal development. As early as 1977, the National Institute on Alcohol Abuse and Alcoholism released the following statement relevant to this syndrome:

> Heavy use of alcohol by women during pregnancy may result in a pattern of abnormalities in the offspring, termed the fetal alcohol syndrome, which consists of specific congenital and behavioral abnormalities. Studies undertaken in animals corroborate the initial observation in humans and also indicate an increased incidence of stillbirths, resorption, and spontaneous abortions. Both the risk and the extent of abnormalities appear to be dose-related, increasing with higher alcohol intake during pregnancy. In human studies, alcohol is an unequivocal factor when the full pattern of the fetal alcohol syndrome is present.[21]

Information summarized in 1987 more clearly characterizes the syndrome. Features of the syndrome include the following: [22]

1. CNS dysfunction, including low intelligence and microcephaly (reduced cranial circumference), mental retardation, and behavioral abnormalities (often presenting as hyperactivity and difficulty with social integration)

2. retarded body growth rate

3. facial abnormalities (short palpebral fissures, short nose, wide-set eyes, and small cheekbones)

4. other anatomical abnormalities (for example, congenital heart defects and malformed eyes and ears)

Either ethanol or its metabolite, acetaldehyde, may inhibit embryonic cell division and proliferation early in pregnancy. Facial development is affected early in pregnancy (up to 4 to 6 weeks), while brain development is affected later in pregnancy. There is also evidence of fetal malnutrition, which is caused by injury to the placenta. Finally, some children with fetal alcohol syndrome exhibit marked deficits in their immune systems, increasing their susceptibility to infections.

In the United States, an estimated 2.6 million infants are born annually following significant intrauterine alcohol exposure.[23] At present, the projected incidence of fetal alcohol syndrome may be as high as 1 in every 300 births, while a "lesser degree of damage, termed *fetal alcohol effects,* may occur in 1 in 100 live births."[23] This would make alcohol ingestion the third leading cause of birth defects with associated mental retardation, following only Down's syndrome and spina bifida; however, fetal alcohol syndrome is the only one of these conditions that is preventable. Indeed, alcohol is the most frequent cause of teratogen-induced mental deficiency known in the Western world.[24]

A study of more than 31,000 pregnancies shows that the consumption of only one or two drinks daily can cause a substantially increased risk of a growth-retarded infant.[25] One drink per day has minimal effect but cannot be considered safe. Fetal alcohol syndrome is thought to occur in 1 out of 3 infants of alcoholic mothers.

Despite these statistics, 20 percent of pregnant women continue to consume alcohol.[26] This obviously places the unborn infant at significant risk of incurring significant damage even before birth. The highest rates of alcohol use during pregnancy occur in women who smoke (37 percent) and in women who are not married (28 percent). As we will see later, cigarette smoking also increases the risk of fetal injury; thus the combination multiplies the risks to the unborn. These facts suggest that special efforts are needed to convince pregnant women who are smokers, unmarried, less educated, or younger to avoid alcohol.

The effects of paternal drinking or alcoholism on the fetus are unknown. More than 25 percent of pregnant women who are moderate-to-heavy drinkers report that their infants' fathers are also heavy drinkers. This factor may or may not be significant.

Alcoholism

Definition of the term *alcoholism* is relatively recent, as is the recognition of alcoholism as a multifaceted disease process.

> At the turn of the century, the term *alcoholism* had not yet been coined. Chronic inebriety, as the condition was known at that time, was widely regarded as a hopeless malady, whose sufferers were seen as doomed to grim outcomes in jails, asylums, or potter's fields.[27]

The founding of Alcoholics Anonymous in 1935 offered a spiritual/ behavioral framework for understanding, accepting, and recovering from the compulsion to use alcohol.[27] It was not until the late 1950s that the American Medical Association recognized the syndrome of alcoholism as an illness. In his book *The Disease Concept of Alcoholism*, E. M. Jellinek presented the hypothesis that alcoholism is a disease.[28]

In the mid-1970s, alcoholism was defined as "a chronic, progressive, and potentially fatal disease. It is characterized by tolerance, and physical dependency, or pathologic organ changes, or both—all the direct or indirect consequences of the alcohol ingested."[29] This definition fails to recognize the biopsychosocial factors that influence the development of alcoholism. Thus, the definition has recently been revised and expanded as follows:

> Alcoholism is a primary, chronic disease with genetic, psychosocial, and environmental factors influencing its development and manifestations. The disease is often progressive and fatal. It is characterized by impaired control over drinking, preoccupation with the drug alcohol, use of alcohol despite adverse consequences, and distortions in thinking, most notably denial. Each of these symptoms may be continuous or periodic.[30]

In this definition, "adverse consequences" involve impairments in such areas as physical health, psychological functioning, interpersonal functioning, and occupational functioning, as well as legal, financial, and spiritual problems.[30] "Denial" refers broadly to a range of psychological maneuvers that decrease awareness of the fact that alcohol use is the cause of a person's problems rather than a solution to those problems. Denial becomes an integral part of the disease and is nearly always a major obstacle to recovery.[30]

Of the 160 million Americans who are old enough to drink legally, 112 million drink.[27,31] As many as 14 million Americans may have serious alcohol problems, and about half that number (7 million) are considered to be alcoholic. The daily consumption of about a half-pint of 80-proof liquor is thought to place a person's health at risk. Approximately 10 percent of the drinking population ingests the equivalent of this quantity of alcohol as beer, wine, or "hard" liquor.

> If cigarette smoking is excluded, alcoholism is by far the most serious drug problem in the United States and most other countries. Measured in terms of accidents, lost productivity, crime, death, or damaged health, the combined social costs of problem drinking in the United States were estimated for 1980 to exceed 89 billion dollars annually. The cost in broken homes, wasted lives, loss to society, and human misery is beyond calculation.[32]

Long-term alcoholism may lead to malnutrition and chronic physiological degeneration. This condition causes a bloated look, flabby muscles, fine tremors, decreased physical capacity and stamina, and increased susceptibility to infections. Although this state of chronic degeneration is not present in the majority of alcoholics who receive adequate nutrition, nutrition alone does not fully protect the brain, the liver, or the digestive tract from damage.[33]

When does alcohol produce a state of physical dependence? When does alcohol harm the body? Clearly, long-term maintenance of high concentrations of alcohol in the body produces a state of physical dependence.[34] Since the body metabolizes about 10 milliliters (one-third of an ounce) of 100 percent alcohol per hour, ingestion of more than that amount will result in alcohol accumulation.

There is a reasonably good correlation between drinking habits, maximum blood concentrations, and the intensity of a withdrawal syndrome. With a low level of dependence, alcohol withdrawal consists of altered sleep patterns, nausea, anxiety, wakefulness, and mild tremors that may last for only a day or so. At higher levels of dependence, an *alcohol withdrawal syndrome* is seen, in which these signs are intensified and accompanied by vomiting, cramps, nightmares, and transient hallucinations. If the hallucinations persist, the syndrome is called *alcoholic hallucinosis*.[34] As the dependence progresses, withdrawal may include confusion, disorientation, agitation, persecutory hallucinations, and severe tremors or seizures. This late stage is termed *alcoholic withdrawal delirium,* or *delirium tremens.* After recovery, depression, sleep deficits, cognitive deficits, and other alterations of brain function may persist for months.

The recent definition of alcoholism calls it a primary disorder, implying that it is not associated with other pathopsychophysiological states. Goodwin states, "A good deal of evidence now indicates that many, if not most, alcoholics *do not* have primary alcoholism. Their alcoholism *is* associated with other psychopathology, including addiction to other drugs."[29] Goodwin further states that 30 to 50 percent of alcoholics meet criteria for major depression; 33 percent have a coexisting anxiety disorder (social phobias in men, agoraphobia in women); many have antisocial personalities (14 percent); some are schizophrenic (3 percent); many (36 percent) are addicted to other drugs. Obviously, dual diagnosis must always be considered.

Drugs Used to Treat Alcoholism

> Since alcoholism involves the ingestion of alcohol, eliminating the taking of alcohol is an obvious therapeutic strategy.[37]

Historically the barbiturates and chloral hydrate (Chapter 3) were mainstays in treating alcohol withdrawal syndrome. More recently the *benzodiazepines* have been extensively utilized and are considered to be the drugs of choice for managing withdrawal. One might question why we would substitute one potentially addictive drug for another. The short duration of action of alcohol and its narrow range of safety make it an extremely dangerous drug. When alcohol ingestion is stopped, it is metabolized within hours, precipitating withdrawal symptoms. Substituting a long-acting drug prevents or suppresses the withdrawal symptoms.[35,36]* The longer-acting drug is then either maintained at a level low enough to allow the person to function or else withdrawn gradually. In general, the longest-acting agents are preferred (especially those with pharmacologically active metabolites, such as chlordiazepoxide [Librium] or diazepam [Valium]).

Disulfiram (Antabuse) has been used to treat alcoholism for a long time. As stated previously, it alters the metabolism of alcohol, allowing acetaldehyde to accumulate. This accumulation results in an *acetaldehyde syndrome* if the patient ingests alcohol within several days of taking disulfiram. If taken daily, disulfiram results in total abstinence in the vast majority of patients. Like any effective drug, it does not work if it is not taken![37]

Haloperidol (Haldol) and other antipsychotic agents (Chapter 11) may be used to treat the hallucinations associated with severe delirium tremens. If seizures occur, haloperidol cannot be used because it lowers the seizure threshold. In addition, there is concern that phenothiazines may increase the liver damage caused by alcohol.

Conditioned-avoidance techniques that include the use of emesis-inducing agents (e.g., apomorphine or Ipecac) have been used to treat alcoholism. The patient takes the emetic agent and then drinks a dose

*See also reference 11, Chapter 4 (page 98).

of alcohol shortly thereafter. When nausea and vomiting occur, the patient associates the drinking of alcohol with the unpleasant reaction. Alcohol thus becomes a conditioned stimulus for the production of nausea and vomiting. Although this technique is decreasing in popularity, treatment with low doses of apomorphine is being tried to reduce the craving for alcohol.[35]

As noted earlier, many alcoholics suffer from a coexisting major depression. Following alcohol withdrawal, the depression may persist and require therapy. Indeed, tricyclic antidepressants (Chapter 8) have been widely used to treat alcoholics during the months following withdrawal. However, there is no evidence that this approach is effective.[35]

In 1989 and 1990, antidepressants that selectively inhibit serotonin reuptake (Chapter 8) were shown to reduce daily alcohol intake in persons in the early stages of alcoholism.[38–40] Two such agents are currently available, one of which, *fluoxetine* (Prozac), is safer and better studied. More recent studies in animals[41,42] and in male alcoholics[43] confirm a reduction in alcohol intake, but in the human studies, the reduction was small (14 percent) and not maintained after the first week. Obviously, more will be written about this intriguing concept of therapy. Fluoxetine is discussed at length in Chapter 8.

In a similar manner, *benzodiazepine antagonists,* such as flumazenil[44] and Ro 19-4603,[45] can block the actions of ethanol and reduce voluntary ethanol consumption in experimental animals. Such actions add support to the hypothesis of a GABA agonist mechanism in the reinforcing property of ethanol and offer hope for developing clinically useful drugs that will attenuate drinking behavior in alcoholics.

Some investigators have tested the hypothesis that there may be a role of the endogenous opioid system (Chapter 10) in modulating the intake of alcohol.[46] In particular, *naltrexone* (a long-acting, orally administered narcotic antagonist) administered to alcoholics over a 12-week period reduced alcohol craving and relapse[47] and potentiated the therapeutic effects of learning coping skills and training to prevent relapse.[48] In 1995, naltrexone was approved by the FDA for use in the treatment of alcoholism.

Techniques for Treating Alcoholism

As stated by Collins,

> contemporary alcoholism treatment is . . . an amalgamation of medical, psychological, psychosocial, and spiritual modalities interacting in a quasi-organized framework to assist the individual in achieving and sustaining lasting, contented sobriety.[27]

It should be emphasized that such treatment can only follow management of alcohol withdrawal symptoms and maintenance of a period of sobriety. Gessner emphasizes that

> heavy chronic consumption of ethanol induces an impairment of memory and cognitive function. At the same time, a great deal of learning is required to maintain abstinent and even more to achieve stable moderate drinking. Accordingly, it is not surprising that one of the best predictors of treatment outcome is the degree of cognitive impairment patients present upon entry into therapy: the greater the impairment the less likely the success of therapy. With abstinence there is a partial reversal of such impairment. Accordingly, an initial period of abstinence is therapeutically desirable, whatever the long-term treatment goals.[49]

Following withdrawal and a period of abstinence, treatment has two goals:[29,50] (1) sobriety and (2) amelioration of psychiatric conditions associated with alcoholism. This allows the therapist to evaluate the individual sober and to diagnose and treat coexisting psychiatric disorders. It also allows the individual time to learn that he or she can cope with life without alcohol.

There are no definitive therapies for alcoholism or for preventing relapse of drinking after an initial period of sobriety. Indeed, such discussion is beyond the scope of this text. Trials of drugs (e.g., fluoxetine, naltrexone, and disulfiram), psychotherapy, cognitive-behavioral therapy, group therapy, Alcoholics Anonymous, aversion therapy, and other methods will continue to be used as treatment. All offer hope and have met with limited to moderate success, but none offers definitive treatment. As stated in a 1987 newsletter, "Detoxification is relatively easy; the most complicated and frustrating part of treatment is preventing relapse."[51]

Since all individuals are different, each person can suffer a unique spectrum of impairments. One person may drink to excess without much damage to his or her physical or vocational health—for example, an executive who is an alcoholic but maintains an adequate diet and has social and family support. On the other hand, an alcoholic's physical health may improve under a program of total abstinence, yet other life problems, such as social, family, and emotional difficulties may not be remedied or may even be worsened. Because of these differences, different prescriptions for treatment and different levels of expectation for success must be employed for each individual. For example, sobriety may be a reasonable expectation for a person whose impairment in life is minimal, while attenuated drinking with modest improvements in health may be all that can be reasonably expected for a more severely impaired alcoholic.

Such individualized treatment has just begun because society has only recently begun to look less scornfully on the alcoholic and to recognize that each alcoholic must have an individual set of therapeutic objectives. The goal of future treatment programs may not necessarily be total abstinence from alcohol for every alcoholic but, rather, treatment of coexisting disorders and a reduction in life problems that are associated with drinking.

Study Questions

1. Describe the relation between alcohol and nonselective CNS depressants.
2. Describe the metabolism of alcohol and how it is altered by disulfiram. How is this alteration applied in the treatment of alcoholism?
3. Describe how alcohol exerts its effect on the CNS.
4. List several of the major physiological and societal problems that are associated with alcohol.
5. Describe the fetal alcohol syndrome. What is a safe level of alcohol intake by a pregnant woman?
6. If a person has developed a physical dependence on alcohol, why might he or she be treated with a benzodiazepine to substitute for the alcohol?
7. Summarize some of the drugs and techniques used in treating alcoholism.
8. What drug offers promise for reducing daily alcohol intake in some alcoholics? Why?
9. Describe the disease concept of alcoholism.
10. How is alcohol involved in the genesis of certain cancers?

Notes

1. J. W. Hanson, K. L. Jones, and D. W. Smith, "Fetal Alcohol Syndrome," *Journal of the American Medical Association* 235 (5 April 1976): 1458–1460.
2. J. Caballeria, M. Frezza, R. Hernandez-Munoz, C. DiPadova, M. A. Korsted, E. Baraona, and C. S. Lieber, "Gastric Origin of the First-Pass Metabolism of Ethanol in Humans: Effect of Gastrectomy," *Gastroenterology* 97 (1989): 1205–1209.
3. M. Frezza, C. DiPadova, G. Pozzato, M. Terpin, E. Baraona, and C. S. Lieber, "High Blood Alcohol Levels in Women. The Role of Decreased Gastric Alcohol Dehydrogenase Activity and First-Pass Metabolism," *New England Journal of Medicine* 322 (1990): 95–99.
4. T. W. Rall, "Hypnotics and Sedatives: Ethanol," in A. G. Gilman, T. W. Rall, A. S. Nies, and P. Taylor, eds., *Goodman and Gilman's The Pharmacological Basis of Therapeutics*, 8th ed. (New York: Pergamon, 1990), p. 379.

5. A. Goldstein, *Addiction: From Biology to Drug Policy* (New York: W. H. Freeman and Company, 1994), pp. 125–127.

6. B. Tabakoff and P. L. Hoffman, "Alcohol: Neurobiology," in J. H. Lowinson, P. Ruiz, R. B. Millman, and J. G. Langrod, eds., *Substance Abuse: A Comprehensive Textbook,* 2nd ed. (Baltimore: Williams & Wilkins, 1992), pp. 152–179.

7. H. H. Samson and R. A. Harris, "Neurobiology of Alcohol Abuse," *Trends in Pharmacological Sciences* 13 (1992): 206–211.

8. K. A. Wafford, D. M. Burnett, N. J. Leidenheimer, D. R. Burt, J. B. Wang, P. Kofuji, T. V. Dunwiddie, R. A. Harris, and J. M. Sikela, "Ethanol Sensitivity of the GABA$_A$ Receptor Expressed in Xenopus Oocytes Requires 8 Amino Acids Contained in the Gamma 2L Subunit," *Neuron* 7 (1991): 27–33.

9. P. Montpied, A. L. Morrow, J. W. Karanian, E. I. Ginns, B. M. Martin, and S. M. Paul, "Prolonged Ethanol Inhalation Decreases GABA$_A$ Receptor Alpha Subunit mRNAs in the Rat Cerebral Cortex," *Molecular Pharmacology* 39 (1991): 157–163.

10. K. J. Buck, L. Hahner, J. Sikela, and R. A. Harris, "Chronic Ethanol Treatment Alters Brain Levels of Gamma-aminobutyric Acid$_A$ Receptor Subunit mRNAs: Relationship to Genetic Differences in Ethanol Withdrawal Seizure Activity," *Journal of Neurochemistry* 57 (1991): 1452–1455.

11. K. J. Buck and R. A. Harris, "Neuroadaptive Responses to Chronic Ethanol," *Alcoholism, Clinical and Experimental Research* 15 (1991): 460–470.

12. R. A. Harris, M. S. Brodie, and T. V. Dunwiddie, "Possible Substrates of Ethanol Reinforcement: GABA and Dopamine," *Annals of the New York Academy of Sciences* 654 (1992): 61–69.

13. S. C. Woods and J. G. Mansfield, "Ethanol and Disinhibition: Physiological and Behavioral Links," in R. Room and S. Collins, eds., *Alcohol and Disinhibition: Nature and Meaning of the Link* (Washington, D.C.: U.S. Government Printing Office, 1983), pp. 4–23.

14. R. G. Niven, "Alcoholism—A Problem in Perspective," *Journal of the American Medical Association* 252 (1984): 1912–1914.

15. M. J. Edkardt and others, "Health Hazards Associated with Alcohol Consumption," *Journal of the American Medical Association* 246 (1981): 648–666.

16. C. X. Poulos and H. Cappell, "Homeostatic Theory of Drug Tolerance: A General Model of Physiologic Adaptation," *Psychological Review* 98 (1991): 390–408.

17. C. S. Lieber, "Alcoholism: Medical Implications," *Annals of the New York Academy of Sciences* 362 (1981): 132–135.

18. S. I. Mufti, H. R. Darban, and R. R. Watson, "Alcohol, Cancer, and Immunomodulation," *Critical Reviews in Oncology/Hematology* 9 (1989): 243–261.

19. S. Palmer, "Diet, Nutrition and Cancer," *Progress in Food and Nutrition Science* 9 (1985): 283–341.

20. R. E. Harris, N. Spritz, and E. L. Wynder, "Studies of Breast Cancer and Alcohol Consumption," *Preventive Medicine* 17 (1988): 676–682.

21. U.S. Department of Health, Education, and Welfare, *Alcohol and Health: Third Special Report to the U.S. Congress* (Washington, D.C.: U.S. Government Printing Office, 1978).

22. National Institute on Alcohol and Alcoholism, *Alcohol and Birth Defects: The Fetal Alcohol Syndrome and Related Disorders,* U.S. Department of Health and Human Services Publication Number ADM 87–1531 (Washington, D.C.: U.S. Government Printing Office, 1987), pp. 6–10.

23. L. P. Finnegan and S. R. Kandall, "Maternal and Neonatal Effects of Alcohol and Drugs," in J. H. Lowinson, P. Ruiz, R. B. Millman, and J. G. Langrod, eds., *Substance Abuse: A Comprehensive Textbook,* 2nd ed. (Baltimore: Williams & Wilkins, 1992), p. 650.

24. T. W. Rall, p. 373.

25. J. L. Mills and others, "Maternal Alcohol Consumption and Birth Weight," *Journal of the American Medical Association* 252 (1984): 1875–1879.

26. M. Serdula, D. F. Williamson, J. S. Kendrick, R. F. Anda, and T. Byers, "Trends in Alcohol Consumption by Pregnant Women," *Journal of the American Medical Association* 265 (1991): 876–879.

27. G. B. Collins, "Contemporary Issues in the Treatment of Alcohol Dependence," *Psychiatric Clinics of North America* 16 (1993), no. 1: 33–48.

28. E. M. Jellinek, *The Disease Concept of Alcoholism* (New Haven: Hillhouse Press, 1960).

29. D. W. Goodwin, "Alcohol: Clinical Aspects," in J. H. Lowinson, P. Ruiz, R. B. Millman, and J. G. Langrod, eds., *Substance Abuse: A Comprehensive Textbook,* 2nd ed. (Baltimore: Williams & Wilkins, 1992), p. 650.

30. R. M. Morse and D. K. Flavin, "The Definition of Alcoholism," *Journal of the American Medical Association* 268 (1992):1012–1014.

31. G. B. Cloninger, S. H. Dunwiddie, and T. Reich, "Epidemiology and Genetics of Alcoholism," *Annual Reviews of Psychiatry* 8 (1989): 331–346.

32. J. H. Jaffe, "Drug Addiction and Drug Abuse," in A. G. Gilman, L. S. Goodman, T. W. Rall, and F. Murad, eds., *Goodman and Gilman's The Pharmacological Basis of Therapeutics,* 7th ed. (New York: Macmillan, 1985), p. 548.

33. U.S. Department of Health and Human Services, *Fifth Special Report to the U.S. Congress on Alcohol and Health* (Washington, D.C.: U.S. Government Printing Office, 1984).

34. J. H. Jaffe, "Drug Addiction and Drug Abuse," in A. G. Gilman, I. W. Rall, A. S. Nies, and P. Taylor, eds., *Goodman and Gilman's The Pharmacological Basis of Therapeutics,* 8th ed. (New York: Pergamon, 1990), pp. 538–539.

35. H. R. Kranzler and B. Orrok, "The Pharmacotherapy of Alcoholism," *Annual Reviews of Psychiatry* 8 (1989): 397–417.

36. O. Nutt, B. Adinoff, and M. Linniola, "Benzodiazepines in the Treatment of Alcoholism," *Recent Developments in Alcoholism* 7 (1989): 283–313.

37. P. K. Gessner, "Alcohols," in C. M. Smith and A. M. Reynard, *Textbook of Pharmacology* (Philadelphia: Saunders, 1992), p. 264.

38. D. A. Gorelick, "Serotonin Uptake Blockers and the Treatment of Alcoholism," *Recent Developments in Alcoholism* 7 (1989): 267–281.

39. C. A. Naranjo, K. E. Kadlee, P. Sanjueze, and D. Woodley-Remus, "Fluoxetine Differentially Alters Alcohol Intake and Other Consummatory Behaviors in Problem Drinkers," *Clinical Pharmacology and Therapeutics* 47 (1990): 490–498.

40. C. A. Naranjo and E. M. Sellers, "Serotonin Uptake Inhibitors Attenuate Ethanol Intake in Problem Drinkers," *Recent Developments in Alcoholism* 7 (1989): 255–266.

41. M. R. Lu, G. C. Wagner, and H. Fisher, "Ethanol Consumption Following Acute Fenfluramine, Fluoxetine, and Dietary Tryptophan," *Pharmacology, Biochemistry and Behavior* 44 (1993): 931–937.

42. T. F. Meert, "Effects of Various Serotonergic Agents on Alcohol Intake and Alcohol Preference in Wistar Rats Selected at Two Different Levels of Alcohol Preference," *Alcohol and Alcoholism* 28 (1993): 157–170.

43. D. A. Gorelick and A. Pareded, "Effect of Fluoxetine on Alcohol Consumption in Male Alcoholics," *Alcoholism, Clinical and Experimental Research* 16 (1992): 261–265.

44. K. J. Buck, H. Heim, and R. A. Harris, "Reversal of Alcohol Dependence and Tolerance by a Single Administration of Flumazenil," *Journal of Pharmacology and Experimental Therapeutics* 257 (1991): 984–989.

45. A. Balakleevsky, G. Colombo, F. Fadda, and G. L. Gessa, "Ro 19-4603, a Benzodiazepine Receptor Inverse Agonist, Attenuates Voluntary Ethanol Consumption in Rats Selectively Bred for High Ethanol Preference," *Alcohol & Alcoholism* 25 (1990): 449–452.

46. J. R. Volpicelli, C. P. O'Brien, A. I. Alterman, and M. Hayshida, "Naltrexone and the Treatment of Alcohol Dependence: Initial Observations," in L. B. Reid, ed., *Opioids, Bulimia, Alcohol Abuse and Alcoholism* (New York: Springer-Verlag, 1990), pp. 195–214.

47. J. R. Volpicelli, I. Alterman, M. Hayashida, and C. P. O'Brien, "Naltrexone in the Treatment of Alcohol Dependence," *Archives of General Psychiatry* 49 (1992): 876–880.

48. S. S. O'Malley, A. J. Jaffe, G. Chang, R. S. Schottenfeld, R. E. Meyer, and B. Rounsaville, "Naltrexone and Coping Skills Therapy for Alcohol Dependence," *Archives of General Psychiatry* 49 (1992): 881–887.

49. P. K. Gessner, "Alcohols," in C. M. Smith and A. M. Reynard, *Textbook of Pharmacology* (Philadelphia: Saunders, 1992), pp. 267–268.

50. R. Castaneda and P. Cushman, "Alcohol Withdrawal: A Review of Clinical Management," *Journal of Clinical Psychiatry* 50(1989): 278–284.

51. "Treatment of Alcoholism, Part I," *The Harvard Medical School Mental Health Letter* 3, no. 12 (June 1987): 1–4.

CHAPTER 6

PSYCHOSTIMULANTS: COCAINE AND AMPHETAMINES

Cocaine and the amphetamines are powerful psychostimulants that markedly affect the mental functioning and behavior of persons who use them. Their effects include excitement, alertness, euphoria, a reduced sense of fatigue, and increased motor activity. Before describing the pharmacology of these drugs, we first distinguish them from other compounds that also stimulate the central nervous system (CNS), elevate mood, or alleviate depression (Table 6.1).

Examples of psychostimulants include the following:

1. cocaine

2. the amphetamines (dextroamphetamine and methamphetamine)

3. amphetamine derivatives used to treat attention deficit hyperactivity disorder (methylphenidate [Ritalin] and pemoline [Cylert])

4. a variety of drugs formerly used to treat obesity pharmacologically (fenfluramine [Pondimin], phentermine [under such trade names as Ionamin, Obe-Nix, Adipex-P, Oby-Trim, and Fastin], and phenmetrazine [Preludin])

All of these drugs are behavioral stimulants, all are behavioral reinforcers, and all are subject to compulsive abuse. In addition, all also have limited (but continuing) therapeutic use, and all have significant side effects and toxicity.

There are two other CNS stimulants. The first is caffeine, the principal psychoactive drug in coffee and other caffeinated beverages; the

TABLE 6.1 Classification of CNS stimulants.

Class	Mechanism of action	Examples
Behavioral stimulants	Augmentation of norepinephrine and dopamine neurotransmitter	Cocaine Amphetamines Methylphenidate (Ritalin) Pemoline (Cylert) Phenmetrazine (Preludin)
Clinical antidepressants	Blockade of norepinephrine reuptake Increased norepinephrine secondary to MAO inhibition Blockade of serotonin reuptake	Imipramine (Tofranil) Amitriptyline (Elavil Tranylcypromine (Parnate) Fluoxetine (Prozac)
Caffeine[a]	Blockade of adenosine receptors	
Nicotine[a]	Stimulation of acetylcholine receptors	

[a]See Chapter 7.

second is nicotine, the principal ingredient in tobacco. The pharmacology of these two drugs is discussed in Chapter 7.

Cocaine and the amphetamines (Figure 6.1) elevate mood, induce euphoria, increase alertness, reduce fatigue, provide a sense of increased energy, decrease appetite, improve task performance, and relieve boredom. Anxiety, insomnia, and irritability are common side effects of cocaine and the amphetamines. At higher doses, irritability and anxiety become more intense, and a pattern of psychotic behavior may appear. Indeed, cocaine and the amphetamines produce remarkably similar behavioral effects. At low doses, the behavioral stimulants evoke an alerting, arousing, or behavior-activating response that is not unlike a normal reaction to an emergency or to stress. Indeed, blood pressure and heart rate increase, pupils dilate, blood flow shifts from skin and internal organs to muscle, and oxygen levels rise, as does the level of glucose in the blood. These effects occur because these drugs augment or potentiate the action of dopamine and norepinephrine both in the body and in the brain. This action mimics the natural release of biological amines (e.g., adrenaline) as part of our normal alerting or activating response, as in a situation evoking a fight/flight/fright response (Appendix III). Indeed, the cocaine or amphetamine experience represents a grossly exaggerated mobilization of our normal fight/flight/fright response.

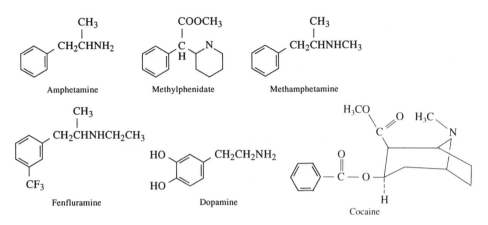

FIGURE 6.1   Structures of amphetamines, dopamine, and cocaine.

COCAINE

Cocaine occurs in the leaves of *Erythroxylon coca*, a tree indigenous to Peru and Bolivia. The drug was used for centuries by the natives for religious, mystical, social, stimulant, and medicinal purposes—most notably to increase endurance, promote a sense of well-being, and alleviate hunger. The usual total daily dose was up to about 200 milligrams. Today, "the relevant clinical issues related to cocaine's history have to do largely with the changes over time in dosage, route of administration, patterns of use, and the technology of cocaine production."[1]

The active alkaloid in *E. coca* was isolated in 1859 and named *cocaine.* In 1884 Freud advocated the use of cocaine to treat depression and to alleviate chronic fatigue. Freud described cocaine as a "magical drug"; he even wrote a "Song of Praise" to it.[2] In the same year, Koller demonstrated cocaine's local anesthetic properties and introduced the drug for use in ophthalmologic surgery. Freud, while using cocaine to relieve his own depression, described cocaine as inducing exhilaration and lasting euphoria, which in no way differs from the normal euphoria of the healthy person.[2] However, he did not immediately perceive its side effects: tolerance, dependence, a state of psychosis, and withdrawal depression.

In America, around 1885, cocaine was incorporated (along with caffeine) in a popular patent medicine later known as the beverage Coca-Cola. By 1891 at least 200 reports of cocaine intoxication and 13 deaths were reported. Until 1903 Coca-Cola contained approximately 60 milligrams of cocaine per 8-ounce serving.[1] In 1914 the Harrison Narcotic Act banned the incorporation of cocaine in patent medicines and beverages.

In 1924 the American Medical Association reviewed 43 deaths of patients who had been under local anesthesia induced by cocaine and attributed 26 of those deaths to cocaine toxicity. Guidelines for the safe use of cocaine were then established.[3]

The use of cocaine rose during the 1920s and then decreased during the 1930s, when amphetamines became available, presumably because amphetamines cost less and produced longer-lasting effects. Thus, cocaine was not used much again until the late 1960s, when tight federal restrictions on amphetamine distribution raised the cost of amphetamines, making cocaine attractive once again. Because their net effects are nearly indistinguishable, cocaine and the amphetamines can be used almost interchangeably as euphoriants. Availability, price, and sociocultural considerations now largely determine the comparative popularity of the two.

In the 1970s cocaine again became popular; in the mid-1980s, the smoking of concentrated preparations of cocaine ("free base" and "crack" cocaine) opened a new era in cocaine abuse characterized by high-dose, rapid-onset effects with the rapid development of drug dependence. How this era of cocaine use will end and what will replace cocaine as a euphoriant and an addicting psychostimulant is open to question.

An estimated 20 to 30 million people in the United States have used cocaine;[4] about 4 million people use it regularly, and about 2 million are "hard core" cocaine users.[5] At its peak use, as many as 800,000 Americans had cocaine daily; today a number closer to 300,000 is likely. This decrease, primarily in recreational users, is a result of the intensive recent campaign against cocaine. However, the number of addicted users has not markedly decreased.

Cocaine addicts are typically young (12 to 39 years of age), dependent on at least three drugs, and male (75 percent); they tend to have coexisting psychopathology (30 percent have anxiety disorders, 67 percent suffer from clinical depression, and 25 percent exhibit paranoia). About 85 to 90 percent are alcohol dependent. Cocaine use is associated with a range of violent premature deaths, including homicides, suicides, and accidents.[1] In addition, more people are using illicit amphetamines (especially methamphetamine), the increased use of which may be negating the positive reductions in cocaine use.

In his later writings, Freud called cocaine the "third scourge" of humanity, after alcohol and heroin. This is perhaps an appropriate description.

Chemistry

Each leaf of *E. coca* contains about 0.5 to 1.0 percent cocaine. When the leaves are soaked and mashed, cocaine is extracted in the form of coca paste (60 to 80 percent cocaine). Because persons who smoke coca paste may experience a high incidence of psychopathological states, extreme toxicity, and severe dependence, coca paste is usually treated to form a hydrochloride salt before it is exported. Then it is diluted (to increase its bulk and decrease its potency) and sold illicitly in powdered form as cocaine hydrochloride ("crystal" or "snow"). Inhaled ("snorted") in this form, a "line" of cocaine hydrochloride provides a dose of about 10 to 25 milligrams into each nostril; thus, a user might sniff about 20 to 50 milligrams of drug at a time.

Until recently the diluted hydrochloride salt preparation was the most common form of cocaine. However, a desire has developed for greater and more potent effects with a more rapid onset. Usually, in pharmacology, such heightened effects are provided only with parenteral (usually intravenous) injection. However, to many people the intravenous use of a recreational drug is objectionable, and so a smokable form was developed. The hydrochloride salt form of the drug is not suitable for smoking, because the drug in this form decomposes at the temperature required to vaporize it.

To resolve this problem, the hydrochloride form is chemically altered to the base form, which is then concentrated by extraction. This is accomplished either by extraction in ether (for "free base") or, more commonly today, by boiling the drug in a solution of baking soda until the water evaporates. The residue from the latter method is a form of cocaine base that is commonly called "crack," from the cracking sound it makes when heated. This base form of cocaine vaporizes at low temperature and can be inhaled by using a heated pipe. Today crack is the preparation used by the vast majority of cocaine addicts. This method yields average doses in the range of 250 milligrams to 1 gram. Because the many effects of cocaine are dose related, the consequences of these higher doses are severe, as will shortly become apparent.

Pharmacokinetics

Cocaine is absorbed from all sites of application, including mucous membranes, the gastrointestinal tract, and the lungs. It is detoxified both in plasma and in the liver. Only small amounts are excreted unchanged. Further pharmacokinetic details follow.

Absorption

The principal routes through which cocaine is taken are oral (chewing), intranasal (snorting), intravenous (mainlining), and by inhalation (smoking or free-basing). Table 6.2 presents some pharmacokinetic data for each method of administration. Taken orally, cocaine hydrochloride is slowly and incompletely absorbed. Absorption occurs over a period of about 1 hour, with about 75 percent of the absorbed drug rapidly metabolized in the liver on its first pass. Therefore, only about 25 percent of orally administered drug reaches the brain, and this occurs over a long period of time, eliminating the feeling of "rush" that follows administration by other routes.

Snorted intranasally, cocaine hydrochloride is poorly absorbed, as the hydrochloride salt poorly crosses the mucosal membranes. Also, because cocaine constricts blood vessels, such vasoconstriction limits its own absorption. However, about 20 to 30 percent of the drug is absorbed, with blood levels peaking within 30 to 60 minutes (Figure 6.2). The pharmacological effects last only about 30 to 60 minutes, although the total amount absorbed declines over about 6 hours.

When cocaine (base) is vaporized and smoked, some particles probably become trapped in the nose while others pass through the nasal pharynx into the trachea and onto lung surfaces, from which absorption is rapid and quite complete. Onset of effects is within seconds, and they persist for 5 to 10 minutes. Only about 6 to 32 percent of the initial amount reaches plasma, the remainder undergoing pyrolysis before inhalation.

Obviously, intravenous injection of cocaine hydrochloride bypasses all the barriers to absorption, placing the drug immediately into the bloodstream. The 30- to 60-second delay in onset of action simply reflects the time it takes the drug to travel from the site of injection to the brain.

Distribution

Cocaine penetrates the brain rapidly; initial brain concentrations far exceed the concentrations in plasma. After it penetrates the brain, cocaine is rapidly redistributed to other tissues. Cocaine freely crosses the placental barrier, achieving levels in the unborn equal to those in the mother.

Elimination

Cocaine has a biological half-life of 30 to 90 minutes, and it is almost completely metabolized by enzymes located both in plasma and in the

TABLE 6.2 Effects of cocaine administration.

Administration		Initial onset of action (s)	Duration of "high" (min)	Average acute dose (mg)	Peak plasma levels (ng/ml)	Purity (percent)	Bioavailability (percent absorbed)
Route	Mode						
Oral	Coca leaf chewing	300–600	45–90	20–50	150	0.5–1	25
Oral	Cocaine HCl	600–1800		100–200	150–200	20–80	20–30
Intranasal	"Snorting" cocaine HCl	120–180	30–45	5 × 30	150	20–80	20–30
Intravenous	Cocaine HCl	30–45	10–20	25–50	300–400	7–100 × 58	100
				>200	1000–1500		
Smoking	Coca paste	8–10	5–10	60–250	300–800	40–85	6–32
	Free base	8–10	5–10	250–1000	800–900	90–100	6–32
	Crack	8–10	5–10	250–1000	?	50–95	6–32

From Gold,[1] table 16.5, p. 209.

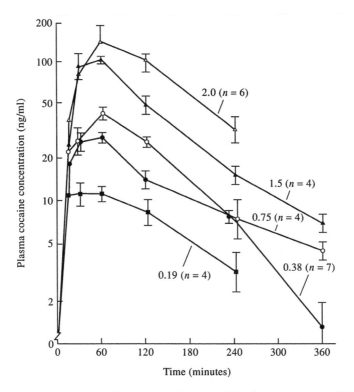

FIGURE 6.2 Time course of plasma cocaine levels following various doses (0.38–2.0 mg/kg) of intranasal cocaine. Points are mean ± S.E. [From J. A. Fleming, R. Byck, and P. G. Barash,[3] fig. 2, p. 520.]

liver. The major metabolite is the inactive compound *benzoylecgonine*, which can be detected in the urine for about 3 days, and much longer (15 to 22 days) in chronic users.[6] A small amount of cocaine is metabolized to an active intermediate (*norcocaine*). Urinary detection of benzoylecgonine forms the basis of drug testing for cocaine use. The persistence of the metabolite in urine implies that high-dose, long-term users might accumulate drug in their body tissues, from which it is later absorbed back into plasma, metabolized, and excreted. In some persons who genetically lack the plasma enzyme that metabolizes cocaine, the duration of action can be prolonged. There is some question as to whether cocaine metabolites can be toxic to the liver under certain circumstances.[3]

Pharmacodynamics

Pharmacologically, cocaine has three prominent actions.

1. It is a potent local anesthetic.
2. It is a powerful constrictor of blood vessels.
3. It is a powerful psychostimulant that has strong reinforcing qualities.

It is the psychostimulant property that contributes to the compulsive abuse of the drug.[7] Therefore, we focus on the actions that lead to its psychostimulation and its behavior-reinforcing properties.

Cocaine has long been known to potentiate the synaptic actions of dopamine, norepinephrine, and serotonin. Such action follows from cocaine's ability to block the active reuptake of these transmitters into the presynaptic nerve terminals from which they were released (Appendix II). By the late 1980s, cocaine's action on the dopaminergic system was known to be crucial to its behavior-reinforcing and psychostimulant properties.[8,9]

> Dopaminergic pathways in the midbrain are emerging as central to many of the behavioral manifestations of cocaine, especially those concerning reinforcement and hyperactivity. The ventral tegmental area of the midbrain . . . gives rise to dopamine-containing neuronal projections which innervate the meso-limbic brain areas, including the medial prefrontal cortex and nucleus accumbens, as well as the amygdala and hippocampus. The activity of cocaine upon the meso-limbic dopamine-terminals is proposed as the key to the reinforcing properties of the drug.[10]

Several recent studies have greatly advanced our understanding of this action on the dopaminergic system.[10–14] These studies showed that both dopamine and cocaine decrease the discharge rate of neurons located in the ventral tegmental area and the nucleus accumbens (Figure 6.3), indicating that dopamine exerts inhibitory effects on the postsynaptic receptors. Cocaine markedly potentiates the dopamine-induced decrease in discharge rate. Mechanistically, the blockade of dopamine reuptake by cocaine increases the extracellular (synaptic) concentration of dopamine, thus potentiating its inhibitory transmitter action.[15] How this inhibitory synaptic transmitter action of dopamine translates into behavioral reinforcement is still unclear, but the mechanism is likely to be extremely complex.[12]

More recently the presynaptic "transporter" protein for dopamine, which is blocked by cocaine, has been cloned and characterized.[16,17]

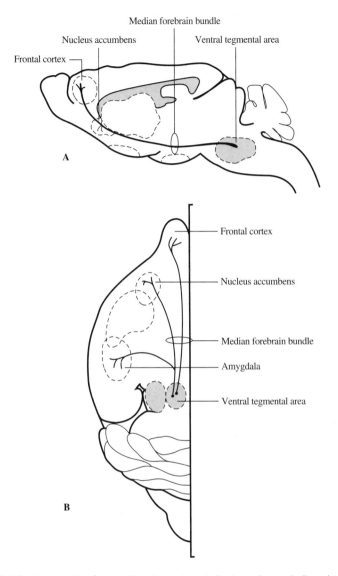

FIGURE 6.3 Schematic of ascending dopaminergic brain pathways believed to mediate the reinforcing effects of cocaine. **(A)** Sagittal or side view. **(B)** Coronal or top view.

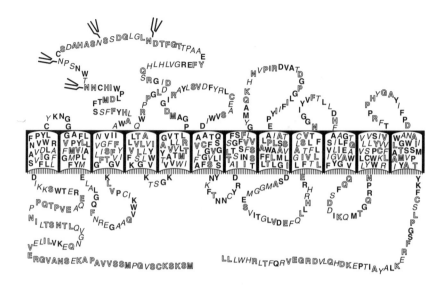

FIGURE 6.4 Schematic representation of the dopamine transporter showing proposed orientation in the plasma membrane, amino acids conserved in GABA, dopamine (DA), and norepinephrine (NE) transporters (dark letters), amino acids conserved in DA and NE transporters (italic letters), or amino acids found only in DA transporters (open letters). [From Shimada and others,[16] fig. 1, p. 577.]

This transporter is a 619-amino-acid protein with 12 putative membrane-spanning regions; both termini of the protein are located in the intracellular cytoplasm of the presynaptic neuron (Figure 6.4). Cocaine binding to this protein probably induces a conformational change in the dopamine-recognition (binding) site that decreases the affinity of dopamine for its receptor.[15] Indeed, it is through such action that cocaine augments the inhibitory response, which is mediated through the ventral tegmental area and the nucleus accumbens. Somehow this in vivo response translates into cocaine's behavioral effects.

At least two of the five (or more) types of dopamine receptors are involved in this action of cocaine.[15] Dopamine$_2$ receptors seem to underlie the positive effects on behavior, the reinforcing effects, the locomotor effects, and the stereotypical behavioral effects observed in animals after cocaine administration. Dopamine$_1$ receptors are less well understood but appear to serve a "permissive" effect in the expression of dopamine-mediated behaviors.[15]

Serotonin also seems to play a role in the actions of cocaine:

> Serotonin depletion increases the efficacy of cocaine as a positive reinforcer, and raises the possibility that the actions of cocaine on serotonin contribute an aversive effect of cocaine that limits its self-administration. In addition . . . the serotonin uptake inhibitor fluoxetine can enhance the discriminative stimulus effects of cocaine.[15]

Finally, the question arises about neuronal mechanisms that might underlie the tolerance that develops with prolonged use of cocaine. Although much remains to be explained, it is clear that chronic exposure of postsynaptic receptors to the increased amounts of dopamine that are available (after its active reuptake has been blocked) leads to both a decrease in the number of postsynaptic dopamine receptors and an increase in the amount of available dopamine transporter protein.[11] As a result, there is decreased receptor sensitivity to dopamine (because fewer receptors are available) and an increased ability of presynaptic neurons to sequester any dopamine in the synaptic space (obviously, in the absence of cocaine). Johanson and Fischman, who reviewed the physiological and adaptive mechanisms of cocaine tolerance, noted that "the extent of tolerance development appears to be limited, i.e., the maximum change was a 2-fold shift. . . . In addition, it (the tolerance) disappears relatively rapidly."[8]

Side Effects of Short-Term, Low-Dose Use

As part of the cocaine-induced fight/flight/fright syndrome, the non-toxic physiological responses include increased alertness, motor hyperactivity, tachycardia, vasoconstriction, hypertension, bronchodilatation, increased body temperature, pupillary dilatation, increased glucose availability, and shifts in blood flow from the internal organs to the muscles. Higher doses of cocaine result in very significant toxicity, which is discussed later.

The enjoyable psychological effects of low to average doses of cocaine (25 to 150 milligrams) begin as soon as cocaine reaches the brain; the exact effects vary depending on the dose, the level of drug tolerance, and the route of administration.

> The major psychological functions affected by cocaine are mood, cognition, drive states such as hunger, sex, and thirst, and consciousness. An immediate and intense euphoria, analogous to a sexual orgasm, occurs and may last seconds, or usually minutes. . . . Other alterations arising from elevation in mood include giddiness, enhanced

self-consciousness, and a forceful boastfulness. The subsequent level of mood is milder euphoria mixed with anxiety, which can last for 60–90 minutes, followed by a more protracted anxious state that spans hours. During acute and subacute intoxication, thoughts typically race and speech becomes talkative and rapid, often pressured, even garrulous, with tangential and incoherent speech.[5]

Appetite is markedly suppressed but later rebounds. Sleep is delayed; fatigue is postponed but later rebounds. Conscious awareness and mental acuity are increased, with later depression. Motor activity is increased, with agitation, restlessness, and a feeling of constant motion. Perhaps most important, cocaine is a potent behavioral reinforcer. A person on cocaine wants to take more cocaine, even instead of such important reinforcers as food.

Cocaine also functions as a discriminative stimulus in several species,[8,15] a fundamental mechanism by which a drug can control behavior. Also, cocaine administration has been reported to be followed by an increase in cocaine craving, "an effect that may, like its positive reinforcing effect, increase the likelihood of additional cocaine consumption."[15] In fact, even when self-administering cocaine is punished, a person on cocaine will still tend to want more of the drug.[8] The craving is made worse by the short action of cocaine. After the "high" ends, anxiety, depression, and paranoia follow. This rapid shift causes the user to crave more drug in an attempt to regain the euphoria felt just minutes ago. Such drug craving becomes intense and "forms a distinct part of the withdrawal syndrome associated with cocaine."[1] At higher doses, all these effects are intensified, as is the depressive rebound that follows. There is a progressive loss of coordination, followed by tremors and eventually seizures. CNS stimulation is followed by depression, dysphoria, anxiety, somnolence, and drug craving.

Although a person's sexual interest may be heightened by using cocaine—high doses of cocaine that are injected or smoked are sometimes described as "orgasmic"—cocaine is not an aphrodisiac: Sexual dysfunction is common in heavy users. Further, when dysfunction is combined with the isolation that cocaine-dependent individuals experience, normal interpersonal, sensual, and sexual interactions are compromised.

Specific medical complications are also associated with the method of administering cocaine. When cocaine is snorted, chronic rhinitis, perforations of the nasal septum, and a loss of the sense of smell can occur. When cocaine is taken intravenously, diseases transmitted by needle (e.g., hepatitis and AIDS) and infectious endocarditis (infections of the heart and its valves) are not uncommon. Finally, smoking crack cocaine can cause pulmonary difficulties and black sputum.

Toxic and Psychotic Effects of Long-Term, High-Dose Use

Although low doses of cocaine cause CNS stimulation that is mostly pleasurable or euphoric, higher doses produce toxic symptoms, including anxiety, sleep deprivation, hypervigilance, suspiciousness, paranoia, and persecutory fears. Persons who use cocaine can have a markedly altered perception of reality, and they can become aggressive or homicidal in response to imagined persecution.[4] These behaviors comprise what is called a *toxic paranoid psychosis.*

Other high-dose, long-term effects of cocaine use include sexual dysfunction, interpersonal conflicts (resulting from the sense of isolation and paranoia), and severe depressive conditions, dysphoria, and bizarre and violent psychotic disorders that can last days or weeks after a person stops using the drug. As summarized by Johanson and Fischman,

> One of the most significant consequences of cocaine abuse is the development of behavioral pathology in chronic users. In its most extreme form, a cocaine psychosis can be produced, characterized by paranoia, impaired reality testing, anxiety, a stereotyped compulsive repetitive pattern of behavior, and vivid visual, auditory and tactile hallucinations including delusions of insects crawling under the skin. More subtle changes in behavior . . . may include irritability, hypervigilance, extreme psychomotor activation, paranoid thinking, impaired interpersonal relations, and disturbances of eating and sleeping.[8]

An acutely toxic dose of cocaine has been estimated to be about 1 to 2 milligrams per kilogram of body weight. Thus, 70 to 150 milligrams of cocaine is a toxic, one-time dose for a 150-pound person. Serious physiological toxicity follows higher doses.

A recent symposium on acute cocaine intoxication addressed the cardiovascular[18] and neurovascular[19] sequelae of cocaine use. Such sequelae include serious complications such as strokes in healthy, young individuals, persistent alterations in blood perfusion of the brain, oxygen deprivation to the heart, cardiac arrhythmias, and seizures.

Chronic cocaine use produces virtually every psychiatric syndrome: affective disorders, schizophrenia-like syndromes, personality disorders, and so on. Rounsaville and coworkers[20] studied 300 cocaine abusers seeking treatment for their substance abuse problem. They found that 56 percent met current criteria and 73 percent met lifetime criteria for the presence of a neuropsychological disorder (major depression, anxiety disorder, bipolar affective disorder, antisocial personality, or history of childhood attention deficit hyperactivity disorder). Thus, toxic symptoms may indicate either high-dose drug toxicities or the onset of symptoms of a coexisting neuropsychological disorder or both. According to one report,

> cocaine addicts, like alcoholics and heroin addicts, often show a certain profile on personality tests—they are reckless, rebellious, and have a low tolerance for frustration and a craving for excitement. In fact, most of them have been, or will be alcoholics or heroin addicts as well. They use opiates and alcohol either to enhance the effects of cocaine or to medicate themselves for unwanted side effects—calming jitters, dulling perceptions, and reducing paranoia to indifference. Intravenous drug users often take cocaine and heroin together in a mixture known as a speedball. Probably more than half of people treated for cocaine abuse are also alcoholic, and the rate of alcoholism in the families of cocaine addicts is high.[21]

Weddington goes on to say that

> with repeated or chronic intoxication, *tolerance* develops. Accompanying a diminishing intensity of euphoria, chronic cocaine users regularly report increasing dysphoria, anxiety, a sense of loss of control with decreased self-esteem, suspiciousness increasing to paranoia, aggressiveness, and confusion. In addition, environmental consequences to cocaine addiction, such as social and family dissolution, financial loss, or legal contingencies, may contribute to an addict's growing dysphoria and despair associated with chronic cocaine abuse.[6]

Fetal Effects

One of the tragedies of the late twentieth century is the birth of hundreds of thousands of infants who have been injured intra utero by drugs and are born into poor nutritional and social environments. Prominent among these drugs is cocaine, a drug that produces infants with "jittery baby syndrome" and infants known as "crack babies." Because of the wide spectrum of fetal effects, a "fetal cocaine syndrome" cannot be well defined, since "most fetal effects may be related to vasoconstriction, hypertension, and infarcts at any time during gestation and in any structure."[22] Indeed, exposure to cocaine at any period in gestation may damage any organ or structure in the unborn child.[22]

To determine possible effects on the fetus, one must examine not only indirect maternal effects on fetal development but also direct teratogenic effects (Figure 6.5).

Indirect effects of cocaine on the fetus result from its vasoconstrictive action in the mother, which decreases blood flow to the uterus and reduces fetal oxygenation. The results of such fetal hypoxia include placental detachment, placental insufficiency, preterm or precipitous labor, fetal death (stillbirths), and low birth weight.[23,24] Lack of oxygen during fetal development can lead to intrauterine growth retardation, small head size (microcephaly), and possible aberrations in brain development. As reviewed by Kain, Rimer, and Barash,[25] virtually any body organ in the neonate can be affected if blood flow to that organ is reduced during fetal development.

Volpe, in his detailed review of the literature on the direct fetal effects of cocaine,[26] notes that the unborn is exposed to cocaine even before fertilization, because cocaine can bind to the sperm of a male cocaine user. As the brain develops, exposure of the fetus to cocaine may promote serious destructive lesions, leading to a neonatal neurological syndrome typified by abnormal sleep patterns, tremors, poor feeding, irritability, occasional seizures, and an increased risk or incidence of sudden infant death syndrome (SIDS).[25]

These conclusions have been disputed.[27] According to this view, the fetal cocaine syndrome is not as clearly defined as the fetal alcohol syndrome (Chapter 5), and cocaine use by the mother "is only one of many undesirable influences in the children's lives. . . . Neglect and abuse by addicted parents are a greater danger." Therefore, babies born into a drug-using environment and possibly into poverty experience little physical or emotional nurturing, and so bonding is incomplete or absent. However, the statistics on cocaine use and newborns are unchallenged, including the fact that "50,000–100,000 babies are born each year to mothers who have used at least some cocaine during pregnancy."[27]

As crack babies enter the school system, they have difficulty developing attachments or dealing effectively with multiple stimuli. They may become either aggressive or withdrawn when they are overstimulated. They have difficulty with unstructured play and a low tolerance for frustration; they also structure input and information poorly. In other words, crack babies of school age show a high incidence of

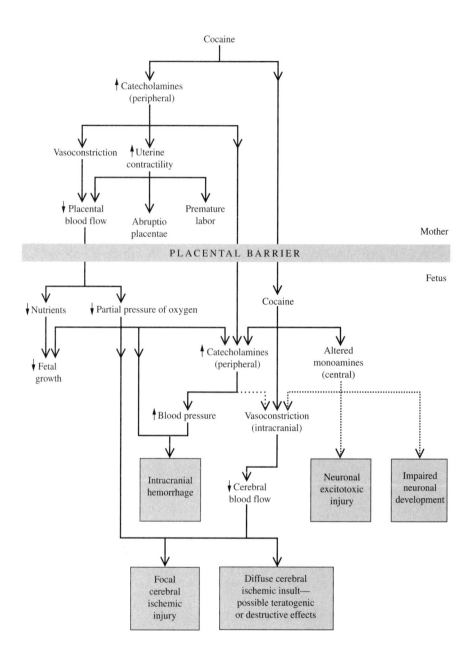

FIGURE 6.5　Deleterious effects of maternal cocaine use on fetuses. Effects that appear plausible on the basis of current information but whose confirmation requires more supporting evidence are indicated by dotted lines. ↑ denotes increased, and ↓ decreased. [From J. J. Volpe, "Effect of Cocaine Use on the Fetus," *New England Journal of Medicine* 327, no. 6 (6 August 1992), fig. 1, p. 401.]

attention deficit hyperactivity disorder (ADHD). This syndrome probably follows from the combined effects of prenatal drug exposure and an early growth period in difficult homes or institutions.

> These children form a *"bio-underclass"*—a cohort of children whose combined physiological damage and extrinsic socioeconomic disadvantage could foredoom them to a life of inferiority. In other words, a generation of children so damaged neurologically and environmentally that their inferiority is determined from birth.[28]

Volpe concludes, "Determining the effect of cocaine on infants may require new techniques of evaluation and years of surveillance. Otherwise, we could seriously underestimate the effects on the infant of a pregnant woman's abuse of cocaine."[26]

We do know that many of these infants, in order to be "normal," require special care and nurturing from the moment of birth, through schooling, and into the early adult years, when deviance or social inferiority becomes more obvious. We have no idea at this time whether adjustment problems (of all sorts) will result from cocaine-aggravated ADHD carried over into adulthood. The societal costs may indeed be enormous.

Treatment of Cocaine Abuse

A variety of psychological, behavioral, and pharmacological approaches have been suggested for treating cocaine abuse,[1,6,8,9,18] but several major problems complicate any attempt at therapy. First is the intensity of both the drug effect and the behavior-reinforcing action of cocaine. Second is the pronounced tendency toward relapse, with cocaine acting as a cue to an increased craving for the drug. Third is the fact that virtually all cocaine addicts have additional drug dependencies and/or psychiatric disorders, including affective disorders, bipolar disorder, borderline personality disorder, antisocial personality disorder, and eating disorders. Given these complications, the needs of the cocaine addict are at least fivefold:

1. immediate abstinence

2. diagnosis of any coexisting disorders

3. determination whether the cocaine addiction is a primary disorder or is secondary to other disorders

4. maintenance of abstinence for long enough to diagnose and begin treatment of coexisting disorders

5. prevention of relapse

Approaches to treatment are many, from classical "12-step" recovery programs resembling that of Alcoholics Anonymous to experimental interventions utilizing psychopharmacotherapy, psychotherapy, or cognitive-behavioral approaches.[6,8] In all cases, abstinence is essential and must be monitored by frequent, random, unannounced urine tests to screen for cocaine and other drugs of abuse.

Gawin and Kleber[29] developed a three-phase model of abstinence symptomatology related to cocaine abuse; the phases, called the "crash," "withdrawal," and "extinction," may have important implications for treatment. The crash phase is quite short (9 hours to 4 days); during this period the user is generally uninterested in abstaining from or using cocaine, appearing quite depressed and somnolent. The withdrawal phase, which lasts 1 to 10 weeks, is the period of maximal relapse potential and drug craving. The extinction phase is of unlimited duration; here patients require continued monitoring because conditioned cues, which must be extinguished, can still trigger craving and result in relapse.

Psychopharmacotherapy could, at least theoretically, be used in treating cocaine abuse for any of four reasons:

1. to antagonize the effects of cocaine at its receptors

2. to produce an aversive (Antabuse-like) reaction if cocaine is taken

3. to treat the coexisting psychiatric disorder

4. to reduce cocaine craving and withdrawal

To date, no specific antagonists are available, nor are any aversive drugs. Therefore, psychopharmacotherapy is aimed at utilizing drugs to attenuate the craving for cocaine. The memory of cocaine euphoria is so powerful that drug craving, even after months or years of abstinence, can produce an overwhelming urge to revert to drug use. Currently the most popular drug for reducing this craving is the antidepressant desipramine[30] (Chapter 8). This drug, through the "desipramine effect," can relieve craving and ameliorate withdrawal. However, the effect is not predictable; any positive effects are short-lived, and any coexisting state of major depression, which is found in about 30 percent of cocaine addicts, may be the primary object of such treatment.

Other agents that have been tried include the antiparkinsonian dopamine receptor blocker *bromocriptine,* the amino acid *tyrosine* (which may increase serotonin levels in the brain), *phenothiazines,* (which work as antipsychotics because they block dopamine receptors), other *antidepressants,* the mood stabilizer *lithium,* the anticonvulsant *carbamazepine,* and many others.

Recently Carroll and coworkers[31] evaluated the effectiveness of cognitive-behavioral treatment (based on relapse prevention principles), clinical management, and desipramine, alone and in randomized combination, in treating ambulatory cocaine abusers. All treatments significantly reduced cocaine use. Desipramine was not as effective as either nonpharmacological treatment, although desipramine as a short-term adjunct appeared to facilitate the effectiveness of psychotherapy. Higher-severity cocaine abusers appeared to respond best to relapse prevention therapy. Lower-intensity approaches (such as desipramine without concomitant psychotherapy) was effective only with less severe abusers. Gold summarizes by advocating prevention as the best treatment:

> Education for prevention actually should begin before a child is conceived. . . . After birth, drug education should begin at home. . . . This . . . should continue when the child begins school, . . . starting with kindergarten and ending in college. Physicians should play a significant role in reducing the cocaine epidemic by never failing to consider the possibility of substance abuse . . . and by inoculating their patients, especially their younger ones, with accurate information about this dangerous and deadly drug.[1]

AMPHETAMINES AND RELATED DRUGS

Amphetamine (see Figure 6.1), the more potent active form dextroamphetamine, the methyl derivative methamphetamine, and several other derivatives (methylphenidate, fenfluramine, pemoline, and others) compose a group of drugs that exert psychostimulant effects closely resembling those of cocaine.

Amphetamine was first synthesized in the late 1880s. It was not used for medicinal purposes until the early 1930s, when it was found to increase blood pressure, stimulate the CNS, and cause bronchodilatation. By 1935 amphetamine was used to treat narcolepsy, a disorder characterized by excessive daytime sleepiness. Like Freud's view of cocaine in the 1880s, it was felt in the 1930s that amphetamine posed little threat to health, an impression that would change within a decade. Between 1935 and 1946, a list of 39 conditions for which amphetamine could be used in treatment was developed, including schizophrenia, morphine addiction, tobacco smoking, heart block, head injury, radiation sickness, hypotension, seasickness, severe hiccups, and caffeine dependence. During World War II, amphetamine was used as an aid to fight fatigue and enhance the performance of servicemen.

Large-scale abuse (usually oral ingestion of amphetamine tablets) began in the late 1940s, primarily by students and truck drivers. Amphetamine continued to be used (and abused) as a diet aid. In the late 1960s, the abuse pattern changed with the advent of injectable forms of amphetamine. These injectable products (by legitimate manufacturers) have been discontinued.

Amphetamine has been used both licitly and illicitly for a wide variety of clinical and recreational purposes. The effects of the amphetamine derivatives are similar to those of amphetamine itself; therefore, amphetamine is discussed at length and the derivatives are compared with it.

Mechanism of Action

The amphetamines exert virtually all of their CNS effects by causing the release of newly synthesized catecholamines (especially dopamine) from presynaptic storage sites in nerve terminals.[32,33] King and Ellinwood[34] review the consequences of this action, which we will summarize here. The behavioral stimulation and increased psychomotor activity appears to follow from stimulation of the dopamine receptors in the mesolimbic system (including the nucleus accumbens). The high-dose stereotypical behavior (including constant repetition of meaningless acts) appears to involve dopamine neurons in the caudate nucleus and putamen of the basal ganglia.

The actions leading to an increase in aggressive behavior are complex. Such action is seen primarily in adults; in children amphetamines are used therapeutically to reduce aggressive behavior and activities characteristic of attention deficit hyperactivity disorder. The neuroanatomic location of these effects is unclear.

Amphetamines, which are potent anorectics (they decrease appetite), have been used clinically in weight loss programs for many years. This action seems to involve the lateral hypothalamus but may also involve serotonin neurons, which, when activated, produce satiety.

Pharmacological Effects

The amphetamines are classified pharmacologically as indirectly acting catecholamine agonists, which exert their peripheral and central actions by causing the release of newly synthesized norepinephrine and dopamine from presynaptic nerve terminals[34] (Appendix III). All the physical and behavioral effects of the amphetamines follow from this action. Note that the release of dopamine increases the amount of dopamine available to the postsynaptic receptor, much as does cocaine, which blocks the presynaptic reuptake of dopamine. Thus, because both drugs have the net effect of increasing the amount of dopamine available, the effects of the two drugs are quite similar.

The pharmacological responses to amphetamine vary with the dose of the drug, the method of administration, and the length of time over which the drug is taken. In general, effects may be categorized as those observed at low to moderate doses (5 to 50 milligrams), usually administered orally, and those observed at high doses (more than approximately 100 milligrams), often administered intravenously.

These dose ranges are not the same for all amphetamines. For example, dextroamphetamine is 3 to 4 times more potent than amphetamine. Low to moderate doses of dextroamphetamine range from 2.5 to 20 milligrams, while high doses are 50 milligrams or more. Because methamphetamine ("speed") is even more potent, dose ranges must be lowered even more.

At low oral doses, all of the amphetamines induce a significant increase in blood pressure, with a reflex slowing of heart rate, a relaxation of bronchial muscle, and a variety of other responses that follow from the body's chemical preparation for the fight/flight/fright response. In the CNS, amphetamine is a potent psychomotor stimulant, producing increased alertness, euphoria, excitement, wakefulness, a reduced sense of fatigue, loss of appetite, mood elevation, increased motor and speech activity, and a feeling of power. Although task performance is improved, dexterity may deteriorate. When short-duration, high-intensity energy output is desired, such as during an athletic competition, a user's performance may be enhanced, despite the fact that his or her dexterity and fine motor skills may be impaired. Amphetamines are excreted in the urine and are easily detectable for up to 48 hours after use.

At moderate doses (20 to 50 milligrams), additional effects of amphetamine include stimulation of respiration, slight tremors, restlessness, a greater increase in motor activity, insomnia, and agitation. In addition, amphetamine prevents fatigue, suppresses appetite, promotes wakefulness, and causes sleep deprivation. Because the biological need for sleep cannot be postponed indefinitely, deep sleep follows when use of the drug is discontinued. Complete recovery of normal sleeping patterns may take many weeks. Indeed, both the prolonged use of low doses of amphetamine and the single use of a high dose of amphetamine are characteristically followed by intense mental depression and fatigue that counterbalance the behavioral stimulation and euphoria produced by the drug.

Persons who chronically use high doses of amphetamine suffer from a different set of drug effects. Stereotypical behaviors include continual, purposeless, repetitive acts, sudden outbursts of aggression and violence, paranoid delusions, and severe anorexia. A state of amphetamine psychosis may develop, which may be indistinguishable from an acute attack of schizophrenia.

In animals, chronic amphetamine administration is associated with persistent depletion of both dopamine and the enzyme tyrosine hydroxylase (Appendix III), which is necessary for the synthesis of dopamine. This suggests that amphetamine may be potentially toxic to dopamine-releasing neurons. Certainly these neurons eventually lose their sensitivity to endogenous dopamine, so that an amphetamine-induced loss of responsiveness to "natural reinforcers" may develop.[34] In other words, the only way to experience positive reinforcement, or reward, may be through the use of the drug (amphetamine or cocaine); natural chemical activity may be ineffective.

Other harmful effects are seen in the deteriorating high-dose user. Psychosis and abnormal mental conditions, weight loss, skin sores, infections resulting from neglected health care, and a variety of other consequences occur because of the actions of the drug itself or because of poor eating habits, lack of sleep, or the use of unsterile equipment for intravenous injections. Most high-dose users show a progressive deterioration in their social, personal, and occupational affairs. Also seen are amphetamine psychosis with paranoid ideation; many addicts must be hospitalized intermittently for treatment of episodes of psychosis.

The toxic dose of amphetamine varies widely. Severe reactions can occur from low doses (20 to 30 milligrams). On the other hand, persons who do not have tolerance have survived doses of 400 to 500 milligrams. Even larger doses are tolerated by chronic users. The slogan "Speed kills" not only refers to a direct fatal effect of single doses of amphetamine but also to the deteriorating mental and physical condition that occurs in the addicted user.

Dependence and Tolerance

As a potent psychomotor stimulant and behavior-reinforcing agent, amphetamine is prone to compulsive abuse (it induces psychological dependence). Dependence is readily induced in both man and laboratory animals and follows a classical positive conditioning model (the positive reward leads to further drug use).

Tolerance rapidly develops and is accompanied by dysphoria, sedation, lassitude, and drug craving. The solution to this state is the taking of more amphetamine in higher and higher doses, which starts a vicious cycle of drug use and withdrawal. At this point, tolerance to the euphoriant effects develops, and periods of prolonged "binging" begin. This tolerance combined with the memory of drug-induced highs leads to further drug intake, social withdrawal, and a focus on procuring drugs.

Therapeutic Uses and Status

The medical uses of amphetamines today are very restricted and often controversial. These uses include

1. treatment of a form of epilepsy called narcolepsy (This application is now rare.)
2. treatment of attention deficit hyperactivity disorder
3. treatment of obesity

Despite the occasional report to the contrary, amphetamines are not of much value in treating major depression (because of the great potential for addiction and the general lack of therapeutic efficacy). Since the use of amphetamines in treating narcolepsy constitutes a specialized neurological use, it will not be discussed here. Here we will focus on the use of amphetamine and its derivatives in treating attention deficit hyperactivity disorder and obesity.

Attention Deficit Hyperactivity Disorder (ADHD)

Amphetamines have been used since about 1936 for treating attention deficit hyperactivity disorder (ADHD). Treatment started historically with the use of amphetamine and dextroamphetamine and has progressed over the years to the use of methylphenidate (Ritalin), pemoline (Cylert), and, more recently, the antidepressant nortriptyline.[35] Along with this evolution has been an evolution of terminology for the disorder: from "minimal brain dysfunction" to "minimal brain disorder" to "hyperactivity syndrome" to "attention deficit disorder" (ADD) to the present ADHD. Although no definitive CNS pathology has been demonstrated (because there is no animal model of ADHD), Levy reviews a dopamine hypothesis of ADHD,[36] invoking a "disorder of polysynaptic dopaminergic circuits, between prefrontal and striate centers." This theory is consistent with our discussion of the mechanism of action of amphetamine and cocaine in the nucleus accumbens.

ADHD, which affects up to 6 percent of school-age children, is characterized by inattentiveness, impulsivity, and hyperactivity that are persistent and sufficiently severe to cause functional impairment at school, at home, and with peers. There is some evidence that the disorder may be inherited.[37]

There is a small but growing belief that symptoms may persist into adulthood in a significant percentage of persons with the childhood disorder.[38] Lie examines the hypothesis that ADHD is a precursor of both criminality and abuse of drugs and alcohol in adults:

> By early adulthood, ADHD appears to remain present in at least one-third of the subjects. Subjects with prior ADHD did not have more mental problems than controls in adolescence and early adulthood, provided they had normal intelligence and no additional disabilities or mental disorders. . . . ADHD combined with delinquency indicates a high rate of subsequent lawbreaking.[39]

Others also feel that ADHD in childhood, and its effective treatment, carries over into adulthood and that effective treatment during childhood leads to better outcome as adults. Conceivably, effective intervention early in childhood may alter the course of ADHD, decreasing the likelihood of developing conduct disorder as an adolescent and antisocial personality disorder with its various complications (e.g., alcohol and drug abuse, criminality) as an adult.

Currently the pharmacological treatment of ADHD is usually discontinued when a child reaches puberty, because adolescents presumably are more prone to the abuse of amphetamine-like psychostimulants. In addition, the possible growth-reducing effects of these drugs may blunt the usual adolescent growth spurt (even with a "summer holiday" from the drug). In some cases, however, continuation of drug therapy may be indicated through adolescence and even into adulthood in some individuals with residual ADHD.[40]

Stimulant drugs improve behavior and learning ability in 50 to 75 percent of children who are correctly diagnosed.[41] The agents differ primarily in terms of their pharmacokinetics (Table 6.3).

Methylphenidate, the most widely used drug for treating ADHD, is of rapid onset and short duration; thus it must be administered at both breakfast and lunchtime. By evening, the blood level drops, allowing for normal sleep. However, the short half-life is a problem in some children who experience an end-of-dose rebound in dysfunctional behavior. Sustained-release preparations of methylphenidate have been disappointing.

Pemoline has a much longer but more variable half-life and is given once a day. Disadvantages include an extremely slow onset of effect and a possibly reduced level of therapeutic efficacy.

TABLE 6.3 Psychostimulants used to treat attention deficit hyperactivity disorder.

Feature	Methylphenidate	Pemoline	Dextro-amphetamine
Elimination half-life	2–3	2–12	6–7
Time to peak plasma concentration (T_{max})	1–3	1–5	3–4
Onset of behavioral effect	1	3–4 weeks	1
Duration of behavioral effect	3–4	Not available	4
Daily dose range			
mg/kg/day	0.6–0.7	0.5–3.0	0.3–1.25
mg/day	10–60	37.5–112.5	5–40

From P. G. Janicak, J. M. Davis, S. H. Preskorn, and F. J. Ayd, Jr., *Principles and Practice of Psychopharmacotherapy* (Baltimore: Williams & Wilkins, 1993), tab. 14.1, p. 493.
Note: All time values are given in hours unless otherwise noted.

Amphetamines, especially dextroamphetamine, are rarely used in treating ADHD today. However, dextroamphetamine can be useful in those children who do not respond to methylphenidate or pemoline.

Antidepressants (Chapter 8) have not been widely used to treat ADHD, but one, nortriptyline, has been studied.[35] In this retrospective study of "nonresponders" to other medications, 84 percent of which had at least one comorbid diagnosis with ADHD, 76 percent were claimed to respond positively to nortriptyline at blood levels of drug ranging from 50 to 150 nanograms per milliliter of plasma. Additional study of nortriptyline in adolescents appears indicated, because antidepressants are not considered to be drugs subject to compulsive abuse (Chapter 8).

Obesity

The amphetamines have widely been used in treating obesity; however, such use has always been extremely controversial. Side effects, dependency, addiction, and the rapid development of tolerance have always been considered impediments to their use. Although small amounts of weight loss (less than 1 pound per week) accompany the use of amphetamine and other dopamine-potentiating agents, this effect is lost after only a few weeks of therapy. As stated in the package insert of each of these compounds:

The natural history of obesity is measured in years, whereas [all studies reviewed] are restricted to a few weeks duration: Thus, the total
impact of drug-induced weight loss over that of diet alone must be
considered clinically limited.

Compounds acting through dopamine-augmented anorexia include
benzphetamine (Didrex), phendimetrazine (Anorex, Oblan, Phendiet,
Wehless), diethylpropion (Tenuate, Tepanol), mazindol (Mazenor,
Sanorex), phentermine (Fastin, Ionamin, Phentrol, Adipex-P, Oby-
Trim), phenylpropanolamine (Dexatrim), and dextroamphetamine/am-
phetamine combination (Obetrol). One researcher stated, "No clinical
need exists for any of these drugs in the treatment of obesity."[42] Thus,
the search has continued for amphetamine-related derivatives that
suppress appetite without the potential for drug abuse and without the
concomitant development of tolerance.

New on the scene are three drugs (fenfluramine, fluoxetine, and
sertraline) that are structurally related to amphetamine but act to
potentiate serotonin neurotransmission rather than dopamine neurotransmission. As mentioned earlier, amphetamine may exert its
anorectic action by augmenting dopamine neurotransmission in the
lateral thalamus; this action, in turn, activates serotonin neurons,
which themselves produce satiety. The three new drugs skip the
dopamine step by augmenting serotonin neurotransmission, thereby
eliminating the dopamine-induced reinforcement of behavior (which
can lead to compulsive abuse and addiction).

Fenfluramine (Pondimin), the best studied of the three seritonergic agents, acts to "partially inhibit the reuptake of serotonin and to release serotonin from nerve ending. This increased serotonin in the
neuronal (synaptic) cleft is believed to reduce food intake."[42]
Furthermore, "fenfluramine combined with phentermine enhanced
the magnitude of weight loss over and above what could be achieved
with the best behavior modification, exercise, and nutrition program,
and the effect continued for nearly 4 years."[42,43]

Weintraub and coworkers[43] conclude that anorexiant medications
can help one lose weight and maintain the weight loss for prolonged
periods of time with little fear of developing abuse patterns of drug
ingestion. The researchers placed weight loss in perspective with the
psychological benefits resulting from the loss of excess fat. Thus, the
combined use of a dopaminergic agent and a serotonergic agent may
lead to yet another era in the pharmacological treatment of obesity.

Fluoxetine and sertraline are serotonin reuptake inhibitors that
have been marketed as clinical antidepressants (Chapter 8). Both of
these drugs can produce satiety and reduce food intake. Tolerance to

this anorectic effect seems to build after several weeks, however. The combination of either of these two agents with phentermine has not yet been reported.

In considering all of this pharmacological therapy, one must remember that obesity is an ongoing, chronic disease. Obesity is rarely cured, palliation is a realistic goal, and weight gain following drug therapy is not necessarily a sign of drug failure but a sign that when drug is not taken, it does not work.[42] Any planned drug therapy must be combined with behavior modification, diet correction, and exercise.

Nasal Decongestants

Nasal decongestants are structurally related to amphetamine. They can alter the synaptic actions of norepinephrine both in the brain and in the peripheral nervous system. Most nasal decongestants are more potent in the peripheral nervous system than in the brain. Representative products include ephedrine, tetrahydrozoline (Tyzine), metaraminol (Aramine), phenylephrine (Neo-Synephrine), pseudo-ephedrine (Sudafed), xylometazoline (Otrivin), nylidrin (Arlidin), propylhexedrine (Benzedrex), phenmetrazine (Preludin), naphazoline (Privine), and oxymetazoline (Afrin).

These compounds differ from one another primarily in terms of the intensity of their effects on the body (heart rate, breathing, and the like) and in the degree to which they stimulate behavior. In general, the responses to these drugs are similar to the peripheral effects of amphetamine; most have very few CNS effects. After use of these decongestants stops, there may be rebound increases in nasal stuffiness, a response that is similar to the stuffy nose that follows the use of cocaine. Ephedrine is the active ingredient in many illicit preparations that are alleged to be amphetamine.

"ICE": A New "Free Base" Form of Methamphetamine

Methamphetamine is more potent than dextroamphetamine and is easily synthesized in clandestine laboratories from inexpensive and readily obtainable chemicals (such as ephedrine), making large amounts of the drug available at low cost. In animals, methamphetamine has been implicated as a neurotoxic agent, although such toxicity has not been demonstrated in humans. Recently much concern has been expressed over a smokable form of potent methamphetamine, a preparation called "ICE."

Like cocaine, methamphetamine hydrochloride is broken down at the temperatures that must be achieved for it to be vaporized for smoking. However, when converted to its base, methamphetamine can be effectively vaporized and inhaled in smoke. This form of methamphetamine is called ICE; it has also been called "crank," "crystal," and "speed." ICE is to methamphetamine as crack is to cocaine, being the free base, smokable form of the parent compound. As with crack, the dose and route of administration create additional problems with abuse and its consequences.

Abuse of ICE began in Hawaii, spread to Japan (where it is called "shabu"), then came to California, and now is traveling eastward.[44,45] As a form of methamphetamine, ICE is between 90 and 100 percent pure. Since it is not injected, smoking can remove the guilt feelings, needle marks, infection risk, obvious evidence of drug use, and "heavy drug" impressions associated with parenteral injection of illegal drugs. Such impressions, however, belie the pharmacological effects and toxicities of the drug.

Pharmacokinetics

Smoking ICE results in its rapid absorption into plasma; this absorption continues over the next 4 hours and then progressively declines in plasma levels thereafter.[46] About 90 percent of smoked ICE eventually reaches plasma. In contrast to the very short duration of effects of cocaine, the biological half-life of methamphetamine is over 11 hours.[47] After distribution to the brain, about 60 percent of the methamphetamine is slowly metabolized in the liver and the end products excreted through the kidneys, along with unmetabolized methamphetamine (about 40 percent is excreted unchanged) and small amounts of the pharmacologically active metabolite amphetamine. Thus, the long action of methamphetamine follows from its slow and incomplete metabolism; in contrast, cocaine is rapidly and completely detoxified by enzymes found in both the plasma and the liver.

Effects and Toxicity

The effects of methamphetamine closely resemble and are frequently indistinguishable from those of cocaine. Both are potent psychomotor stimulants and positive reinforcers, with self-administration being extremely difficult to control and modify. Repeated high doses of methamphetamine are associated with violent behavior and paranoid psychosis. Such doses cause long-lasting decreases in dopamine and serotonin in the brain. These changes appear to be irreversible, since the chemical effects can persist for more than a year after drug administration. This toxic effect is directed at the neurons that manufacture dopamine and serotonin, and the biochemical changes do not appear to be expressed in gross behavioral changes. Permanent neurochemical alterations, however, may be expressed as alterations in sleep, sexual function, depression, movement disorders, or schizophrenia.

As discussed earlier, prolonged cocaine use can result in psychoses resembling paranoid schizophrenia. A similar pattern of acute delusional and psychotic behavior occurs after smoking ICE. However, unlike cocaine, ICE-induced psychosis can persist for days or weeks and can occur much earlier.[48]

Fatalities reported to date have resulted from cardiac toxicity manifested as either pulmonary edema or heart failure.[49] Undoubtedly, more information on methamphetamine toxicity will come to light as the use of ICE replaces crack cocaine.

Study Questions

1. Compare and contrast cocaine and amphetamine.
2. Explain the actions of cocaine and amphetamine in light of the fight/flight/fright syndrome.
3. What is crack? What is ICE?
4. Describe the three major actions of cocaine.
5. Discuss the effects of cocaine on the fetus.
6. Describe the behavioral states that are observed in high-dose amphetamine users.
7. Describe the effects of amphetamine on neurotransmitters.
8. Why might amphetaminelike drugs be useful in treating children who have attention deficit hyperactivity disorder (ADHD)?
9. Compare and contrast the psychostimulants with the clinical antidepressants.
10. What is meant by the phrase "Speed kills"?

Notes

1. M. S. Gold, "Cocaine (and Crack): Clinical Aspects," in J. H. Lowinson, P. Ruiz, R. B. Millman, and J. G. Langrod, eds., *Substance Abuse: A Comprehensive Textbook*, 2nd ed. (Baltimore: Williams & Wilkins, 1992), p. 205.
2. S. Freud, "Über Coca (On Cocaine)," in R. Byck, ed., *Cocaine Papers* (New York: Stonehill, 1974), pp. 49–73.

3. J. A. Fleming, R. Byck, and P. G. Barash, "Pharmacology and Therapeutic Applications of Cocaine," *Anesthesiology* 73 (1990): 518–531.

4. J. H. Jaffe, "Drug Addiction and Drug Abuse," in A. G. Gilman, T. W. Rall, A. S. Nies, and P. Taylor, eds., *Goodman and Gilman's The Pharmacological Basis of Therapeutics*, 8th ed. (New York: Pergamon, 1990), pp. 539–545.

5. M. S. Gold, N. S. Miller, and J. M. Jonas, "Cocaine (and Crack): Neurobiology," in J. H. Lowinson, P. Ruiz, R. B. Millman, and J. G. Langrod, eds., *Substance Abuse: A Comprehensive Textbook*, 2nd ed. (Baltimore: Williams & Wilkins, 1992), p. 226.

6. W. W. Weddington, "Cocaine: Diagnosis and Treatment," *Psychiatric Clinics of North America* 16, no. 1 (1993): 88.

7. D. Clouet, K. Asqhar, and R. Brown, eds., *Mechanisms of Cocaine Abuse and Toxicity*, NIDA Research Monograph 88 (Rockville, Md.: National Institute on Drug Abuse, 1988).

8. C.-E. Johanson and M. W. Fischman, "The Pharmacology of Cocaine Related to Its Abuse," *Pharmacological Reviews* 41 (1989): 35.

9. F. H. Gawin, "Cocaine Addiction, Psychology, and Neurophysiology," *Science* 251, no. 3 (1991): 1580–1586.

10. J.-T. Qiao, P. M. Dougherty, R. C. Wiggins, and N. Dafny, "Effects of Microiontophoretic Application of Cocaine, Alone and with Receptor Antagonists, upon the Neurons of the Medial Prefrontal Cortex, Nucleus Accumbens and Caudate Nucleus of Rats," *Neuropharmacology* 29 (1990): 379–385.

11. S. L. Peterson, S. A. Olsta, and R. T. Matthews, "Cocaine Enhances Medial Prefrontal Cortex Neuron Response to Ventral Tegmental Area Activation," *Brain Research Bulletin* 24 (1990): 267–273.

12. L. C. Einhorn, P. A. Johansen, and F. J. White, "Electrophysiological Effects of Cocaine in the Mesoaccumbens Dopamine System: Studies in the Ventral Tegmental Area," *Journal of Neuroscience* 8 (1988): 100–112.

13. M. G. Lacey, N. B. Mercuri, and R. A. North, "Actions of Cocaine on Rat Dopaminergic Neurons *in Vitro*," *British Journal of Pharmacology* 99 (1990): 731–735.

14. N. Uchimura and R. A. North, "Actions of Cocaine on Rat Nucleus Accumbens Neurons *in Vitro*," *British Journal of Pharmacology* 99 (1990): 736–740.

15. W. L. Woolverton and K. M. Johnson, "Neurobiology of Cocaine Abuse," *Trends in Pharmacological Sciences* 13 (1992): 193–200.

16. S. Shimada, S. Kitayama, C.-L. Lin, A. Patel, E. Nanthakumar, P. Gregor, M. Kuhar, and G. Uhl, "Cloning and Expression of a Cocaine-Sensitive Dopamine Transporter Complementary DNA," *Science* 254 (1991): 576–578.

17. J. E. Kilty, D. Lorang, and S. G. Amara, "Cloning and Expression of a Cocaine-Sensitive Rat Dopamine Transporter," *Science* 254 (1991): 578–580.

18. L. R. Goldfrank and R. S. Hoffman, "The Cardiovascular Effects of Cocaine—Update 1992," in H. Sorer, ed., *Acute Cocaine Intoxication:*

Current Methods of Treatment, NIDA Research Monograph 123, Pub. No. 93-3498 (Rockville, Md.: National Institutes of Health, 1993), pp. 70–109.

19. B. L. Miller, F. Chiang, L. McGill, T. Sadow, M. A. Goldberg, and I. Mena, "Cerebrovascular Complications from Cocaine: Possible Long-Term Sequelae," in H. Sorer, ed., *Acute Cocaine Intoxication: Current Methods of Treatment,* NIDA Research Monograph 123, Pub. No. 93-3498 (Rockville, Md.: National Institutes of Health, 1993): 129–146.

20. B. J. Rounsaville, S. F. Anton, K. Carroll, D. Budde, B. A. Prusoff, and F. Gawin, "Psychiatric Diagnoses of Treatment-Seeking Cocaine Abusers," *Archives of General Psychiatry* 48 (1991), 43–51.

21. "Update on Cocaine, Part II," *The Harvard Mental Health Letter* 10, no. 3 (September 1993): 2.

22. M. A. Plessinger and J. R. Woods, Jr., "Maternal, Placental, and Fetal Pathophysiology of Cocaine Exposure during Pregnancy," *Clinical Obstetrics and Gynecology* 36 (1993): 267–278.

23. I. J. Chasnoff, W. J. Burns, S. H. Schnoll, and K. A. Burns, "Cocaine Use in Pregnancy," *New England Journal of Medicine* 313 (1985): 666–669.

24. I. J. Chasnoff, C. E. Hunt, and D. Kaplan, "Prenatal Cocaine Exposure as Associated with Respiratory Pattern Abnormalities," *American Journal of Diseases of Childhood* 143 (1989): 583–587.

25. Z. N. Kain, S. Rimar, and P. G. Barash, "Cocaine Abuse in the Parturient and Effects on the Fetus and Neonate," *Anesthesia and Analgesia* 77 (1993): 835–845.

26. J. J. Volpe, "Effects of Cocaine Use on the Fetus," *New England Journal of Medicine* 327, no. 6 (6 August 1992): 399–407.

27. "Update on Cocaine, Part I," in *The Harvard Mental Health Letter* 10, no. 2 (August 1993): 3.

28. M. C. Rist, "The Shadow Children," *The American School Board Journal* (January 1990): 19–24.

29. F. H. Gawin and H. D. Kleber, "Abstinence Symptomatology and Psychiatric Diagnoses in Cocaine Abusers," *Archives of General Psychiatry* 43 (1986): 107–113.

30. F. H. Gawin, H. D. Kleber, R. Byck, B. J. Rounsaville, T. R. Kosten, P. I. Jatlow, and C. Morgan, "Desipramine Facilitation of Initial Cocaine Abstinence," *Archives of General Psychiatry* 46 (1989): 117–121.

31. K. M. Carroll, B. J. Bruce, J. Rounsaville, L. T. Gordon, C. Nich, P. Jatlaw, R. M. Bisighini, and F. H. Gawin, "Psychotherapy and Pharmacotherapy for Ambulatory Cocaine Abusers," *Archives of General Psychiatry* 51 (1994): 177–187.

32. L. H. Gold, M. A. Gold, and G. F. Koob, "Neurochemical Mechanisms Involved in Behavioral Effects of Amphetamines and Related Designer Drugs," in K. Asqhar and E. DeSouza, eds., *Pharmacology and Toxicology of Amphetamine and Related Designer Drugs,* NIDA Research Monograph 94 (Rockville, Md.: National Institute on Drug Abuse, 1989), pp. 101–126.

33. P. M. Groves, L. J. Ryan, M. Diana, S. Y. Young, and L. J. Fisher, "Neuronal Actions of Amphetamine in the Rat Brain," in K.Saqhar and E. DeSouza,

eds., *Pharmacology and Toxicology of Amphetamine and Related Designer Drugs*, NIDA Research Monograph 94 (Rockville, Md.: National Institute on Drug Abuse, 1989), pp. 127–145.

34. G. R. King and E. H. Ellinwood, Jr., "Amphetamines and Other Stimulants," in J. H. Lowinson, P. Ruiz, R. B. Millman, and J. G. Langrod, eds., *Substance Abuse: A Comprehensive Textbook*, 2nd ed. (Baltimore: Williams & Wilkins, 1992), pp. 247–266.

35. T. E. Wilens, J. Biederman, D. E. Geist, R. Steingard, and T. Spencer, "Nortriptyline in the Treatment of ADHD: A Chart Review of 58 Cases," *Journal of the American Academy of Child and Adolescent Psychiatry* 32 (1993): 343–349.

36. F. Levy, "The Dopamine Theory of Attention Deficit Hyperactivity Disorder," *Australian and New Zealand Journal of Psychiatry* 25 (1991): 277–283.

37. J. Biederman and others, "A Family Study of Patients with Attention Deficit Disorder and Normal Controls," *Journal of Psychiatry Research* 20 (1986): 263–274.

38. G. Weiss, L. Hechtman, T. Milroy, and T. Perlman, "Psychiatric Status of Hyperactives as Adults: A Controlled Prospective 15-Year Follow-up of 63 Hyperactive Children," *Journal of the American Academy of Child and Adolescent Psychiatry* 24 (1985): 211–220.

39. N. Lie, "Follow-ups of Children with Attention Deficit Hyperactivity Disorder (ADHD): Review of Literature," *Acta Psychiatrica Scandinavica* 368 (1992): 1–40.

40. P. H. Wender, *The Hyperactive Child, Adolescent, and Adult: Attention Deficit Disorder through the Lifespan* (New York: Oxford University Press, 1987).

41. D. Jacobitz, A. Sroufe, M. Stewart, and N. Leffert, "Treatment of Attentional and Hyperactivity Problems in Children with Sympathomimetic Drugs: A Comprehensive Review," *Journal of the American Academy of Child and Adolescent Psychiatry* 29 (1990): 677–688.

42. G. A. Bray, "Use and Abuse of Appetite-Suppressant Drugs in the Treatment of Obesity," *Annals of Internal Medicine* 119 (1993): 708–709.

43. M. Weintraub, P. R. Sundaresan, M. Madan, B. Schuster, A. Balder, L. Lasagna, and C. Cox, "Long-Term Weight Control Study: I–VII," *Clinical Pharmacology and Therapeutics* 51 (1992): 581–646.

44. T. A. Nestor, W. I. Tamamoto, T. H. Kam, and T. Schultz, "Crystal Methamphetamine-Induced Acute Pulmonary Edema: A Case Report," *Hawaii Medical Journal* 48 (1989): 457–458.

45. R. W. Derlet and B. Heischober, "Methamphetamine: Stimulant of the 1990s?" *Western Journal of Medicine* 153 (1990): 625–628.

46. R. M. Perez, W. R. White, S. A. McDonald, J. M. Hill, and A. R. Jeffcoat, "Clinical Effects of Methamphetamine Vapor Inhalation," *Life Sciences* 49 (1991): 953–959.

47. C. E. Cook, A. R. Jeffcoat, J. M. Hill, D. E. Pugh, P. K. Patetta, B. M. Sadler, W. R. White, and M. Perez-Reyes, "Pharmacokinetics of Methamphetamine Self-Administration to Human Subjects by Smoking S- (+)-Meth-

amphetamine Hydrochloride," *Drug Metabolism and Disposition: The Biological Fate of Chemicals* 21 (1993): 717–723.

48. American Society for Pharmacology and Experimental Therapeutics and the Committee on Problems of Drug Dependence, "Anticipating a New ICE Age: The Pharmacology and Abuse Implications of Methamphetamine," presented at a symposium held on March 6, 1990, in publication.

49. R. Hong, E. Matsuyama, and K. Nur, "Cardiomyopathy Associated with the Smoking of Crystal," *Journal of the American Medical Association* 265 (1991): 1152-1154.

CHAPTER 7

PSYCHOSTIMULANTS: CAFFEINE AND NICOTINE

CAFFEINE

Caffeine, the most popular and widely consumed drug in the world, is found in significant concentrations in coffee, tea, cola drinks, chocolate candy, and cocoa.[1] As shown in Table 7.1, the average cup of coffee contains about 50 to 150 milligrams of caffeine. A 12-ounce bottle of cola contains between 35 and 55 milligrams of caffeine, much of which is added as a supplement by the manufacturer. The caffeine content of chocolate may be as high as 25 milligrams per ounce. The annual consumption of coffee alone in the United States is estimated at about 15 million pounds, with the daily per capita intake of caffeine averaging between 170 and 200 milligrams.[2] Eighty percent of adults consume between three and five cups of coffee every day.

Why is there such massive consumption of a legal, widely used, and socially acceptable psychoactive drug? Certainly, caffeine must be reinforcing; otherwise there would be no compulsion to ingest the drug. If caffeine is reinforcing, does the reinforcement mechanism involve the mesolimbic system described for cocaine and the amphetamines, or is its behavioral reinforcement exerted through another mechanism? Also, given the almost universal dependence on caffeinated beverages, what is caffeine's potential for inducing physical dependency?

TABLE 7.1 Caffeine content in beverages, foods, and medicines.

Item	Caffeine content	
	Average (mg)	Range
Coffee (5-ounce cup)	100	50–150
Tea (5-ounce cup)	50	25–90
Cocoa (5-ounce cup)	5	2–20
Chocolate (semisweet, baking) (1 ounce)	25	15–30
Chocolate milk (1 ounce)	5	1–10
Cola drink (12 ounces)	40	35–55
OTC stimulants (No Doz, Vivarin)	100+	
OTC analgesics (Excedrin)	65	
(Anacin, Midol, Vanquish)	33	
OTC cold remedies (Coryban-D, Triaminicin)	30	
OTC diuretics (Aqua-ban)	100	

Note: OTC, over the counter.

Pharmacokinetics

Taken orally, caffeine is rapidly absorbed; significant blood levels of caffeine are reached in 30 to 45 minutes. Complete absorption occurs over the next 90 minutes, with levels in plasma peaking in about 2 hours.

Caffeine is freely and equally distributed throughout all the water in the body. Thus, caffeine is found in almost equal concentrations in all parts of the body and the brain. Most caffeine is metabolized by the liver before it is excreted by the kidneys. Only about 10 percent of the drug is excreted unchanged (that is, without being metabolized). The half-life of caffeine is about 3.5 to 5 hours in most adults; it is longer in infants, pregnant women, and the elderly, and shorter in smokers. Like all psychoactive drugs, caffeine freely crosses the placenta to the fetus. Eskenazi states:

> Caffeine has a longer half-life in the human fetus than in the adult because the fetus does not have the liver enzymes for detoxifying caffeine. The half-life of caffeine in the pregnant woman increases from 3 to 10 hours by the latter part of pregnancy.[3]

Concentrations of caffeine in breast milk equal or may even exceed the level that exists in the mother's plasma.

Pharmacological Effects

Caffeine is an effective psychostimulant, ingested to "obtain a rewarding effect, usually described as feeling more alert and competent."[4] The cortex, being more sensitive to caffeine than are brain stem structures, is affected first. Only at toxic doses of caffeine is the spinal cord stimulated. As a result of cerebral cortical stimulation, the earliest behavioral effects of caffeine include increased mental alertness, a faster and clearer flow of thought, wakefulness, and restlessness. Fatigue is reduced and the need for sleep is delayed.

This increased mental awareness may result in sustained intellectual effort for prolonged periods of time without the disruption of coordinated intellectual or motor activity that usually follows an alteration in the function of the medulla (such as occurs with amphetamines or cocaine). However, tasks that involve delicate muscular coordination and accurate timing or arithmetic skills may be adversely affected.[5] The effects on the cerebral cortex occur after oral doses that are as small as 100 or 200 milligrams, that is, one to two cups of coffee. Heavy consumption (12 or more cups a day, or 1.5 grams of caffeine) can cause more intense effects, such as agitation, anxiety, tremors, rapid breathing, and insomnia.

Only after massive doses (probably 2 to 5 grams) does the spinal cord become stimulated. The lethal dose of caffeine is about 10 grams, which is equivalent to 100 cups of coffee. Thus, death from caffeine is highly unlikely, and the drug is usually considered to be relatively nontoxic. The syndrome of "caffeinism" is discussed in the section on side effects.

Caffeine has a slight stimulant action on the heart, increasing cardiac contractility and output and dilating the coronary arteries. It should be noted, however, that caffeine exerts an opposite effect on the cerebral blood vessels; it constricts these vessels, thus decreasing blood flow to the brain. Such action can afford striking relief from headaches, especially migraines. Cardiac arrhythmias after ingesting caffeine are not uncommon, although they are rarely serious.

Other actions of caffeine include bronchial relaxation (an antiasthmatic effect), increased secretion of gastric acid, and increased urine output.

Mechanism of Action

Today the mechanism of action of caffeine is being clarified. As proposed in the early 1980s[6] and recently reviewed by Greden and Walters[7] and by Daly,[8] caffeine's dose-related behavioral stimulant ef-

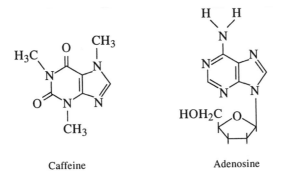

FIGURE 7.1   Structures of caffeine and adenosine.

fects follow from its attachment to, and blockade of, adenosine receptors in the CNS.[9] Caffeine is therefore considered a competitive antagonist of adenosine at its receptors, which are located on cell membranes both in the CNS and in the peripheral nervous system.[10] Thus, to understand the pharmacology of caffeine, we should examine the role of adenosine in the brain.

Adenosine is an *autacoid** that acts on specific receptors on the surface of cells to produce behavioral sedation, to regulate the delivery of oxygen to cells, to dilate cerebral and coronary blood vessels, to produce bronchospasm (asthma), and to regulate other metabolic processes. There do not appear to be discrete adenosinergic pathways in the CNS; instead, adenosine, through attachment to caffeine-sensitive receptors, inhibits the release of many classes of neurotransmitters, including norepinephrine, dopamine, acetylcholine, glutamate, and GABA.[7,8] The blockade of adenosine receptors by caffeine therefore increases the turnover of such neurotransmitters. Especially prominent is an increase in the activity of dopamine systems, as indicated by potentiation of the CNS effects of cocaine and the amphetamines and by the weak behavioral reinforcing effects of the drug.[8] Although ventral tegmental activity increases after caffeine has been ingested, nucleus accumbens activity is not markedly affected.[8]

Blockade of adenosine receptors by caffeine (note the structural similarity between caffeine and adenosine in Figure 7.1) would thus

---

*The term *autacoid,* derived from the Greek *autos* ("self") and *akos* ("medicine" or "remedy"), refers to a variety of locally acting, hormonelike or neurotransmitter-like substances that regulate cellular functions. Studies involving adenosine and caffeine suggest a neuromodulatory role for adenosine, indicating that adenosine-releasing neurons constitute an important CNS depressant system that is blocked by caffeine.[11]

account for the variety of caffeine's behavioral effects.[8] At the levels obtained after drinking a few cups of coffee, caffeine occupies 50 percent of adenosine receptors, antagonizing adenosine-induced neuronal inhibition.[12]

The mild reinforcing effects induced by caffeine upon reward and pleasure centers in the brain do not appear to be direct.[13,14] Rather, the action is probably exerted through a blockade of the normal adenosine-induced inhibitory modulation of dopaminergic activity in the meso-limbic system.

Shi and coworkers[15] note that chronic administration of very high doses of caffeine (100 mg/kg/day) to mice increased the density of cerebral cortical adenosine receptors (adenosine-1 receptors), implying that chronic ingestion may increase the numbers of receptors in order to overcome their chronic drug-induced blockade (a possible mechanism of adenosine tolerance). Also affected, however, were beta receptors (reduced in density), serotonin receptors (increased in density), cholinergic receptors (increased in density),and GABA receptors (increased in density). Thus, besides being an adenosine antagonist, caffeine may cause a wide range of biochemical alterations in the CNS.[15]

Side Effects

Despite some early reports, there is now little evidence that caffeine plays a role in the cause of cancer in humans.[16] Similarly, early reports indicated that caffeine use by women might be associated with the formation or enlargement of benign (noncancerous) lumps (fibrocystic lesions) in the breasts, but current thought is that no causative relationship exists.[17] However, it seems prudent to advise patients with known fibrocystic lesions to try a caffeine-free diet to determine whether the lesions shrink or become less painful.[18]

Caffeinism

Caffeinism is a clinical syndrome produced by the overuse of caffeine. It is usually characterized by both CNS and peripheral symptoms. The former include anxiety, insomnia, and mood changes. Peripheral symptoms include tachycardia, hypertension, cardiac arrhythmias, and gastrointestinal disturbances. Caffeinism is usually dose related, with doses higher than about 500 to 1000 milligrams per day causing the most unpleasant effects.[7,11] Cessation of caffeine ingestion resolves these symptoms.

Panic Attacks

Patients who have a history of panic disorders may be particularly sensitive to the effects of caffeine. Indeed, in a 1985 study,[19] moderate doses of caffeine (about 4 to 5 cups of coffee) precipitated panic attacks in about half of the subjects. Here the implications are twofold: (1) In a person who experiences panic attacks, caffeine should be investigated as a possible, treatable cause, and (2) any person who has a history of panic attacks should be counseled to avoid caffeine-containing products or, at least, to use them in moderation and to be alert for signs of drug-induced precipitation of an attack. Greden and Walters[7] state that caffeine does not cause panic attacks in normal individuals. However, in persons predisposed to panic disorders, the peripheral and the CNS effects of caffeine can be exaggerated.

Cardiovascular Risks

The cardiovascular side effects of caffeine have been presented. Although they are not harmful to most individuals, these effects of caffeine might be detrimental to a subpopulation of heart patients. Despite some views to the contrary, "the use of caffeinated coffee and the total intake of caffeine does not appreciably increase the risk of coronary artery disease or stroke."[20]

A conservative view is that caffeine should be used in moderation by people who are at risk for heart disease (that is, males, smokers, and people who have a family history of heart disease, obesity, hypertension, or elevated blood cholesterol levels). Also, it should be noted that the consumption of decaffeinated coffee may be associated with a "marginally significant" increase in the risk of coronary artery disease: "There seems to be little merit in switching from caffeinated coffee to decaffeinated coffee as a means of reducing the risk of cardiovascular disease."[20]

Reproductive Effects

> Is caffeine safe during pregnancy? Caffeine, the most widely used psychotropic drug, is consumed by at least 75% of pregnant women via caffeinated beverages. In spite of its widespread use, the safety of this habit during pregnancy is unresolved.[3]

For over 30 years, it has been known that, in very large doses, caffeine (due to its structural relation to DNA purine bases) may induce chromosomal aberrations in a variety of nonhuman species.[21,22] In 1980, mainly on the basis of data from animal studies, the U.S. Food and Drug Administration cautioned pregnant women to minimize their intake of caffeine.

Data in this area have always been both conflicting and controversial. Indeed, in 1993 the *Journal of the American Medical Association* published two studies on this issue having contradictory conclusions. The first reported that caffeine was relatively safe in moderate doses (less than 300 milligrams per day, or less than 3 medium-sized cups of coffee per day; see Table 7.1).[23] At higher levels, an increased incidence of intrauterine growth retardation was seen. The second study reported that low doses of caffeine (about 160 milligrams per day) in the first trimester of pregnancy increased the risk of intrauterine growth retardation; high consumption (greater than 300 milligrams per day), even in the month before pregnancy, "nearly doubled the risk of spontaneous abortion."[24]

In conclusion,

> the weight of evidence indicates that high levels of caffeine intake (>300 mg/d) during pregnancy are potentially harmful. . . . We cannot conclude that lower levels are safe, given that studies have conflicting results and exposure assessment is problematic.[3]

It should be noted that a pregnant woman who reduces her caffeine intake may be too late to prevent adverse consequences. Pregnancy is usually quite advanced (about 8 to 10 weeks) by the time it is confirmed, and caffeine exposure even before pregnancy may be harmful.[24] Thus, women even considering having a baby should limit their caffeine intake. Likewise, breast-feeding mothers should avoid caffeine, as drug present in the infant's diet may harm neurodevelopment. The "prudent course is to avoid caffeine during pregnancy, beginning (if possible) even before conception"[4] and continuing throughout the period of breast-feeding.

Tolerance and Dependence

Chronic use of caffeine "is often associated with habituation and tolerance, and . . . discontinuation may produce a withdrawal syndrome."[7] In one study, "those who drank the most coffee complained of headache, drowsiness, fatigue, and a generally negative mood state on awakening the morning after placebo had been drunk, but not the morning after caffeine."[4] These are certainly signs of mild withdrawal. Other reported withdrawal signs include impaired intellectual and motor performance, difficulty with concentration, drug (caffeine) craving, and other psychological complaints.[25] As noted earlier, caffeine may cause an increase in the number of adenosine receptors, a situation associated with an increased sensitivity to adenosine.[12] Since about 80 percent of American adults consume more than 200 milligrams of caffeine daily, there is almost universal dependence on caffeine. However, this seems to be of minimal consequence because "no toxic effects of any kind have been associated with modest use of caffeine. . . . And, when caffeine is used on a long-term basis—unlike alcohol or tobacco—it causes no evident organ damage."[4]

It is also generally agreed that caffeine can induce a degree of tolerance, which probably has both pharmacological and adaptive origins (Chapter 1). Habitual drinkers of caffeine, compared with nondrinkers, have less difficulty sleeping at comparable blood levels of caffeine.[4] Chronic users certainly become less sensitive to the drug, an effect that is independent of the blood level of the drug; this finding suggests that there is decreased receptor sensitivity and tolerance.

NICOTINE

Together with caffeine and ethyl alcohol, nicotine is one of the three most widely used psychoactive drugs in our society. Despite the fact that nicotine has little or no therapeutic application in medicine, its potency, its widespread use, and its toxicity give it considerable importance. Recent evidence indicates that nicotine and the other ingredients in tobacco are responsible for a wide variety of health problems and the deaths of more than 1000 Americans every day![26]

From the end of World War II to the mid-1960s, cigarette smoking was considered chic and was associated with few ill effects. Today, after almost 30 years of U.S. government reports on the adverse health consequences of cigarettes, cigarette smoking is being increasingly shunned both in the United States[27,28] and throughout the Americas.[29] Thirty years ago celebrities and athletes appeared in cigarette commercials; today they are rarely seen smoking. The impression that cigarette smoking is healthful, youthful, and adventurous is conveyed only by unknown actors in print advertisements that are accompanied by mandated health warnings. Nevertheless, tobacco advertising continues to be "deceptive, alluring, and pitched to minors and children."[26]

On the positive side, half of all persons who have ever smoked cigarettes have quit, and the proportion of American adults who smoke has fallen from 50 percent in 1965 to 29 percent in 1989. About one million potential deaths have been averted or postponed by persons who have quit smoking. Millions more deaths will be avoided or post-poned during the 1990s.[27]

On the negative side, individual cigarette consumption has risen substantially (from 14 to 22 cigarettes per day among male smokers and from 7 to 17 cigarettes per day among female smokers between 1949 and 1978). The typical chronic cigarette smoker smokes 10 to 50 cigarettes per day. This increase in average consumption may be re-lated to a reduction in nicotine content, which has caused addicted smokers to smoke more heavily in order to maintain a constant level of nicotine in the blood.

Among young people, the proportion of high school students who smoke cigarettes fell from 30 to 20 percent between the late 1970s and 1990. These numbers do not include high school dropouts, 75 percent of whom were smokers in 1990. Those young smokers create a huge population of less-educated individuals who will eventually suffer poor health and mortality as a direct consequence of their cigarette habit. As stated by the surgeon general, "Smoking will continue as the lead-ing cause of preventable, premature death for many years to come."[27]

In this discussion, it is important to note that nicotine, the primary active ingredient in tobacco, is only 1 of about 4000 compounds re-leased by the burning of cigarette tobacco. Nicotine accounts only for the acute pharmacological effects of smoking and the dependence on cigarettes. The adverse, long-term cardiovascular, pulmonary, and car-cinogenic effects of cigarettes are related to the many compounds con-tained in the product.

Pharmacokinetics

According to Jarvik and Schneider, "Nicotine is readily absorbed from every site on or in the body, including the lungs, buccal and nasal mucosa, skin, and gastrointestinal tract."[30] This easy and complete absorption forms the basis for the recreational abuse of smoked or chewed tobacco, as well as the medical use of nicotine in gums and transdermal skin patches.

Nicotine is suspended in cigarette smoke in the form of minute particles ("tars"), and it is quickly absorbed into the bloodstream from the lungs when the smoke is inhaled. Most cigarettes contain between 0.5 and 2.0 milligrams of nicotine, depending on the brand. Approxi-mately 20 percent (between 0.1 and 0.4 milligrams) of the nicotine in a cigarette is actually inhaled and absorbed into the smoker's blood-stream. Indeed, the physiological effects of smoking a single cigarette can be closely duplicated by the intravenous injection of these

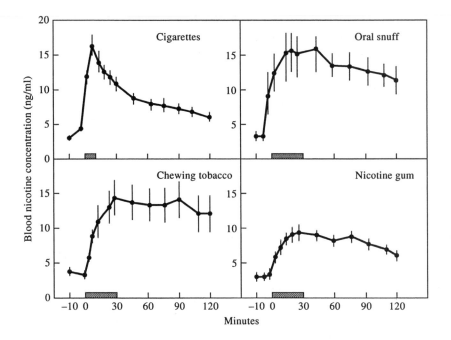

FIGURE 7.2 Blood nicotine concentrations during and after the use of cigarettes, oral snuff, chewing tobacco, and nicotine gum (two 2-milligram pieces). Data represent average values for 10 subjects: vertical bars indicate S.E. Shaded bars above the time axis indicate the period of tobacco or nicotine gum exposure. [From N. L. Benowitz, H. Porchet, L. Skeiner, and P. Jacob III, "Nicotine Absorption and Cardiovascular Effects with Smokeless Tobacco Use: Comparison with Cigarettes and Nicotine Gum," *Clinical Pharmacology and Therapeutics* 44 (1988): 24.]

amounts of nicotine. This amount of nicotine is well below the lethal dose of the drug, which is considered to be approximately 60 milligrams. Furthermore, the smoker can readily avoid acute toxicity, because inhalation as a route of administration offers exceptional controllability of the dose.[31] The user-controlled frequency of breaths, the depth of inhalation, the time the smoke is held in the lungs, and the total number of cigarettes smoked all allow the smoker to regulate the rate of drug intake and thus control the blood level of nicotine.

When nicotine is administered orally in the form of snuff, chewing tobacco, or gum, blood levels of nicotine are comparable to those achieved by smoking (Figure 7.2).

Nicotine is quickly and thoroughly distributed throughout the body, rapidly penetrating the brain, crossing the placental barrier, and appearing in all bodily fluids, including breast milk. Indeed, the breast-fed infant may have a blood level of nicotine as high as that of the mother. The liver metabolizes approximately 80 to 90 percent of the nicotine administered to a person either orally or by smoking before it is excreted by the kidneys. The elimination half-life of nicotine in a chronic smoker is about 2 hours, necessitating frequent administration of drug to avoid withdrawal symptoms (which are invariably felt upon wakening in the morning).

Pharmacological Effects

Nicotine appears to be the only pharmacologically active drug in tobacco smoke apart from carcinogenic tars. It exerts powerful effects on the brain, the spinal cord, the peripheral nervous system, the heart, and various other body structures.

Nicotine stimulates specific acetylcholine receptors ("nicotinic" receptors) in the CNS, including the cerebral cortex, producing increases in psychomotor activity,[32] cognitive function,[33] sensorimotor performance, attention, and memory consolidation.[34] The drug can also induce tremors and, in toxic overdosage, convulsions. As with all stimulant drugs, a period of depression follows.

In the early stages of smoking, nicotine causes nausea and vomiting by stimulating both the vomiting center in the brain stem and the sensory receptors in the stomach. Tolerance to this effect develops rapidly. Nicotine stimulates the hypothalamus to release a hormone, antidiuretic hormone (ADH), that causes fluid retention. Nicotine reduces the activity of afferent nerve fibers coming from the muscles, leading to a reduction in muscle tone. This action may be involved (at least partially) in the relaxation that a person may experience as a result of smoking. Nicotine also reduces weight gain, probably by reducing appetite.

Nicotine exerts a potent reinforcing action, especially in the early phases of drug use. The reinforcing action of nicotine probably involves indirect activation of midbrain dopamine neurons.[33] This is discussed further in the next section.

In the veteran smoker, the reinforcing action appears to diminish, and the user smokes primarily to relieve or avoid withdrawal symptoms. In the later stages, smokers adjust their nicotine intake to maintain nicotine levels between about 30 to 40 nanograms of nicotine per milliliter of plasma.[30] Because of nicotine's short half-life, there is a very low residual level of nicotine in the blood and brain after a night's sleep. In essence, the smoker wakes each morning in a state of drug withdrawal: "The first cigarette of the morning has a powerful (rein-forcing) effect because it brings relief of withdrawal discomfort. Thereafter, each cigarette produces a sharp increase in the nicotine concentration bathing the brain."[31]

In addition to its effects on the CNS, normal doses of nicotine can increase heart rate, blood pressure, and cardiac contractility. In non-atherosclerotic coronary arteries, nicotine initiates vasodilatation, in-creasing blood flow to meet the increased oxygen demand of the heart muscle. In atherosclerotic coronary arteries (which cannot dilate), however, cardiac ischemia can result when the oxygen supply fails to meet the oxygen demand created by the drug's cardiac stimulation. This occurrence can precipitate angina or myocardial infarction (a heart attack).

Mechanism of Action

Nicotine exerts most of its CNS and peripheral effects by activating acetylcholine receptors of the nicotinic type. In the peripheral nervous system, these receptors are found on nerve axons (sensory and motor) and on many synaptic junctions, including those at autonomic ganglia. The activation of these receptors causes the increases in blood pres-sure and heart rate; it causes release of epinephrine (adrenaline) from the adrenal glands (producing the symptoms characteristic of the fight/flight/fright response), and it increases the tone and activity of the gastrointestinal tract.

In the CNS, the nicotine-sensitive acetylcholine receptors are lo-cated in

> the medial habenula and interpeduncular nucleus, thalamus, and projection areas in layers III and IV of the cerebral cortex, and, most importantly for reinforcement, in the substantia nigra and ventral tegmental area, where they are associated with the cell bodies of dopaminergic neurons. The projections from the ventral tegmental area to the nucleus accumbens are important for the mediation of re-ward with the release of dopamine. . . . Nicotinic receptors are found on presynaptic dopaminergic and serotonergic neurons, which ex-plains how nicotine may release these neurotransmitters.[30]

Therefore, nicotine's reinforcing action resembles that of cocaine and the amphetamines, except that nicotine's action is indirect, resulting in a lower level of dopaminergic stimulation in the reinforcement areas of the brain.

Tolerance and Dependence

Nicotine does not appear to induce any pronounced degree of biological tolerance. Indeed, as discussed above, smokers seem to learn how to dose themselves so as to maintain a blood level of nicotine within a reasonably narrow range (30 to 40 nanograms per milliliter). To achieve this can take anywhere from 10 to 50 cigarettes per day, as a result of the many variables associated with self-dosing through inhalation.

Nicotine clearly induces both physiological and psychological dependence. Indeed, as early as 1988, the surgeon general of the United States made the following conclusions:

> Cigarettes and other forms of tobacco are addicting.
>
> Nicotine is the drug in tobacco that causes addiction.
>
> The pharmacologic and behavioral processes that determine tobacco addiction are similar to those that determine addiction to drugs such as heroin and cocaine.
>
> More than 300,000 cigarette-addicted Americans die yearly as a consequence of their addiction.[31]

Today, this number has increased to 435,000 deaths per year.[35]

Elaborating on the costs of cigarette addiction, Cocores wrote,

> The national health insurance crisis and the national deficit are both, in part, a product of nicotine dependence, costing America $52 billion annually. The right of a minority to use nicotine compromises the rights of nonusers to clean air; lower risk of lung cancer and emphysema; lower health, life, and disability insurance premiums; and lower state and federal taxes.[26]

Withdrawal from cigarettes is characterized by an abstinence syndrome. This includes a craving for nicotine, irritability, anxiety, anger, difficulty in concentrating, restlessness, impatience, increased appetite, and insomnia.[36] The period of withdrawal may be intense and persistent, often lasting for many months.[36] The difficulty in handling cigarette dependence is illustrated by the fact that cigarette smokers who seek treatment for other drug and alcohol problems often find it harder to quit cigarette smoking than to give up the other drugs. Even in the late 1800s

> Freud . . . continued his cigar habit (20/day) until death, in spite of an endless series of operations for mouth and jaw cancer (the jaw was eventually totally removed), persistent heart problems that were exacerbated by smoking, and numerous attempts at quitting.[37]

Currently a topic of heated discussion is the addictive potential of nicotine. Most government and university authorities consider nicotine to be addicting according to accepted criteria.[38,39] In contrast, scientists associated with the tobacco industry have written that cigarettes are a *"resource* that provides smokers with needed psychological benefits (increased mental alertness, anxiety reduction, coping with stress)."[40] They argue that smoking "habituation" does not meet the criteria of addiction. Interested readers can read the arguments for and against the addictive potential of nicotine,[38–41] although they should consider the bias and financial support of the various authors.

Toxicity

The toxic substances in cigarette smoke are nicotine, carbon monoxide, and tars.[42] It is estimated that more than 435,000 persons in the United States die annually from tobacco use. Of these, 82,000 deaths are caused by noncancerous lung diseases, 110,000 deaths are caused by lung cancer, 30,000 deaths are caused by cancers of other body organs, and more than 200,000 deaths result from heart and vascular diseases. A person's life is shortened 14 minutes for every cigarette smoked. In other words, a person who smokes two packs of cigarettes a day for 20 years loses an estimated 8 years of his or her life. More than 50 million people (one out of every five Americans) alive today will die prematurely from the effects of smoking cigarettes. Cigarette smoking, the nation's greatest public health hazard, is, ironically, the nation's most preventable cause of premature death, illness, and disability.[43] Internationally, similar statistics are appearing; according to a current estimate, global tobacco use is responsible for nearly 2.5 million deaths per year.[44] A 1992 government report details the growing problem of cigarette toxicity in the Americas; for instance, over 100,000 deaths every year are attributable to cigarette smoking in Latin America and the Caribbean.[29]

In 1964, the first surgeon general's report on the health consequences of smoking was released. It cited cigarette smoking as a cause of cancer and other serious diseases. The major conclusions from the more than 20 surgeon general's reports on smoking are summarized in Tables 7.2 and 7.3. In sum, they present the following five conclusions:

1. The prevalence of smoking among adults decreased from 40 percent in 1965 to 29 percent in 1987. Nearly half of all living adults who ever smoked have quit.

TABLE 7.2 Surgeon general's reports on smoking and health, 1964–1988.

Year	Subject/Highlights
1964	First official report of the federal government on smoking and health. Concluded that cigarette smoking is a health hazard of sufficient importance in the United States to warrant appropriate remedial action. Concluded that cigarette smoking is a cause of lung cancer in men and a suspected cause of lung cancer in women. Identified many other causal relationships and associations between smoking and diseases.
1967	Confirmed and strengthened conclusions of 1964 report. Stated that "the case for cigarette smoking as the principal cause of lung cancer is overwhelming." Found that evidence "strongly suggests that cigarette smoking can cause death from coronary heart disease." 1964 report had described this relationship as an "association." Also concluded that "cigarette smoking is the most important of the causes of chronic non-neoplastic bronchiopulmonary diseases in the United States." Identified measures of morbidity associated with smoking.
1968	Updated information presented in 1967 report. Estimated smoking-related loss of life expectancy among young men as 8 years for "heavy smokers" (over 2 packs per day) and 4 years for "light smokers" (less than $^{1}/_{2}$ pack per day).
1969	Also supplemented 1967 report. Confirmed association between maternal smoking and low infant birth weight. Identified evidence of increased incidence of prematurity, spontaneous abortion, stillbirth, and neonatal death.
1971	Reviewed entire field of smoking and health, with emphasis on most recent literature. Discussed new data indicating associations between smoking and peripheral vascular disease, atherosclerosis of the aorta and coronary arteries, increased incidence and severity of respiratory infections, and increased mortality from cerebrovascular disease and nonsyphilitic aortic aneurysm. Concluded that smoking is associated with cancers of the oral cavity and esophagus. Found that "maternal smoking during pregnancy exerts a retarding influence on fetal growth."
1972	Examined evidence on immunological effects of tobacco and tobacco smoke, harmful constituents of tobacco smoke, and "public exposure to air pollution from tobacco smoke." Found tobacco and tobacco smoke antigenic in humans and animals; tobacco may impair protective mechanisms of immune system; nonsmokers' exposure to tobacco smoke may exacerbate allergic symptoms; carbon monoxide in smoke-filled rooms may harm health of persons with chronic lung or heart disease; tobacco smoke contains hundreds of compounds, several of which have been shown to act as carcinogens, tumor initiators, and tumor promoters. Identified carbon monoxide, nicotine, and tar as smoke constituents most likely to produce health hazards of smoking.
1973	Presented evidence on health effects of smoking pipes, cigars, and "little cigars." Found mortality rates of pipe and cigar smokers higher than those of nonsmokers but lower than those of cigarette smokers. Found that cigarette smoking impairs exercise performance in healthy young men. Presented additional evidence on smoking as risk factor in peripheral vascular disease and problems of pregnancy.

TABLE 7.2 Surgeon general's reports on smoking, 1964–1988 *(continued).*

Year	Subject/Highlights
1974	Tenth anniversary report. Reviewed and strengthened evidence on major hazards of smoking. Reviewed evidence on association between smoking and atherosclerotic brain infarction and on synergistic effect of smoking and asbestos exposure in causing lung cancer.
1975	Updated information on health effects of involuntary (passive) smoking. Noted evidence linking parental smoking to bronchitis and pneumonia in children during the first year of life.
1976	Compiled selected chapters from 1971–75 reports.
1977–78	Combined two-year report focused on smoking-related health problems unique to women. Cited studies showing that use of oral contraceptives potentiates harmful effects of smoking on the cardiovascular system.
1979	Fifteenth anniversary report. Presented most comprehensive review of health effects of smoking ever published, and first surgeon general's report to carefully examine behavioral, pharmacological, and social factors influencing smoking. Also first report to consider role of adult and youth education in promoting nonsmoking. First report to review health consequences of smokeless tobacco. Many new sections including one identifying smoking as "one of the primary causes of drug interactions in humans."
1980	Devoted to health consequences of smoking for women. Reviewed evidence that strengthened previous findings and permitted new ones. Noted projections that lung cancer would surpass breast cancer as leading cause of cancer mortality in women. Identified trend toward increased smoking by adolescent females.
1981	Examined health consequences of "the changing cigarette," i.e., lower tar and nicotine cigarettes. Concluded that lower-yield cigarettes reduced risk of lung cancer but found no conclusive evidence that they reduced risk of cardiovascular disease, chronic obstructive pulmonary disease, and fetal damage. Noted possible risks from additives and their products of combustion. Discussed compensatory smoking behaviors that might reduce potential risk reductions of lower-yield cigarettes. Emphasized that there is no safe cigarette and that any risk reduction associated with lower-yield cigarettes would be small compared with benefits of quitting smoking.
1982	Reviewed and extended understanding of the health consequences of smoking as cause or contributory factor of numerous cancers. Included first surgeon general's report consideration of emerging epidemiological evidence of increased lung cancer risk in nonsmoking wives of smoking husbands. Did not find evidence sufficient to conclude that relationship was causal but labeled it "a possible serious public health problem." Discussed potential for low-cost smoking cessation interventions.
1983	Examined health consequences of smoking for cardiovascular disease. Concluded that cigarette smoking is one of three major independent causes of coronary heart disease (CHD) and, given its prevalence, "should be considered the most important of the known modifiable risk factors for CHD." Discussed relationships between smoking and other forms of cardiovascular disease.

TABLE 7.2 Surgeon general's reports on smoking, 1964–1988. *(concluded)*

Year	Subject/Highlights
1984	Reviewed evidence on smoking and chronic obstructive lung disease (COLD). Concluded that smoking is the major cause of COLD, accounting for 80 to 90 percent of COLD deaths in the United States. Noted that COLD morbidity has greater social impact than COLD mortality because of extended disability periods of COLD victims.
1985	Examined relationship between smoking and hazardous substances in the workplace. Found that for the majority of smokers, smoking is a greater cause of death and disability than their workplace environment. Risk of lung cancer from asbestos exposure characterized as multiplicative with smoking exposure. Observed special importance of smoking prevention among blue collar workers because of their greater exposure to workplace hazards and their higher incidence of smoking.
1986	Focused on involuntary smoking, concluding that "involuntary smoking is a cause of disease, including lung cancer, in healthy nonsmokers." Also found that, compared with the children of nonsmokers, children of smokers have higher incidence of respiratory infections and symptoms and reduced rates of increase in lung function. Presented detailed examination of growth in restrictions on smoking in public places and workplaces. Concluded that simple separation of smokers and nonsmokers within same airspace reduces but does not eliminate exposure to environmental tobacco smoke.
1987	Special report of advisory committee appointed by the surgeon general to study the health consequences of smokeless tobacco. Concluded that use of smokeless tobacco can cause cancer in humans and can lead to nicotine addiction.
1988	Established nicotine as a highly addictive substance, comparable in its physiological and psychological properties to other addictive substances of abuse.

From Levin.[33]

2. Between 1964 and 1985, approximately three-quarters of a million smoking-related deaths were avoided or postponed as a result of decisions to quit smoking or not to start.

3. The prevalence of smoking remains higher among blacks, blue collar workers, and less-educated persons than in the overall population. The decline in smoking has been substantially slower among women than among men.

4. Smoking begins primarily during childhood and adolescence. The age of initiation has fallen over time, particularly among females. Smoking among high school seniors leveled off from 1980 through 1987 after previous years of decline.

5. Smoking is responsible for more than one of every six deaths in the United States. Smoking remains the single most important preventable cause of death in our society.[45,46]

Cardiac Disease

Carbon monoxide decreases the amount of oxygen delivered to the heart muscle, while nicotine increases the amount of work that the heart must do (by increasing the heart rate and blood pressure). Both carbon monoxide and nicotine increase the incidence of atherosclerosis* (narrowing) and thrombosis (clotting) in the coronary arteries. These three actions (and others as well) seem to underlie the five-fold to nineteenfold increase in the risk of death from coronary heart disease in smokers as compared to nonsmokers. If a smoker has pre-existing hypertension or diabetes, the risk is even greater.

Pulmonary Disease

In the lungs, chronic smoking results in a smoker's syndrome, characterized by difficulty in breathing, wheezing, chest pain, lung congestion, and increased susceptibility to infections of the respiratory tract. Cigarette smoking impairs ventilation and greatly increases the risk of emphysema (a form of irreversible lung damage). About nine million Americans suffer from cigarette-induced chronic bronchitis and emphysema.

Cancer

The relation between smoking and cancer is now beyond question. Cigarette smoking is the major cause of lung cancer in both men and women, causing approximately 112,000 deaths in the United States every year. Smoking is also a major cause of cancers of the mouth, voice box, and throat. Concomitant alcohol ingestion greatly increases the incidence of these problems. In addition, cigarette smoking is a primary cause of many of the nearly 10,000 deaths every year that result from bladder cancer, as well as a primary cause of pancreatic cancer. The 1989 surgeon general's report also implicated cigarette

---

*Atherosclerosis first appears as fatty deposits inside large arteries and progresses to occlusion of the arteries throughout the body; the result is clinically manifested as strokes or peripheral vascular ischemic disease. In a large study of arteries collected from young men who had died of violent causes, a history of cigarette smoking was associated with a threefold to fourfold increase in atherosclerosis of the coronary arteries and abdominal aorta.[47] This was the first report of cigarette-induced, severe atherosclerosis in persons under 25 years of age. It emphasizes that in males, cigarette-induced atherosclerosis begins at a young age, and it reinforces the fact that smoking must be controlled for the long-range prevention of adult vascular disease.

TABLE 7.3 Summary of the principal effects of cigarette smoking.

Effect	Year first discussed in surgeon general's report	Knowledge in 1989
MORTALITY AND MORBIDITY		
Overall mortality, increased in men	1964	Overall mortality increased in men and women
Overall morbidity, increased	1967	Overall morbidity increased
CARDIOVASCULAR SYSTEM		
Coronary heart disease, mortality increased in men	1964	Major cause of coronary heart disease in men and women
Cerebrovascular disease (stroke), mortality increased	1964	Cause of cerebrovascular disease (stroke)
Atherosclerotic aortic aneurysm, mortality increased	1967	Increased mortality from atherosclerotic aortic aneurysm
Atherosclerotic peripheral vascular disease, risk factor	1971	Cause and most important risk factor for atherosclerotic peripheral vascular disease
CANCER		
Lung cancer, the major cause in men	1964	Major cause of lung cancer in men and women
Laryngeal cancer, a cause in men	1964	Major cause of laryngeal cancer in men and women
Oral cancer (lip), a cause (pipe smoking)	1964	Major cause of cancer of the oral cavity (lip, tongue, mouth, pharynx)
Esophageal cancer, association	1964	Major cause of esophageal cancer
Bladder cancer, association	1964	Contributory factor for bladder cancer
Pancreatic cancer, increased mortality	1967	Contributory factor for pancreatic cancer

Renal cancer, increased mortality	1968	Contributory factor for renal cancer
Gastric cancer, association	1982	Association with gastric cancer
Cervical cancer, possible association	1982	Association with cervical cancer
PULMONARY SYSTEM		
Chronic bronchitis, major cause	1964	Major cause of chronic bronchitis
Emphysema, increased mortality	1964	Major cause of emphysema
WOMEN		
Low-birth-weight babies, association	1964	Cause of intrauterine growth retardation
Unsuccessful pregnancy, association	1980	Probable cause of unsuccessful pregnancies
MISCELLANEOUS		
Tobacco habit, related to psychological and social drives	1964	Addictiveness of cigarette smoking and other forms of tobacco use
Involuntary smoking, irritant effect	1972	Cause of disease, including lung cancer, in healthy nonsmokers
Peptic ulcer disease, association	1964	Probable cause of peptic ulcer disease
Occupational interactions, adverse effect	1971	Adverse occupational interactions that increase the risk of cancer
Alcohol interactions, adverse effect	1971	Adverse interactions with alcohol that increase the risk of cancer
Drug interactions, adverse effect	1979	Adverse drug interactions
Nonmalignant oral disease, association	1969	Association with nonmalignant oral disease
Smokeless tobacco, association with oral cancer	1979	Smokeless tobacco a cause of oral cancer

From the U.S. Department of Health and Human Services.[34]

smoking in cancer of the uterine cervix. How cancer is caused by the compounds in cigarette smoke is unclear, but at least 23 of the more than 2000 compounds identified in cigarette tar have been classified as carcinogenic. Of all cancer deaths in the United States, 30 percent (154,000 annually) would be prevented if people stopped smoking.[48]

Historically, society has focused on the adverse effects of smoking on men, but some recent reports have focused on women.[49] More women now die from cigarette-induced lung cancer than from breast cancer, and cigarettes are now the leading cause of cancer-related deaths in women. Women who smoke also suffer higher incidences of coronary heart disease and heart attacks than do women who do not smoke.

In addition to the direct effects of cigarettes on smokers, the environmental pollution caused by smokers can have adverse consequences for nonsmokers.[48,49] Indeed, an estimated 4000 Americans die annually from lung cancer caused by other persons' smoking (so-called passive smoke). A 1986 government report estimated that an additional 37,000 deaths every year follow from heart disease contracted as a result of inhaling passive smoke.[50] More recently, Wells recalculated earlier data and estimated that in 1985 there were 62,000 deaths due to coronary artery disease caused by passive smoking.[51] Wells further concluded that nonsmokers exposed to passive smoking have a coronary death rate 20 to 70 percent higher than do nonsmokers not exposed to passive smoking.

Effects during Pregnancy

There is now irrefutable evidence that cigarette smoking adversely affects the developing fetus.[52] Cigarettes increase the rates of spontaneous abortion, stillbirth, and early postpartum death. In 1988, 2552 infant deaths were attributed to maternal smoking. Pregnant women who smoke have approximately twice the number of stillborn infants as do nonsmoking mothers, with a direct relation between the number of cigarettes smoked every day and the percentage of stillbirths. There is evidence that infants born of nonsmoking mothers may be heavier than those born of smoking mothers. Cigarette smoking reduces oxygen delivery to the developing fetus, causing fetal hypoxia, which can result in long-term, irreversible intellectual and physical deficiencies. Nicotine is thus contraindicated during pregnancy; indeed, cigarettes are contraindicated for all women who might become pregnant and all women who breast-feed.

Governmental Response

To address these severe effects on health, the warning placed on cigarette packs and advertisements in 1970 ("Warning: The Surgeon General has determined that cigarette smoking is dangerous to your health") has been replaced by four new statements that are used on a rotating basis. These warnings read as follows:

> Surgeon General's Warning: Smoking causes lung cancer, heart disease, and emphysema.

> Surgeon General's Warning: Quitting smoking now greatly reduces serious risks to your health.

> Surgeon General's Warning: Smoking by pregnant women may result in fetal injury and premature birth.

> Surgeon General's Warning: Cigarette smoke contains carbon monoxide.

Although these statements are an improvement over the old warning, they greatly understate the toxicity of cigarettes and the health consequences of habitual cigarette smoking. On an encouraging note, tighter controls have been placed on smoking in recent years, with government and private agencies establishing workplaces that are smokefree; ideally, these smokefree areas will be expanded to include all public places.

Negative factors in the effort to control cigarette smoking include the following:

1. the continued denial by cigarette manufacturers of cigarette-induced toxicity and addictive potential

2. the promotion of smoking among impressionable youth

3. smoking by youth

4. contradictions in government policy

These contradictions include income from taxes on cigarettes but expenditures for the subsidization of tobacco growing and for the social and health consequences that result from long-term cigarette use.

Because of the addictive potential of cigarettes and nicotine, the surgeon general's dream of a smokeless society will probably not be realized anytime soon; even the goal of a smoking rate of 15 percent of the U.S. population by the year 2000 may be unattainable. Further progress in smoking reduction and treatment can only be achieved through governmental actions that are consistent with the data and warnings of its own expert advisors.

Recently, Henningfield, Kozlowski, and Benowitz proposed labeling cigarettes much as food products are labeled with nutritional information.[53] The proposed label would include an improved warning statement and information on the yields of nicotine, tar, carbon monoxide, and harmful chemicals, as well as information about nicotine delivery. Hopefully, such information would increase health consciousness among smokers and increase the motivation to quit smoking.

Therapy for Nicotine Dependence

Therapy for nicotine dependence, like therapy for all drug dependence syndromes, involves withdrawal, diagnosis, therapy for coexisting disorders, reduction in drug craving, and prevention of relapse. The pharmacological involvement usually "involves medical detoxification (i.e., transdermal nicotine patch plus a tricyclic antidepressant) and psychotherapy (i.e., behavioral and cognitive relapse prevention therapy) side-by-side."[26]

Smoking cigarettes with a lower nicotine content usually fails to help persons cut down their nicotine consumption, because they merely smoke more cigarettes. Attempts to free persons from nicotine dependence by substituting nicotine-free cigarettes also fail.

The first nicotine-containing replacement for cigarettes was the prescription chewing gum Nicorette, each piece containing 2 or 4 milligrams of nicotine in a slow-release resin complex.[37] The gum supplies the nicotine, and the user can control his or her intake to avoid withdrawal symptoms. The gum can be used as a first step, allowing the person to tackle the psychological dependence and social components of smoking without altering learned patterns of blood level dosing. Later, gum consumption can be slowly reduced.

Perhaps a better alternative is to eventually replace the gum consumption with transdermal nicotine patch therapy, which takes away the self-medication component and provides a more consistent blood level of nicotine than can be achieved with the gum. Because the patches each last 24 hours, they reduce morning craving. The patches are also available at various dose levels, which allow a step-down dosage regime. Recently Fiore and coworkers determined that individuals wearing the nicotine patch were more than twice as likely to quit smoking and maintain abstinence than were individuals wearing a placebo patch.[54]

Besides nicotine replacement and nicotine reduction therapies, other drugs can be used to reduce craving or relieve withdrawal symptoms such as anxiety or depression. Clonidine (Catapres), through a

CNS action, has been shown to reduce the release of norepinephrine and epinephrine (adrenaline). As a consequence, it reduces blood pressure (it is clinically marketed as an antihypertensive drug) and also reduces craving and withdrawal symptoms in heavy cigarette smokers, doubling (from 30 to 60 percent) the number of individuals who remain abstinent for 6 months or more.[37] The mechanism of the action of clonidine is unknown, but there is now a growing literature in the field of pain control and anesthesia indicating that clonidine is an effective pain reliever when injected directly into the spinal canal.[55,56] Such action may be related intimately to its use as an aid in drug withdrawal syndromes.

Other drugs for the relief of withdrawal symptoms include the antidepressants (Chapter 8) and the anxiolytics (Chapter 4). Of the latter group of drugs, buspirone may hold the most promise. The symposium chaired by Fiore details therapeutic strategies for quitting smoking.[35]

Study Questions

1. Differentiate the CNS stimulant actions of caffeine from those of amphetamines or cocaine.
2. Describe the mechanism of action of caffeine. How does this mechanism explain the clinical effects of the drug?
3. What is the relation between panic attacks and caffeine?
4. Discuss the effects of caffeine on the cardiovascular system.
5. What evidence is there for and against the use of caffeine by women who are pregnant or breast-feeding?
6. Discuss the political, health, and economic contradictions that are related to tobacco.
7. List some of the statistics that are relevant to the health effects of cigarettes.
8. Separate the acute effects of nicotine from the long-term effects of smoking. Discuss the long-term problems faced by persons who smoke cigarettes.
9. Are cigarettes addicting or are they merely habit-forming? Defend your position.
10. Discuss the clinical uses and limitations of Nicorette gum.

Notes

1. D. Grady, "Don't Get Jittery over Caffeine," *Discover* 7, no. 7 (1986): 73–79.
2. G. L. Clementz and J. W. Dailey, "Psychotropic Effects of Caffeine," *American Family Physician* 37 (1988): 167–172.

3. B. Eskenazi, "Caffeine during Pregnancy: Grounds for Concern," *Journal of the American Medical Association* 270 (1993): 2973–2974.

4. A. Goldstein, *Addiction: From Biology to Drug Policy* (New York: W. H. Freeman and Company, 1994), pp. 179–189.

5. T. W. Rall, "Drugs Used in the Treatment of Asthma," in A. G. Gilman, T. W. Rall, A. S. Nies, and P. Taylor, eds., *Goodman and Gilman's The Pharmacological Basis of Therapeutics*, 8th ed. (New York: Pergamon, 1990), pp. 618–637.

6. T. V. Dunwiddie, "The Physiological Role of Adenosine in the Central Nervous System," *International Review of Neurobiology* 27 (1985): 63–139.

7. J. F. Greden and A. Walters, "Caffeine," in J. H. Lowinson, P. Ruiz, R. B. Millman, and J. G. Langrod, eds., *Substance Abuse: A Comprehensive Textbook*, 2nd ed. (Baltimore: Williams & Wilkins, 1992), pp. 357–370.

8. J. W. Daly, "Mechanism of Action of Caffeine," in S. Garattini, ed., *Caffeine, Coffee, and Health* (New York: Raven Press, 1993).

9. G. B. Kaplan, D. J. Greenblatt, M. A. Kent, M. M. Cotreau, G. Arcelin, and R. I. Shader, "Caffeine-Induced Behavioral Stimulation is Dose-Dependent and Associated with A1 Adenosine Receptor Occupancy," *Neuropsychopharmacology* 6 (1992): 145–153.

10. I. Biaggioni, S. Paul, A. Puckett, and C. Arzubiaga, "Caffeine and Theophylline as Adenosine Antagonists in Humans," *Journal of Pharmacology & Experimental Therapeutics* 258 (1991): 588–593.

11. P. J. Marangos and J. P. Boulenger, "Basic and Clinical Aspects of Adenosinergic Neuromodulation," *Neuroscience and Biobehavioral Reviews* 9 (1988): 421–430.

12. S. H. Snyder and P. Sklar, "Behavioral and Molecular Actions of Caffeine: Focus on Adenosine," *Journal of Psychiatric Research* 18 (1984): 91–106.

13. L. H. Gold, M. A. Geyer, and G. F. Koob, "Neurochemical Mechanisms Involved in Behavioral Effects of Amphetamines and Related Designer Drugs," *NIDA Research Monograph* 94 (1989): 101–126.

14. L. Pulvirenti, N. R. Swerdlow, and G. F. Koob, "Nucleus Accumbens NMDA Antagonist Decreases Locomotor Activity Produced by Cocaine, Heroin, or Accumbens Dopamine, but Not Caffeine," *Pharmacology, Biochemistry and Behavior* 40 (1991): 841–845.

15. D. Shi, O. Nokodijevic, K. A. Jacobson, and J. W. Daly, "Chronic Caffeine Alters the Density of Adenosine, Adrenergic, Cholinergic, GABA, and Serotonin Receptors and Calcium Channels in Mouse Brain," *Cellular & Molecular Neurobiology* 13 (1993): 247–261.

16. H. M. Phelps and C. E. Phelps, "Caffeine Ingestion and Breast Cancer. A Negative Correlation," *Cancer* 61 (1988): 1051–1054.

17. W. Levinson and P. M. Dunn, "Nonassociation of Caffeine and Fibrocystic Breast Disease," *Archives of Internal Medicine* 146 (1986): 1773–1775.

18. L. C. Russell, "Caffeine Restriction as Initial Treatment for Breast Pain," *Nurse Practitioner* 14 (1989): 36–37.

19. D. S. Charney, G. R. Heniger, and P. L. Jatlow, "Increased Anxiogenic Effects of Caffeine in Panic Disorders," *Archives of General Psychiatry* 42 (1985): 233–243.

20. D. E. Grobbee, E. B. Rimm, E. Giovannucci, G. Colditz, M. Stampfer, and W. Willett, "Coffee, Caffeine, and Cardiovascular Disease in Men," *New England Journal of Medicine* 323 (1990): 1026–1032.

21. M. S. Morris and L. Weinstein, "Caffeine and the Fetus: Is Trouble Brewing?" *American Journal of Obstetrics and Gynecology* 140 (1981): 607–610.

22. L. Dlugosz and M. S. Bracken, "Reproductive Effects of Caffeine: A Review and Theoretical Analysis," *Epidemiology Review* 14 (1992): 83–100.

23. J. L. Mills and others, "Moderate Caffeine Use and the Risk of Spontaneous Abortion and Intrauterine Growth Retardation," *Journal of the American Medical Association* 269 (1993): 593–597.

24. C. Infante-Rivard, A. Fernandez, R. Gauthier, M. David, and G.-E. Rivard, "Fetal Loss Associated with Caffeine Intake before and during Pregnancy," *Journal of the American Medical Association* 270 (1993): 2940–2943.

25. R. R. Griffiths, S. M. Evans, S. J. Heishman, K. L. Preston, C. A. Sannerud, B. Wolf, and P. P. Woodson, "Low–Dose Caffeine Physical Dependence in Humans," *Journal of Pharmacology and Experimental Therapeutics* 255 (1990): 1123–1132.

26. J. Cocores, "Nicotine Dependence: Diagnosis and Treatment," *Psychiatric Clinics of North America* 16 (1993): 49.

27. U.S. Department of Health and Human Services, *Reducing the Health Consequences of Smoking: 25 Years of Progress. A Report of the Surgeon General* (Rockville, Md.: U.S. Department of Health and Human Services, 1989), p. iv.

28. U. S. Department of Health and Human Services, *The Health Benefits of Smoking Cessation. A Report of the Surgeon General* (Rockville, Md.: U.S. Department of Health and Human Services, 1990).

29. U. S. Department of Health and Human Services, *Smoking and Health in the Americas*, DHHS Publication No. (CDC)92-8419 (Atlanta, Ga: U.S. Department of Health and Human Services, Centers for Disease Control, Office on Smoking and Health, 1992).

30. M. E. Jarvik and N. G. Schneider, "Nicotine," in J. H. Lowinson, P. Ruiz, R. B. Millman, and J. G. Langrod, eds., *Substance Abuse: A Comprehensive Textbook*, 2nd ed. (Baltimore: Williams & Wilkins, 1992), pp. 339–340.

31. U.S. Department of Health and Human Services, *The Health Consequences of Smoking: Nicotine Addiction. A Report of the Surgeon General* (Rockville, Md.: U.S. Department of Health and Human Services, 1988), p. 9.

32. N. Sherwood, J. S. Kerr, and I. Hindmarch, "Psychomotor Performance in Smokers Following Single and Repeated Doses of Nicotine Gum," *Psychopharmacology* 108 (1992): 432–436.

33. E. D. Levin, "Nicotine Systems and Cognitive Function," *Psychopharmacology* 108 (1992): 417–431.

34. D. M. Warburton, J. M. Rusted, and J. Fowler, "A Comparison of the Attentional and Consolidation Hypothesis for the Facilitation of Memory by Nicotine," *Psychopharmacology* 108 (1992): 443–447.

35. M. C. Fiore, "Trends in Cigarette Smoking in the United States: The Epidemiology of Tobacco Use," *The Medical Clinics of North America* 76 (March 1992): 289–304.

36. J. R. Hughes, S. W. Gust, K. Skoog, R. M. Keenan, and J. W. Fenwick, "Symptoms of Tobacco Withdrawal: A Replication and Extension," *Archives of General Psychiatry* 48 (1991): 52–59.

37. P. K. Gessner, "Substance Abuse Treatment," in C. M. Smith and A. M. Reynard, eds., *Textbook of Pharmacology* (Philadelphia: Saunders, 1992), p. 1160.

38. R. West, "Nicotine Addiction: A Re-analysis of the Arguments," *Psychopharmacology* 108 (1992): 408–410.

39. J. R. Hughes, "Smoking Is a Drug Dependence: A Reply to Robinson and Pritchard," *Psychopharmacology* 113 (1993): 282–283.

40. J. H. Robinson and W. S. Pritchard, "The Role of Nicotine in Tobacco Use," *Psychopharmacology* 108 (1992): 397–407.

41. J. H. Robinson and W. S. Pritchard, "The Meaning of Addiction: Reply to West," *Psychopharmacology* 108 (1992): 411–416.

42. M. E. Jarvik, "Biological Factors Underlying the Smoking Habit," in M. E. Jarvik, J. W. Cullen, E. R. Gritz, T. M. Vogt, and L. J. West, eds., *Research on Smoking Behavior*, National Institute on Drug Abuse Research Monograph 17 (Washington, D.C.: U.S. Government Printing Office, 1977), pp. 122–146.

43. W. Pollin, in M. E. Jarvik, J. W. Cullen, E. R. Gritz, T. M. Vogt, and L. J. West, eds., *Research on Smoking Behavior*, National Institute on Drug Abuse Research Monograph 17 (Washington, D.C.: U. S. Government Printing Office, 1977), pp. v–vi.

44. M. Barry, "The Influence of the U.S. Tobacco Industry on the Health, Economy, and Environment of Developing Countries," *New England Journal of Medicine* 324 (1991): 917–920.

45. U.S. Department of Health and Human Services, *Reducing the Health Consequences of Smoking*, pp. 16–17.

46. Ibid., pp. 98–99.

47. Pathobiological Determinants of Atherosclerosis in Youth (PDAY) Research Group, "Relationship of Atherosclerosis in Young Men to Serum Lipoprotein Cholesterol Concentrations and Smoking," *Journal of the American Medical Association* 264 (1990): 3018–3024.

48. P. A. Newcomb and P. P. Carbone, "The Health Consequences of Smoking: Cancer," *The Medical Clinics of North America* 76 (March 1992): 305–332.

49. U.S. Department of Health, Education and Welfare, *The Health Consequences of Smoking for Women. A Report of the Surgeon General* (Washington, D.C.: U.S. Government Printing Office, 1980).

50. U.S. Department of Health and Human Services, *The Health Consequences of Involuntary Smoking. A Report of the Surgeon General* (Washington, D.C.: U.S. Government Printing Office, 1986).

51. A. J. Wells, "Passive Smoking as a Cause of Heart Disease," *Journal of the American College of Cardiology* 24 (1994): 546–554.

52. U.S. Department of Health and Human Services, *Reducing the Health Consequences of Smoking*, pp. 71–76.

53. J. E. Henningfield, L. T. Kozlowski, and N. L. Benowitz, "A Proposal to Develop Meaningful Labeling for Cigarettes," *Journal of the American Medical Association* 272 (27 July 1994): 312–314.

54. M. C. Fiore, S. S. Smith, D. E. Jorenby, and T. B. Baker, "The Effectiveness of the Nicotine Patch for Smoking Cessation," *Journal of the American Medical Association* 271 (22/29 June 1994): 1940–1947.

55. M. DeKock, B. Crochet, C. Morimont, and J. L. Scholtes, "Intravenous or Epidural Clonidine for Intra- and Postoperative Analgesia," *Anesthesiology* 79 (1993): 525–531.

56. D. B. Quan, D. L. Wandres, and D. J. Schroeder, "Clonidine in Pain Management," *Annals of Pharmacotherapy* 27 (1993): 313–315.

CHAPTER 8

PHARMACOTHERAPY OF MOOD DISORDERS: DRUGS FOR TREATING MAJOR DEPRESSION

Major depressive disorder and *bipolar disorder* are mood (or affect) disorders, in contrast to schizophrenia, which is a thought disorder. Mood disorders are characterized by extreme or prolonged disturbances of mood, such as sadness and apathy on the one hand or elation on the other. The occurrence of manic symptoms distinguishes bipolar disorders from depressive, or unipolar, disorders. Because of this difference, pharmacological therapy for the two conditions is quite different, but overlap does exist because of the anxiety component often seen in depressive disorder and the depressive component of bipolar disorder. In this and the next chapter, however, we will treat the two disorders as largely separate entities. This chapter will focus on the drugs used to treat depressive disorder (the antidepressants), while Chapter 9 will focus on the drugs used to treat bipolar disorder (lithium and the anticonvulsants carbamazepine and valproic acid).

Episodes of depression are characterized by dysphoria, or loss of interest or pleasure in all (or almost all) of a person's usual activities or pastimes. Accompanying this condition are feelings of intense sadness and despair; diminished energy; decreased sexual drive; mental slowing and loss of concentration; pessimism; feelings of helplessness, worthlessness, or self-reproach; inappropriate guilt; recurrent thoughts of death, suicide, and hopelessness; blunted affect; anorexia; fatigue; and insomnia. Anxiety almost invariably occurs in persons who are depressed, which can lead to a misdiagnosis and inappropriate or improper treatment. About 15 percent of persons suffering from depression die by suicide.[1,2]

Certainly, sadness is a normal human emotion in response to various life events. However, depression that has no known cause or unremitting depression that interferes with normal activity is pathological. One report states that "nearly 8 percent of the U.S. population will develop a mood disorder at some time during their lives; nearly 5 percent of the population will develop major depression, occurring twice as often in women as in men."[2]

Another report states:

> Depression afflicts about 5% of the adult population in the United States at any given time. . . . Over a lifetime, about 30% of the adult population will have suffered from depression. Also, if left untreated, 25% to 30% of adult depressives will commit suicide. . . . More than 50% of suicides saw a physician in the month before their death. These patients, however, were not diagnosed as being depressed. Data . . . from 1991 show that there were 30,000 reported suicides. It is the 8th leading cause of death in the U.S.[3]

Major depression typically has an onset in individuals in their middle to late twenties, although it can occur at any age, even in the elderly. More than 50 percent of persons experiencing an episode of major depression have recurrences, with the average number of episodes being five or six in a lifetime. It is now clear that

> depression is a disease resulting from biochemical changes in the brain. It is undertreated. Surveys . . . show that about 70% of depressed patients do NOT get treatment for their disease. . . . The vast majority of people respond to the excellent treatments that we have available. About 85% can be treated successfully.[3]

Patients who experience episodes of major depression respond to the various types of antidepressants, to monoamine oxidase inhibitors, and, in severe or drug-resistant cases, to electroconvulsive shock therapy (ECT) and psychotherapy.

Patients who experience reactive, or exogenous, depression seldom display evidence of a psychosis and do not appear to possess a genetic or biochemical origin for their depression. Anxiety, agitation, and substance abuse are often present in these patients. The antidepressant drugs are rarely appropriate for treating such persons and certainly should not be a treatment of first and only choice. Professional counseling frequently resolves the problems associated with reactive depression, often without any drug therapy.

Mechanism of Action

Attempts to identify the underlying causes of major depressive disorders have led to inconclusive results.[4,5] Most investigators agree that a neurochemical imbalance is involved and, in some cases, genetically determined. Pharmacological evidence points to an involvement of at least two and perhaps three biological amines in the brain (norepinephrine, serotonin, and possibly dopamine).

The biological amine theory of mania and depression was first postulated in the mid-1960s. According to this theory, depression is caused by a functional deficit of specific transmitters at certain sites in the brain, while mania results from a functional excess of the same transmitters.

Several bits of evidence support this claim. First, reserpine, an older drug that induces severe emotional depression, concomitantly depletes norepinephrine and serotonin from the neurons that release them. Second, the antidepressant drugs exert important actions on both of these transmitters to potentiate their neurotransmitter action. Third, strong evidence for the genetic predisposition toward depression has led to the belief that major depressive episodes may include an abnormally low functioning of the neurotransmission of norepinephrine and serotonin or of the receptors for these transmitters.

Although reasonable correlations have been found between drug-induced increases in the levels of norepinephrine and serotonin and positive, mood-elevating effects in persons who are depressed, several limitations and inconsistencies in this pattern have also been seen. One major difficulty is that the time course of action is vastly different for the biochemical effect and the clinical response. Although neurotransmission of norepinephrine and serotonin is augmented soon after the drug is taken, the clinical antidepressant effect may not appear for two weeks or longer. Thus, increasing the amounts of neurotransmitter may only be an initial step in relieving depression. A more complex series of cellular events may then occur that eventually results in secondary, adaptive changes.

A second problem in correlating antidepressive activity with levels of neurotransmitters is that cocaine and the amphetamines augment biological amine neurotransmission (Chapter 6), but they are not effective as antidepressants, even though they can induce a manic paranoia or psychosis. Perhaps the preference of amphetamines and cocaine for dopamine neurons (rather than for norepinephrine and serotonin neurons) accounts for this discrepancy. According to Baldessarini:

A few tentative generalizations may be made from these observations, together with the clinical and behavioral effects of antidepressant drugs. First, blockade of *dopamine* transport seems to be associated with *stimulant* rather than antidepressant activity. Second, inhibition of *serotonin* uptake may well contribute to antidepressant activity. Finally, inhibitory actions on the uptake of *norepinephrine* seem to correspond with antidepressant activity. However, there is increasing doubt that inhibition of the uptake of norepinephrine or serotonin *per se* is a sufficient explanation for the antidepressant action of these drugs.[5]

Postsynaptic receptor desensitization is a new refinement of the biological amine theory. This hypothesis posits that depression, rather than being the result of a hypoadrenergic (norepinephrine) state, may be due to a hyperresponsiveness of postsynaptic receptors caused by the decreased availability of norepinephrine.[6] Thus, by blocking norepinephrine reuptake, presynaptic activity normalizes (normal amounts of transmitter become available at the receptor), and slowly the postsynaptic receptors down-regulate to a normal level of responsiveness. Such an adaptive change accounts for the slow onset of clinical effect yet allows for an action subsequent to blockade of reuptake.

The serotonin hypothesis is a recent variation of the receptor desensitization theory. This hypothesis holds that blocking the reuptake of serotonin is more clinically efficacious than blocking the reuptake of norepinephrine. Furthermore, the adaptive changes in serotonin receptors would explain the slow onset of clinical antidepressant effect. While the older, traditional antidepressants are generally more potent at blocking reuptake of norepinephrine, the newer, "second generation" antidepressants are generally more selective and more effective at blocking the reuptake of serotonin. Paul states:

> Alterations in serotonin neurotransmission have been postulated to be involved in a variety of neuropsychiatric disorders including depression, generalized anxiety disorder, and obsessive-compulsive disorder, although the precise role of serotonin in either the etiology or the pathogenesis of these disorders is still unclear. . . . Augmentation of serotonergic neurotransmission may mediate, at least in part, the therapeutic actions of a variety of psychotherapeutic drugs, including antidepressants. . . . Virtually all effective antidepressant treatments augment serotonergic neurotransmission, and, therefore, the serotonergic system may represent a "final common pathway" underlying the therapeutic effects of these drugs.[7]

The symposium edited by Paul extensively reviews the role of serotonin in the action of the antidepressants,[7] concluding that the different types of antidepressant treatments all enhance the neurotransmission of serotonin,* albeit via different mechanisms. As summarized in that symposium by Blier, de Montigny, and Chaput:

> Tricyclic antidepressant drugs and electroconvulsive shock treatment sensitize postsynaptic neurons to serotonin. Monoamine oxidase inhibitors enhance the availability of releasable serotonin. Serotonin reuptake blockers increase the efficacy of serotonin neurons by desensitizing serotonin autoreceptors located on serotonin nerve terminals.[9]

Until 1991 there was little information on the structure and regulation of the presynaptic reuptake transporter for serotonin. It was thought that the transporter might be analogous to the dopamine transporter, which is blocked by cocaine (Chapter 6). Then, in 1991, Blakely and coworkers[10] and Hoffman and coworkers[11] isolated and cloned a complementary DNA sequence that predicted a 653-amino-acid protein with 12 to 13 putative transmembrane domains. It strongly resembles the GABA, dopamine, and norepinephrine transporters, but it is significantly different from the postsynaptic serotonin receptor, which is not affected by antidepressant drugs. The latter receptor is a 420-amino-acid chain with 7 membrane-spanning regions.[11]

Shortly after the presynaptic serotonin transporter was identified, the activity of this transporter was shown to be regulated by a cyclic nucleotide called cyclic adenosine monophosphate (cAMP).[12,13] Thus, this protein, being subject to regulation, may fall under the influence of abnormal and as yet uncharacterized regulatory effects during episodes of depressive illness.[14,15] With such plasticity in the serotonin system,[16] perhaps we will eventually identify specific serotonergic alterations that underlie major depression.

Table 8.1 compares how effectively various antidepressant drugs block the reuptake of norepinephrine, serotonin, and dopamine (in an experimental model) and calculates the selectivity for serotonin over norepinephrine. Most of the newer drugs (fluoxetine, sertraline, paroxetine, clomipramine, and venlafaxine) have serotonin selectivity; one new drug (bupropion) does not. Janicak and others review other, less-accepted hypotheses concerning the action of antidepressant drugs.[6]

---

*Harrington and coworkers[8] discuss the molecular biology of serotonin receptors. While these receptors are likely the site of action of drugs used to treat migraine headache, they are not a major site of antidepressant drug action. Rather, the antidepressants block the presynaptic serotonin transporter protein, which is structurally and functionally distinct from the postsynaptic serotonin receptor.

TABLE 8.1 Potency and selectivity of various antidepressants.

| Drug | Potency[a] | | | Selectivity[b] |
	Norepinephrine	Serotonin	Dopamine	
Amitriptyline	4.2	1.5	0.043	0.36[c]
Amoxapine	23	0.21	0.053	0.0091
Bupropion	0.043	0.0064	0.16	0.15
Clomipramine	3.6	18	0.057	5.3[d]
Desipramine	110	0.29	0.019	0.0026
Doxepin	5.3	0.36	0.018	0.067
Fluoxetine	0.36	8.3	0.063	23
Imipramine	7.7	2.4	0.020	0.31
Maprotiline	14	0.030	0.034	0.0021
Nortriptyline	25	0.38	0.059	0.015
Paroxetine	3.0	136	0.059	45
Protriptyline	100	0.36	0.054	0.0036
Sertraline	0.46	29	0.38	64
Trazodone	0.020	0.53	0.0070	26
Trimipramine	0.20	0.040	0.029	0.20
REFERENCE COMPOUND				
d-amphetamine[e]	2.00	—	1.2	

From Richelson,[3] tab. 2, p. 468, with permission.
[a]$10^{-7} \times 1/K_i$, where K_i = inhibitor constant in molarity.
[b]Ratio of potency of serotonin uptake blockade to potency of norephinephrine uptake blockade.
[c]Indicates that amitriptyline as about 2.8 (1/0.36) times more potent at blocking uptake of norepinephrine than uptake of serotonin.
[d]Indicates that clomipramine is about 5 times more potent at blocking uptake of serotonin than uptake of norepinephrine.
[e]This is not an antidepressant but is shown here for comparison.

Evolution of Antidepressant Drug Therapy

The pharmacological treatment of endogenous depression began in the early 1950s, first with the recognition of the antidepressant effects of iproniazid (a *monoamine oxidase inhibitor,* or MAO inhibitor) and later with the availability of the first *tricyclic antidepressant* (TCA), imipramine. Through the 1960s, analogues of these drugs were developed and marketed. By the late 1970s, seven TCAs and three MAO inhibitors were available. By 1980, it was conceded that these drugs were therapeutically useful for patients with depression but that about one-third of the patients treated did not respond adequately. In addition, adverse reactions associated with the TCAs (sedation, dry mouth,

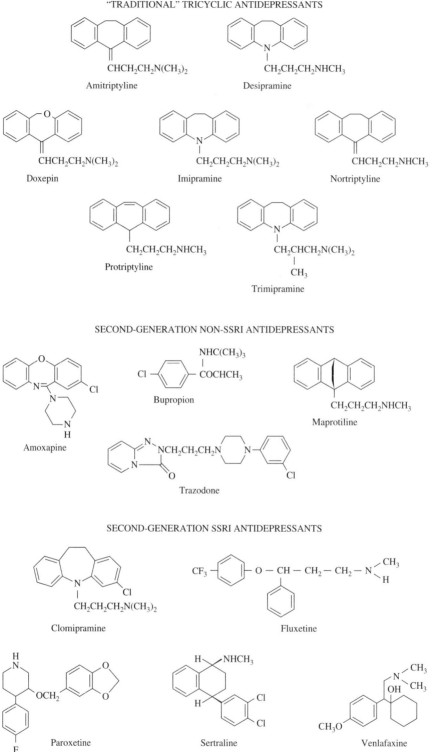

FIGURE 8.1 Chemical structures of antidepressants.

hypotension, and changes in cardiac conduction) and the MAO inhibitors (tyramine-associated hypertensive reactions) limited their use in many patients.

In the 1980s, new drugs were introduced for treating depression, the so-called second-generation antidepressants. These included trazodone, amoxapine, maprotiline, and bupropion. None offered significant increases in therapeutic efficacy, but they had a lower incidence of certain side effects (the dry mouth due to anticholinergic actions and cardiac conduction problems). However, these drugs had side effects of their own, as will be detailed later in this chapter.

The most recent additions to the antidepressant agents are the *serotonin-specific reuptake inhibitors* (SSRIs): fluoxetine, sertraline, paroxetine, and, most recently, venlafaxine. These drugs seem to be as effective as earlier antidepressants in managing mild to moderate depression, but they are not very effective in treating severely depressed patients.[17] The SSRIs have little effect on cardiac conduction, but they have other side effects that are not insignificant.

Despite these advances in drug development, about 20 percent of patients with depression fail to respond to antidepressant drug therapy; others cannot tolerate the side effects of the drugs. Thus, the search continues to identify new pharmacological agents for treating depression.

We can classify the clinical antidepressants by their chemical structure (Figure 8.1) or their mechanism of action:

1. tricyclic antidepressants, the actions of which include the blockade of the active presynaptic reuptake of norepinephrine and/or serotonin

2. second-generation antidepressants, which are structurally dissimilar to the TCAs but otherwise exert similar effects; newer serotonin-specific reuptake inhibitors

3. monoamine oxidase inhibitors, which increase the amounts of norepinephrine, dopamine, and serotonin available for release, as a result of drug-induced inhibition of the enzyme that normally metabolizes the transmitter

In addition to the pharmacological approach to treating major depression, electroconvulsive therapy (ECT), although not publicized as a major method of treatment, has proven effective.

Tricyclic Antidepressants

The term *tricyclic antidepressant* describes a class of drugs that all have a three-ring molecular core (see Figure 8.1) and relieve depression in

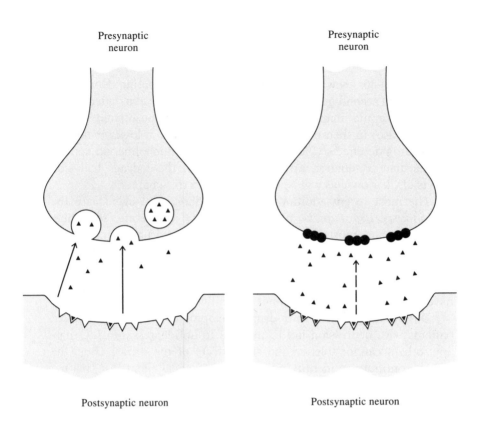

Presynaptic neuron

Presynaptic neuron

Postsynaptic neuron

Postsynaptic neuron

▲ Norepinephrine or serotonin

● Tricyclic antidepressant drug

FIGURE 8.2   Normal mechanism of inactivation of norepinephrine or serotonin by presynaptic uptake (*left*) and its inhibition by tricyclic antidepressant drugs (*right*). [From S. H. Snyder, *Drugs and the Brain* (New York: Scientific American Library, 1986), p. 106.]

persons who experience major depressive illness.[5] TCAs are generally considered to be the drugs of first choice for treating major depression despite two facts: (1) The SSRIs, which are widely promoted and effective, can substitute as drugs of first choice, and (2) the TCAs are effective in only about two-thirds of depressed patients.

Imipramine, the first of the TCAs, was first studied for antipsychotic effect, but a mood-elevating effect was noted. Two of the marketed drugs (desipramine and nortriptyline) are the active intermediate metabolites of imipramine and amitriptyline, respectively. In fact, these active intermediates may actually be responsible for much of the antidepressant effect of imipramine and amitriptyline.

All the TCAs probably attach to and inhibit the presynaptic serotonin transporter protein. This protein is responsible for the active neuronal reuptake of serotonin into the presynaptic nerve terminals from which it was originally released (Figure 8.2). The TCAs, however, are not ideal for clinical use because they have a slow onset of action, their effectiveness is unreliable, they all cause bothersome side effects, and their overdoses are difficult to manage.

Because TCAs do not produce euphoria or other pleasurable effects and have few discernible psychological effects in normal patients, they have no recreational or behavior-reinforcing value. Thus abuse and psychological dependence are not a concern. The choice of drug is determined by effectiveness, tolerance of side effects, and duration of action. TCAs elevate mood, increase physical activity, improve appetite and sleep patterns, and reduce morbid preoccupation. They are useful in treating patients who are experiencing acute episodes of depression as well as in preventing relapses, serving as maintenance therapy for persons who are prone to major depressive episodes.

Pharmacological Effects

Central Nervous System   The therapeutic and side effects of the TCAs all result from drug-induced blockade of histamine, acetylcholine, dopamine, and norepinephrine receptors (Table 8.2). The blockade of serotonin and norepinephrine receptors, as well as the down regulation of these receptors, accounts for therapeutic effectiveness. The blockade of acetylcholine receptors produces dry mouth, confusion, and blurred vision. Because most TCAs are fairly potent blockers of the histamine receptors, drowsiness frequently occurs. Blockade of the norepinephrine receptors can result in hypotension, particularly when the patient rises from a recumbent position. Blockade of the dopamine receptors can produce parkinsonianlike movement disorders as a bothersome side effect.

In the patient on long-term therapy with TCAs, tolerance develops to most of these side effects; however, choosing a particular drug with an awareness of its side effects can turn a disadvantage into a therapeutic advantage. For example, amitriptyline and doxepin are the most sedating of the TCAs, making them useful in treating individuals with agitation as well as depression or where improved sleep is desirable. Table 8.3 lists the clinical consequences that can follow blockade of each type of receptor.

TABLE 8.2 Affinity of antidepressants for neurotransmitter receptors of human brain.

Drug	Histamine (H$_1$)[a]	Acetylcholine (Muscarinic)	Norepinephrine (α_1-Adrenoceptor)	Dopamine (D$_2$)
Amitriptyline	91	5.6	3.7	0.10
Amoxapine	4.0	0.10	2.00	0.62
Bupropion	0.015	0.0021	0.022	0.00048
Clomipramine	3.2	2.7	2.63	0.53
Desipramine	0.91	0.50	0.77	0.030
Doxepin	420	1.2	4.2	0.042
Fluoxetine	0.016	0.050	0.0169	0.015
Imipramine	9.1	1.1	1.1	0.050
Maprotiline	50	0.18	1.1	0.29
Nortriptyline	10	0.7	1.7	0.083
Paroxetine	0.0045	0.93	0.029	0.0031
Protriptyline	4.0	4.0	0.77	0.043
Sertraline	0.0041	0.16	0.27	0.0093
Trazodone	0.29	0.00031	2.8	0.026
Trimipramine	370	1.7	4.2	0.56
REFERENCE COMPOUNDS[b]				
Diphenhydramine	7.1	—	—	—
Atropine	—	42	—	—
Phentolamine	—	—	6.7	—
Haloperidol	—	—	—	26

From Richelson,[3] tab. 3, p. 469, with permission.
[a]$10^{-7} \times 1/K_d$, where K_d = equilibrium dissociation constant in molarity.
[b]These are not antidepressants but are shown here for comparison.

Of additional importance are the possible effects of TCAs on memory and cognitive function. Here, one must distinguish between the direct effects of these drugs on cognition, which are related to their intrinsic properties, and indirect effects, which result from the improvement in mood.[18] TCAs with either sedative effects or anticholinergic effects can directly impair attention, motor speed, dexterity, and memory.[19] Relatively nonsedating compounds with low degrees of anticholinergic side effects cause very little impairment of psychomotor or memory functions. These results should not be surprising, since sedatives (such as barbiturates) and anticholinergics (such as scopolamine) profoundly impair memory and cognitive ability. The

TABLE 8.3 Pharmacological properties of antidepressants and possible clinical consequences.

Property	Possible Clinical Consequences
Blockade of norepinephrine uptake at nerve endings	Tremors Tachycardia Erectile and ejaculatory dysfunction Blockade of the antihypertensive effects of guanethidine (Ismelin and Esimil and guanadrel (Hylorel) Augmentation of pressor effects of sympathomimetic amines
Blockade of serotonin uptake at nerve endings	Gastrointestinal disturbances Increase or decrease in anxiety (dose dependent) Sexual dysfunction Extrapyramidal side effects Interactions with L-tryptophan, monoamine oxidase inhibitors, and fenfluramine
Blockade of dopamine uptake at nerve endings	Psychomotor activation Antiparkinsonian effect Aggravation of psychosis
Blockade of histamine H_1 receptors	Potentiation of central depressant drugs Sedation drowsiness Weight gain Hypotension
Blockade of acetylcholine receptors	Blurred vision Dry mouth Sinus tachycardia Constipation Urinary retention
Blockade of norepinephrine receptors	Memory dysfunction Potentiation of the antihypertensive effect of prazosin (Minipress), terazosin (Hytrin), doxazosin (Cardura), labetalol (Normodyne) Postural hypotension, dizziness Reflex tachycardia
Blockade of dopamine D_2 receptors	Extrapyramidal movement disorders Endocrine changes Sexual dysfunction (males)

From Richelson,[3] tab. 4, p. 471, with permission.

TABLE 8.4 Drugs used in affective disorders: Antidepressants.

Drug name Generic (trade)	Sedative activity	Anticholinergic activity[a]	Elimination half-life (hr)	Reuptake inhibition		
				Norepinephrine	Serotonin	Dopamine
TRICYCLIC COMPOUNDS						
Imipramine (Tofranil)	Moderate	Moderate	5–20	++	+	0
Desipramine (Norpramin)	Low	Low	12–75	+++	0	0
Trimipramine (Surmontil)	High	High	8–10	+	0	0
Protriptyline (Vivactil)	Low	Moderate	55–125	++	+/−	0
Nortriptyline (Pamelor, Aventil)	Moderate	Low	15–35	++	+	0
Amitriptyline (Elavil)	High	High	20–35	+	++	0
Doxepin (Adapin, Sinequan)	High	High	8–24	++	+	0
SECOND-GENERATION COMPOUNDS						
Amoxapine (Asendin)[b]	Low	Low	8–10	++	0	0
Maprotiline (Ludiomil)	Moderate	Moderate	27–58	++	0	0
Trazodone (Desyrel)	Moderate	Low	6–13	0	++	0
Fluoxetine (Prozac)	None	None	24–96	0	+++	0
Bupropion (Wellbutrin)	None	None	14	+/−	0	++
Sertraline (Zoloft)	None	None	26	0	+++	0
Paroxetine (Paxil)	None	None	24	+	+++	0
Clomipramine (Anafranil)	None	None	19–37	+	+++	0
Venlafaxine (Effexor)	None	None	3–11	++	+++	0
MAO INHIBITORS: IRREVERSIBLE						
Phenelzine (Nardil)	Low	None	2–4[c]	0	0	0
Isocarboxazid (Marplan)	None	None	1–3[c]	0	0	0
Tranylcypromine (Parnate)	None	None	1–3[c]	0	0	0
MAO INHIBITORS: REVERSIBLE						
Moclobemide (NA)[d]	None	Low	1–3[c]	0	0	0
Brofaramine (NA)	None	Low	12–15[c]	0	0	0
Cimoxatone (NA)	None	Low	9–16[c]	0	0	0

[a]Anticholinergic side effects include dry mouth, blurred vision, tachycardia, urinary retention, and constipation. [b]Also has antipsychotic effects due to blockage of dopamine receptors (Chapter 7). [c]Half-life does not correlate with clinical effect (see text). [d]Trade name not available; not available for use in the United States.
0 = no effect; + = mild effect; ++ = moderate effect; +++ = strong effect.

elderly appear to be somewhat more susceptible to the anticholinergic-induced impairment of memory, although such impairments are "mild and are not similar to those of Alzheimer's patients."[20]

In contrast to these direct effects, relief from depression indirectly improves attention, cognition, and memory.[21] This will be elaborated upon in the discussion of second-generation antidepressants.

Peripheral Nervous System   The TCAs exert a variety of effects on the peripheral nervous system (Tables 8.2 and 8.4; summary in Table 8.3). Here, the effects of TCAs on the heart deserve special mention, since there is both cardiac depression and increased electrical irritability (as evidenced by cardiac arrhythmias). Cardiac depression can be life threatening when an overdose is taken, as in suicide attempts. In such a situation, the patient commonly exhibits excitement, delirium, and convulsions, followed by respiratory depression and coma, which can persist for several days. Cardiac arrhythmias can lead to ventricular fibrillation, cardiac arrest, and death. These arrhythmias are extremely difficult to treat. Thus all TCAs can be lethal in doses that are commonly available to depressed patients. For this reason, "it is unwise to dispense more than a week's supply of an antidepressant to an acutely depressed patient."[5]

Pharmacokinetics

The TCAs are well absorbed when they are administered orally. Because most of them have relatively long half-lives (Table 8.4), they should only be taken once a day at bedtime to minimize unwanted side effects, especially the persistent sedation. The TCAs are metabolized in the liver, and as discussed above, two TCAs are converted into pharmacologically active intermediates that are detoxified later (Figure 8.3). This combination of a pharmacologically active drug and active metabolite results in a clinical effect lasting up to 4 days and even longer in elderly patients.

Drug Administration

The initial treatment period is usually 4 to 8 weeks, which is necessary to make a reasonable evaluation of the patient. Excessive sedation can occur during the first few weeks of therapy, and this effect can reduce patient compliance. Thus if the treatment is ineffective, patients should be evaluated to determine whether the drug was ineffective or not taken. Here therapeutic monitoring (by determining blood levels of drug) is useful.

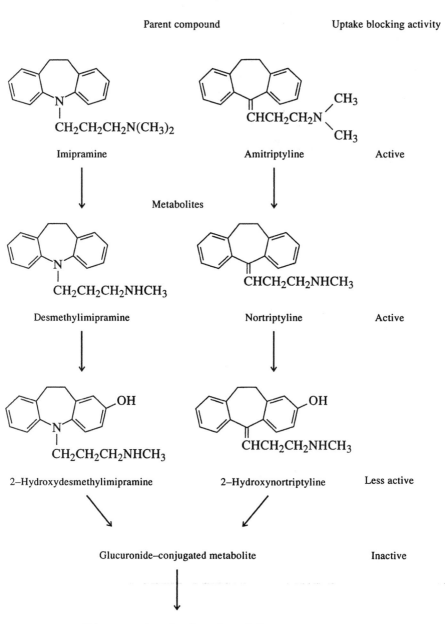

FIGURE 8.3 Metabolism of imipramine and amitriptyline. Note that the two active intermediates are marketed clinically.

For patients undergoing long-term therapy, continuous administration of low doses is usually preferred. Therapy usually continues for
at least 4 to 5 months after the initial clinical response. At this point
the dosage may be reduced or discontinued completely. If signs of relapse are observed, the initial dosage should be reinstituted. In elderly
patients, drugs with short half-lives and inactive metabolites should be
used (see Table 8.4). In addition, elderly patients should be administered markedly reduced dosages and be closely supervised. Elderly patients who have cardiac disease are especially susceptible to serious
side effects.

Drug interactions involving the TCAs are commonplace and potentially serious. These drugs markedly potentiate the effects of alcohol,
and deaths have resulted from drinking a normally harmless amount
of alcohol. Other dangerous interactions involve TCAs and drugs used
to treat high blood pressure, arthritis, epilepsy, and parkinsonism.
Awareness of these problems and close monitoring of the patient are
essential.

Therapeutically, major depression is a primary indication for prescribing TCAs. TCAs are also effective in treating children who experience enuresis (bed-wetting); they have also been tried in patients who
have other problems, including anorexia nervosa, bulimia, obsessive-
compulsive disorders, panic disorder, chronic pain, migraine headaches, post-traumatic stress disorder, and even peptic ulcer disease
(from the blockade of histamine$_1$ receptors).[22]

Second-Generation (Atypical) Antidepressants

As noted, in the 1980s it was hoped that structurally different agents
might overcome some of the disadvantages of the TCAs (slow onset of
action, limited efficacy, and significant side effects). Early efforts (late
1970s to mid-1980s) produced the so-called *second-generation* or
atypical antidepressants. Their pharmacokinetic data and a comparison with standard TCAs are listed in Tables 8.4 and 8.5, respectively.
Further efforts produced the serotonin-specific reuptake inhibitors
(SSRIs), which are described later.

The Non-SSRIs

Maprotiline (Ludiomil) was one of the first clinically available antidepressants that modified the basic tricyclic structure (Figure 8.1). It
has a long half-life, blocks norepinephrine uptake, and is as efficacious
as imipramine (the "gold standard" of tricyclic antidepressants).
However, it offers few, if any, therapeutic advantages. A major limita-

TABLE 8.5 Advantages and disadvantages of second-generation antidepressants compared to tricyclic antidepressants.

Drug	Advantages	Disadvantages
Maprotiline	Sedating and may be useful for agitation Does not antagonize anti-hypertensive effects of clonidine	Increased incidence of seizures Increased lethality in overdose Has long half-life, therefore accumulates Increased incidence of rashes
Amoxapine	Low in sedative effects Low in anticholinergic effects Possibly effective for monotherapy for psychotic depression Has possible rapid onset	Can promote parkinsonian side effects and tardive dyskinesia Cannot separate antidepressant from "antipsychotic" effect Increased lethality in overdose
Trazodone	Relatively safe in overdose Sedating (may be useful in controlling agitation and hostility in geriatric patients) Useful as a hypnotic in conjunction with MAO inhibitors	Efficacy not clearly established May induce or exacerbate ventricular arrhythmia Can promote priapism
Fluoxetine	Low in sedative, anticholinergic, and hypotensive side effects Does not promote weight gain, maybe helps weight loss No prolonging of cardiac conduction Effective in obsessive-compulsive disorders	Causes anxiety, nausea, and insomnia Has long half-life, therefore accumulates Unknown efficacy in panic Possibly has indirect dopamine blocking effects Has pharmacokinetic interactions with tricyclics and benzodiazepines
Bupropion	Low in sedative, hypotensive, and anticholinergic side effects Does not promote weight gain Lack of ECG changes	Tends to "overstimulate," with insomnia, terror Not effective for panic; unknown effectiveness for obsessive-compulsive disorders Increased incidence of seizures in bulimia May induce perceptual abnormalities and psychosis Causes increase in prolactin

tion of maprotiline is that it tends (albeit rarely) to cause seizures, presumably due to the accumulation of active metabolites. Allain and coworkers[23] reported that maprotiline did not cause deterioration in cognitive functions.

Amoxapine (Asendin) was another early antidepressant agent that was structurally different from the tricyclics. It is as effective as imipramine, although amoxapine may be slightly more effective in relieving anxiety and agitation. Amoxapine exhibits a high incidence of serious parkinsonianlike, neuroleptic side effects (it blocks dopamine receptors), sometimes even after therapy has stopped. Amoxapine can be lethal when an overdose is taken. It has been used in closely monitored patients who suffer from panic disorder.[24]

Trazodone (Desyrel) is yet another chemically unique antidepressant. It is as therapeutically efficacious as the TCAs.[25] Its mechanism of antidepressant action is unclear because it is not a potent reuptake blocker of either norepinephrine or serotonin. However, it does block a subclass of serotonin receptors (the serotonin$_2$ receptor), and it appears to "down-regulate either the norepinephrine or serotonin receptors."[26] Trazodone has a short onset of action ($^1/_2$ to 1 week), but 2 to 5 weeks are still required to produce an optimal effect. Drowsiness, its most common side effect, occurs in about 20 percent of all patients. In rare instances, priapism (prolonged and painful penile erections) limits its use in males. The effect of trazodone on cognitive functions is controversial; one report indicated sedation and psychomotor impairments,[27] while another report noted no detriment in depressed patients' cognitive skills.[28]

Bupropion (Wellbutrin) was withheld from distribution for several years because of serious side effects. It is now available as an antidepressant that is sometimes effective in depressed individuals who do not respond to other agents. Bupropion differs from the other antidepressants in that it selectively inhibits dopamine reuptake (a cocainelike action), but it does not seem to exert a reinforcing action in animals. Although bupropion is effective in treating depression, it is not effective in treating panic disorders. Because of its potentiation of dopamine, it has been successfully used to treat children with attention deficit disorders.[29] Side effects of bupropion include behavioral stimulation, anxiety, restlessness, tremor, and insomnia. Its potential for compulsive abuse is unclear because the drug may resemble the behavioral stimulants more than it resembles the antidepressants. More serious side effects include the induction of psychosis de novo and generalized seizures. A recent report noted that patients suffering sexual dysfunction as a side effect of fluoxetine (discussed below) may recover their capacity for orgasm and feel greater sexual satisfaction without becoming depressed again if they are switched to bupropion.[30]

The SSRIs

As discussed earlier, there is correlation between diminished serotonin neurotransmission and episodes of major depression. This fact suggests that drugs potentiating serotonin neurotransmission by inhibiting its active presynaptic reuptake may be clinically useful in treating major depression. This assumes, of course, that a cause-and-effect relationship exists and that the correlation is not just coincidental.

Today, five SSRIs are clinically available for use in treating major depression (see Figure 8.1). Others are likely to follow as other pharmaceutical manufacturers enter the marketplace. The five drugs include (in descending order of selectivity) sertraline, paroxetine, fluoxetine, clomipramine, and venlafaxine.

Fluoxetine (Prozac), which became clinically available in the United States in 1988 as the first SSRI, has now become the most widely prescribed of all the antidepressant drugs. Fluoxetine is the first second-generation antidepressant to be considered a first-to-be-prescribed antidepressant (not just for patients who have failed other drug therapy), particularly for patients who do not have severe depression. Its efficacy is comparable to that of the TCAs, but its side effects are fewer; in particular, it does not cause serious cardiac problems in overdosage.

Fluoxetine has a long half-life (1 to 4 days), and its active metabolite (norfluoxetine) has a half-life of about 1 to 3 weeks. The antidepressant action thus tends to build with repeated doses over time, presumably because the blood levels of both the parent compound and its active metabolite continue to build. Indeed, it takes many weeks to reach steady-state levels of drug and active metabolite in the blood. This may at least partially explain the slow onset of both peak therapeutic effect and the late onset of side effects with the drug. With time, doses are stabilized at a low daily level. As a result of the long half-lives of fluoxetine and norfluoxetine, a 5-week drugfree interval is recommended between cessation of fluoxetine administration and the initiation of another drug therapy.

The relation between the clinical effects, blood levels, and daily doses of fluoxetine is still unclear.

Fluoxetine is also used to treat persons who suffer from obsessive-compulsive disorder.[31-33] Although we are still uncertain about the neurochemistry of depression, obsessive-compulsive disorder appears to involve a dysfunction of the neurotransmission of serotonin.[34,35] Indeed, the mainstay of pharmacological treatment of persons who suffer from obsessive-compulsive disorder continues to be antidepressant drugs that block serotonin reuptake, especially fluoxetine and clomipramine (discussed below).

In addition, fluoxetine in very low doses has been effective in treating patients who experience panic disorder;[36,37] the drug is administered either alone or in combination with the benzodiazepine derivative alprazolam (Xanax).[34,38] This application is particularly useful in individuals who either are depressed or have experienced undesirable weight gain on other drugs. Side effects, which can include worsening of the attacks or the precipitation of mania, must be considered. It is important to keep dosage as low as possible and to rapidly remove nonresponders from therapy with the drug.

As discussed in Chapter 6, the long-term pharmacological treatment of obesity has, until recently, been disappointing. Now two pharmacological approaches are showing excellent results as adjuvant therapy to nonpharmacological interventions. First is the combination of fenfluramine and phentermine, discussed in Chapter 6. Second is the use of SSRIs to produce satiety, reduce caloric intake, and assist with weight loss.

In 1987 researchers at the Lilly Research Laboratories first demonstrated the efficacy and safety of fluoxetine in treating obesity.[39] Several studies since then have confirmed this observation, demonstrating that fluoxetine reduces eating binges in nondepressed, obese individuals, and that this reduced food intake accounts for the weight loss that follows use of the drug.[40–43]

Finally, fluoxetine and other serotonin-potentiating antidepressants appear to be modestly effective in reducing alcohol consumption in heavy drinkers, which suggests an innovative approach to moderating the alcohol intake of problem drinkers.[44–47] More recent data, however, question the usefulness of this effect, since the observed 14 percent reduction in alcohol intake occurred only in the first week, with no significant effects in later weeks.[48] Chapter 5 discusses in more detail drugs used to treat alcoholism.

A recent article in *Newsweek* discussed unapproved uses of Prozac (fluoxetine) for treating multiple disorders, such as mood swings, speaker's anxiety, premenstrual syndrome, and others.[49] Today Prozac has probably attained the popularity that Librium and Valium attained in the 1960s.

Side effects of fluoxetine include nervousness, anxiety, sexual dysfunction, insomnia, nausea, loss of appetite, motor restlessness, and muscle rigidity. How therapeutically limiting these side effects are is still being evaluated. It is generally agreed that fluoxetine does not adversely affect memory and cognition.[28] Indeed, fluoxetine and other SSRIs may relieve memory disorders resulting from depression or alcohol abuse.[18]

Sertraline (Zoloft) was the second SSRI approved for clinical use in the United States. It is at least as effective as TCAs in patients with moderate to severe depression, even in patients with coexisting disorders. It is quite effective and well tolerated in the elderly.

Sertraline is about 4 to 5 times more potent than fluoxetine in blocking serotonin reuptake and is more selective. Importantly, steady-state levels of the drug in plasma are achieved within 5 to 7 days, and its metabolites are less cumulative and less pharmacologically active. Sertraline may also be useful in treating obsessive-compulsive disorder, comparable in efficacy to other SSRIs. "[Sertraline] has significantly fewer anticholinergic, antihistaminic, and cardiovascular adverse effects than the TCAs; as well as a low risk of toxicity in overdose."[50]

Paroxetine (Paxil) was the third SSRI available for clinical use in treating depression. Therapeutically, it is comparable to the TCAs in efficacy, being clearly superior to placebo. Paroxetine is effective "in the presence or absence of anxiety, agitation, retardation, and reactive and endogenous features. . . . [It] is highly effective in reducing anxiety, a common symptom in depressive illness."[25]

Like sertraline, paroxetine is more selective than fluoxetine in blocking serotonin reuptake. Also, paroxetine's metabolites are relatively inactive, and steady state is achieved within about 7 days. The metabolic half-life is about 24 hours. A recent symposium edited by Boyer and Feighner is devoted solely to the use of paroxetine as an antidepressant.[51]

Clomipramine (Anafranil), long used in Europe and Canada to treat obsessive-compulsive disorder, was introduced in the United States in 1990 for this purpose. About 40 to 75 percent of patients with obsessive-compulsive disorder respond favorably but are seldom completely cured. Behavioral therapy helps maximize the response. The drug has also been used around the world in the treatment of depression, panic disorder, and phobic disorders. Clomipramine appears to be about equal to the TCAs in both its efficacy and its profile of side effects. It is one of the most selective inhibitors of serotonin reuptake.

In 1994, *venlafaxine* (Effexor) was introduced as the fifth antidepressant that is thought to exert its effect by blockading active serotonin reuptake. Structurally dissimilar to other antidepressants (see Figure 8.1), it also blocks the active reuptake of norepinephrine, with little effect on dopamine reuptake.[52] It has little or no activity at cholinergic, histamine, or adrenergic receptors, and it does not inhibit monoamine oxidase enzyme. Effects on cardiac conduction are minimal.[53] Thus, side effects are expected to be low, although this fact remains to be demonstrated. The primary metabolite of venlafaxine is pharmacologically active; the secondary metabolites are less so. The half-lives of the parent compound and the primary metabolite are 3 to 5 hours and 9 to 11 hours, respectively. Its clinical effectiveness compares favorably with that of other SSRIs. One study reports that venlafaxine produces improvements in psychomotor and cognitive function,[54] likely due to the relief of depression and the absence of sedation and anticholinergic effect.

In 1995 *fluvoxamine*[55] (Luvox), a structural derivative of fluoxetine, became available in the United States for the treatment of obsessive compulsive disorder. Other SSRI agents, including citalopram, will likely be introduced for the treatment and preventive maintenance of major depression, panic disorder, and OCD.[34]

Monoamine Oxidase Inhibitors

The traditional monoamine oxidase (MAO) inhibitors have long been considered alternative drugs for treating major depressive illnesses; their limitations include their serious side effects and their limited efficacy. Introduced during the late 1950s, they have a checkered and controversial history. Soon after their introduction, they were noted to have serious, frequently fatal interactions with certain foods and medicines. The latter included adrenalinelike drugs found in nasal sprays, antiasthma medications, cold medicines, cocaine, and so on. Foods included those that contain tyramine, a by-product of fermentation; among such foods are many cheeses, wines, beers, liver, and some beans. As a result of the interaction, blood pressure increases severely, occasionally enough to be fatal. Thus, for about 20 years these drugs were considered dangerous. However, with strict dietary restrictions, they can be used safely. Today these drugs are experiencing a resurgence in use for several reasons.

1. With appropriate dietary restrictions, they can be as safe or safer than TCAs.

2. They can work in many patients who respond poorly to both TCAs and SSRIs.

3. They may be the drugs of choice for atypical depression, which presents primarily with anxiety and phobic symptoms, masked depression (such as hypochondriasis), anorexia nervosa, and bulimia.

Monoamine oxidase (MAO) is an enzyme that breaks down normal neurotransmitters in the body, including norepinephrine and serotonin (Appendix II). There are two types of the enzyme: MAO-A (here, the "good" MAO) is found in norepinephrine and serotonin nerve terminals. MAO-B (here, the "bad" MAO) is found in dopamine-secreting neurons. Pharmacologically, drug-induced inhibition of MAO-A is presumably responsible for the antidepressant activity, while inhibition of MAO-B is responsible for side effects, including the serious drug interactions discussed above.

Drug-induced blockade of MAO (especially MAO-A) allows large amounts of transmitters to accumulate in the nerve terminals. As a result, more transmitter is released when the neurons are stimulated. Three MAO inhibitors have been available for many years, and all three are both nonselective and irreversible in their inhibition of both MAO-A and MAO-B. Short-acting, reversible MAO-A inhibitors are newer and as yet clinically unavailable.

Irreversible MAO Inhibitors

The three MAO inhibitors currently available (phenelzine, tranylcypromine, and isocarboxazid) all block both MAO-A and MAO-B irreversibly. Irreversible effects are unusual in pharmacology; most drugs discussed to this point exert reversible actions, usually by competing for receptors with naturally occurring neurotransmitters. The irreversible MAO inhibitors form a chemical bond with part of the MAO enzyme, a bond that cannot be broken; enzyme function returns only as new enzyme is biosynthesized.

Pharmacokinetics and Mechanism of Action   As shown in Table 8.4, the elimination half-life of tranylcypromine is about 2 hours. This rapid rate of elimination results in a rapid decline in plasma levels of the drug (Figure 8.4A) but not in the degree of MAO inhibition (Figure 8.4B). The reason for this lack of correlation is that after tranylcypromine is absorbed, it is metabolized to a reactive intermediate compound. This compound then binds irreversibly with MAO-A and MAO-B in a tight covalent bond. Excess drug that is not converted to the intermediate compound is rapidly metabolized and then excreted.[56] This course of events is illustrated in Figure 8.4B. Here, the upper graph reflects the rapid rise and fall in the blood (plasma) levels of tranylcypromine given orally 3 times a day for 7 days. There is little drug accumulation because the liver rapidly metabolizes the drug. The irreversible inhibition of MAO occurs slowly; a level of 70 percent inhibition is reached by day 7. After the patient stops taking the drug, MAO activity returns very slowly, reflecting the synthesis of new, biologically active enzyme.

Efficacy   The nonselective, irreversible MAO inhibitors were the first clinically effective drugs for treating major depression, preceding the TCAs by about 10 years. Their fall from favor was not from lack of

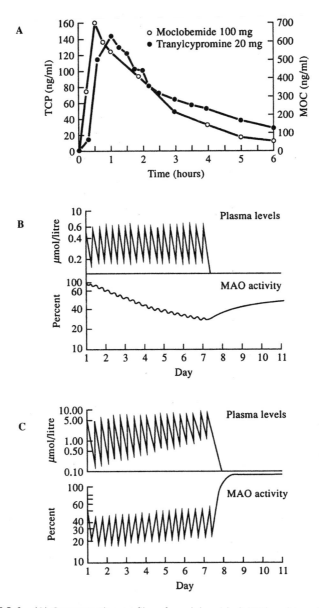

FIGURE 8.4 (**A**) Concentration profiles of moclobemide (MOC) and tranylcypromine (TCP) after an oral dose. (**B**) Tranylcypromine (10 mg three times a day) plasma levels and MAO activity. (**C**) Moclobemide (150 mg three times a day) plasma levels and MAO activity. [From R. Amrien and others.[56]]

efficacy but from fear of adverse reactions. Indeed, their efficacy seems to be comparable to that of the TCAs. Importantly, MAO inhibitors can be effective in patients in whom therapy with TCAs and SSRIs has failed. Therefore, when administered with dietary counseling, these drugs can be used relatively safely. Needed, however, are reversible MAO inhibitors with shorter durations of clinical action and an increased margin of safety.

Reversible MAO-A Inhibitors

Several short-acting, selective, reversible MAO inhibitors have been developed, but they have not yet been released for clinical use. The one that has been best studied is *moclobemide*. This agent, and others also under study, are highly selective in their ability to reversibly inhibit MAO-A. Thus, they are much safer than the irreversible MAO inhibitors, having minimal interaction with the tyramine in food.[57]

These agents are as effective as the TCAs, with more rapid onset of antidepressant action and fewer side effects. If these promising early results are maintained, these drugs may become treatments for depression.

Figure 8.4 demonstrates that the half-lives and plasma decay curves of moclobemide and tranylcypromine are virtually identical. With moclobemide (administered orally 3 times a day for 7 days), however, the inhibition of MAO is correlated with the plasma concentration of the drug (Figure 8.4C). With each dose, MAO activity fell and then returned as the drug was metabolized and its plasma level fell. When therapy ended, MAO activity rapidly returned to normal. This pattern is like that of most drugs; unlike tranylcypromine, moclobemide does not form an irreversible, covalent bond. Figure 8.4C shows that MAO inhibition is at a maximum after just one dose of moclobemide. Drug effects can be controlled easily, plasma concentration parallels pharmacological effects, and the effect has a short duration with no aftereffects. Because of the specificity of enzyme blockade (MAO-A), side effects are minimal.

Allain and coworkers[23] reported that moclobemide not only caused no deterioration in cognitive functions but also appeared to improve vigilance, attention, and some crucial components of memory. These improvements may be related to inhibition of MAO-A as well as to the lack of any anticholinergic action.

In conclusion, the newer, selective, reversible MAO-A inhibitors offer distinct advantages over the older agents. Presumably clinical usefulness and tolerability will be increased. Indeed, one author has referred to these agents as the "gentle MAO inhibitors."[57]

Study Questions

1. Differentiate between major depressive disorder and bipolar disorder.
2. What is the correlation between depression and the biological amine transmitters in the brain?
3. Differentiate cocaine and the amphetamines from clinical antidepressants.
4. What might account for the 2- to 3-week therapeutic delay that occurs when a patient takes a tricyclic antidepressant?
5. Compare and contrast imipramine and fluoxetine.
6. Discuss what happens when a patient overdoses on a tricyclic antidepressant. Identify the patients who are at risk, the dose of the drug, the side effects, and the treatment.
7. How does MAO inhibition result in antidepressant activity?
8. Compare and contrast tranylcypromine and moclobemide.
9. What is the presynaptic serotonin transporter? How is this related to antidepressant drug action?

Notes

1. American Medical Association, "Drugs Used in Mood Disorders," in *Drug Evaluations, Annual 1994* (Milwaukee, Wis.: American Medical Association, 1993), pp. 287–318.
2. U.S. Congress, Office of Technology Assessment, *The Biology of Mental Disorders*, OTA-BA-538 (Washington, D.C.: U.S. Government Printing Office, September 1992), pp. 8, 56.
3. E. Richelson, "Treatment of Acute Depression," *The Psychiatric Clinics of North America* 16 (September 1993): 462.
4. H. P. Rang and M. M. Dale, "Drugs Used in Affective Disorders," in H. P. Rang and M. M. Dale, eds., *Pharmacology*, 2nd ed. (Edinburgh: Churchill Livingstone, 1991), pp. 660–665.
5. R. J. Baldessarini, "Drugs and the Treatment of Psychiatric Disorders," in A. G. Gilman, T. W. Rall, A. S. Nies, and P. Taylor, eds., *Goodman and Gilman's The Pharmacological Basis of Therapeutics*, 8th ed. (New York: Pergamon, 1990), p. 408.
6. P. G. Janicak, J. M. Davis, S. H. Preskorn, and F. J. Ayd, Jr., *Principles and Practice of Psychopharmacotherapy* (Baltimore: Williams & Wilkins, 1993), pp. 211–219.
7. S. M. Paul, "Introduction: Serotonin and Its Effects on Human Behavior," *Journal of Clinical Psychiatry* 51, no. 4, suppl. (April 1990): 3.
8. M. A. Harrington, P. Zhong, S. J. Garlow, and R. D. Ciaranello, "Molecular Biology of Serotonin Receptors," *Journal of Clinical Psychiatry* 53, suppl. (October 1992): 8–27.
9. P. Blier, C. de Montigny, and Y. Chaput, "A Role for the Serotonin System in the Mechanism of Action of Antidepressant Treatments: Preclinical Evidence," *Journal of Clinical Psychiatry* 51, no. 4, suppl. (April 1990):

14–21.

10. R. D. Blakely, H. E. Berson, R. T. Fremeau, Jr., M. G. Caron, M. M. Peek, H. K. Prince, and C. C. Bradley, "Cloning and Expression of a Functional Serotonin Transporter from Rat Brain," *Nature* 354 (1991): 66–70.

11. B. J. Hoffman, E. Mezey, and M. J. Brownstein, "Cloning of a Serotonin Transporter Affected by Antidepressants," *Science* 254 (1991): 579–580.

12. D. R. Cool, F. H. Leibach, V. K. Bhalla, V. B. Mahesh, and V. Ganapathy, "Expression and Cyclic AMP-Dependent Regulation of a High Affinity Serotonin Transporter in the Human Placental Choriocarcinoma Cell Line (JAR)," *Journal of Biological Chemistry* 266 (1991): 15750–15757.

13. S. C. King, A. A. Tiller, A. S. Chang, and D. M. Lam, "Differential Regulation of the Imipramine-Sensitive Serotonin Transporter by cAMP in Human JAR Choriocarcinoma Cells, Rat PC12 Pheochromocytoma Cells, and C33-14-B1 Transgenic Mouse Fibroblast Cells," *Biochemical & Biophysical Research Communications* 183 (1992): 487–491.

14. S. C. Risch and C. B. Nemeroff, "Neurochemical Alterations of Serotonergic Neuronal Systems in Depression," *Journal of Clinical Psychiatry* 53, suppl. (October 1992): 3–7.

15. S. Ramamoorthy, A. L. Bauman, K. R. Moore, H. Han, T. Yang-Feng, A. S. Chang, V. Ganapathy, and R. D. Blakely, "Antidepressant- and Cocaine-Sensitive Human Serotonin Transporter: Molecular Cloning, Expression, and Chromosomal Localization," *Proceedings of the National Academy of Sciences USA* 90 (1993): 2542–2546.

16. E. C. Azmitia and P. M. Whitaker-Azmitia, "Awakening the Sleeping Giant: Anatomy and Plasticity of the Brain Serotonergic System," *Journal of Clinical Psychiatry* 52, suppl. (December 1991): 4–16.

17. T. C. Cantu, J. S. Korek, and A. J. Romanoski, "Focus on Venlafaxine: A New Option for the Treatment of Depression," *Hospital Formulary* 29 (1994): 25–33.

18. J. M. Danion, "Antidepresseurs et Memoire," *Encephale* 19, spec. no. 2 (July 1993): 417–422.

19. H. V. Curran, M. Sakulsriprong, and M. Lader, "Antidepressants and Human Memory: An Investigation of Four Drugs with Different Sedative and Anticholinergic Profiles," *Psychopharmacology* 95 (1988): 520–527.

20. B. A. Marcopulos and R. E. Graves, "Antidepressant Effect on Memory in Depressed Older Persons," *Journal of Clinical and Experimental Neuropsychology* 12 (1990): 655–663.

21. B. Spring, A. J. Gelenberg, R. Garvin, and S. Thompson, "Amitriptyline, Clovoxamine and Cognitive Function: A Placebo-Controlled Comparison in Depressed Outpatients," *Psychopharmacology* 108 (1992): 327–332.

22. P. J. Orsulak and D. Waller, "Antidepressant Drugs: Additional Clinical Uses," *Journal of Family Practice* 28 (1989): 209–216.

23. H. Allain, A. Liery, F. Brunet-Bourgin, C. Mirabaud, P. Trebon, F. LeCoz, and J. M. Gandon, "Antidepressants and Cognition: Comparative Effects of Moclobemide, Viloxazine, and Maprotiline," *Psychopharmacology* 106, suppl. (1992): S56–S61.

24. D. D. Gold, "Management of Panic Disorder: Case Reports Support a

Potential Role for Amoxapine," *Hospital Formulary* 25 (1990): 1178–1184.

25. Janicak, Davis, Preskorn, and Ayd, *Principles and Practice of Psychopharmacotherapy*, pp. 230–232.

26. J. A. Roth, "Antidepressants—Drugs Used in the Treatment of Mood Disorders," in C. M. Smith and A. M. Reynard, eds., *Textbook of Pharmacology* (Philadelphia: Saunders, 1992), p. 317.

27. M. Sakulsripong, H. V. Curran, and M. Lader, "Does Tolerance Develop to the Sedative and Amnesic Effects of Antidepressants? A Comparison of Amitriptyline, Trazodone and Placebo," *European Journal of Clinical Pharmacology* 40 (1991): 43–48.

28. J. L. Fudge, P. J. Perry, M. J. Garvey, and M. W. Kelly, "A Comparison of the Effect of Fluoxetine and Trazodone on the Cognitive Functioning of Depressed Outpatients," *Journal of Affective Disorders* 18 (1990): 275–280.

29. C. D. Casat, D. Z. Pleasants, D. H. Schroeder, and D. W. Parler, "Bupropion in Children with Attention-Deficit Disorder," *Psychopharmacology Bulletin* 25 (1989): 198–201.

30. W. Parks and others, "Improvement in Fluoxetine-Associated Sexual Dysfunction in Patients Switched to Bupropion," *Journal of Clinical Psychiatry* 54 (1993): 459–465.

31. M. A. Jenike, "Drug Treatment of Obsessive-Compulsive Disorder," in M. A. Jenike, L. Baer, and W. E. Minichiello, eds., *Obsessive-Compulsive Disorders: Theory and Management*, 2nd ed. (Chicago: Year Book Medical Publishers, 1990), pp. 249–265.

32. M. A. Jenike, I. Baer, and J. H. Greist, "Clomipramine versus Fluoxetine in Obsessive-Compulsive Disorder: A Retrospective Comparison of Side Effects and Efficacy," *Journal of Clinical Psychopharmacology* 10 (1990): 122–124.

33. R. A. Dominguez, "Serotonergic Antidepressants and Their Efficacy in Obsessive Compulsive Disorder," *Journal of Clinical Psychiatry* 53, suppl. (October 1992): 56–59.

34. D. L. Murphy and T. A. Pigott, "A Comparative Examination of a Role for Serotonin in Obsessive-Compulsive Disorder, Panic Disorder, and Anxiety," *The Journal of Clinical Psychiatry* 51, no. 4, suppl. (April 1990): 53–59.

35. J. H. Greist, J. W. Jefferson, K. A. Kobak, D. J. Katzelnick, and R. C. Serlin, "Efficacy and Tolerability of Serotonin Transport Inhibitors in Obsessive Compulsive Disorder," *Archives of General Psychiatry* 52 (1995): 53–60.

36. L. Solyom, C. Solyom, and B. Ledwidge, "Fluoxetine in Panic Disorder," *Canadian Journal of Psychiatry* 36 (1991): 378–380.

37. F. R. Schneier, M. R. Liebowitz, S. O. Davies, J. Fairbanks, E. Hollander, R. Campeas, and D. F. Klein, "Fluoxetine in Panic Disorder," *Journal of Clinical Psychopharmacology* 10 (1990): 119–121.

38. J. C. Ballenger, G. Burrows, R. DuPont, I. M. Lesser, R. Noyes, J. Pecknold, A. Rifkin, and R. Swinson, "Alprazolam in Panic Disorder and Agoraphobia: Results from a Multicenter Trial. I: Efficacy in Short Term Treatment," in J. C. Ballenger, ed., *Clinical Aspects of Panic Disorder, Frontiers in Clinical Neuroscience*, vol. 9 (New York: Wiley, 1990), pp.

219–237.

39. L. R. Levine, S. Rosenblatt, and J. Bosomworth, "Use of a Serotonin Re-uptake Inhibitor, Fluoxetine, in the Treatment of Obesity," *International Journal of Obesity* 11, Suppl. 3 (1987): 185–190.

40. S. D. Wise, "Clinical Studies with Fluoxetine in Obesity," *American Journal of Clinical Nutrition* 55, Suppl. 1 (1992): 181S–184S.

41. H. Pijl, H. P. Koppeschaar, F. L. Willekens, I. Op-de-Kamp, H. D. Veldhuis, and A. E. Meinders, "Effect of Serotonin Re-uptake Inhibition by Fluoxetine on Body Weight and Spontaneous Food Choice in Obesity," *International Journal of Obesity* 15 (1991): 237–242.

42. J. McGuirk and T. Silverstone, "The Effect of the 5-HT Reuptake Inhibitor Fluoxetine on Food Intake and Body Weight in Healthy Male Subjects," *International Journal of Obesity* 14 (1990): 361–372.

43. M. D. Marcus, R. R. Wing, L. Ewing, E. Kern, M. McDermott, and W. Gooding, "A Double-Blind, Placebo-Controlled Trial of Fluoxetine plus Behavior Modification in the Treatment of Obese Binge-Eaters and Non-Binge Eaters," *American Journal of Psychiatry* 147 (1990): 876–881.

44. C. A. Niranjo and E. M. Sellers, "Serotonin Uptake Inhibitors Attenuate Ethanol Intake in Problem Drinkers," *Recent Developments in Alcoholism* 7 (1989): 255–266.

45. K. Gill and Z. Amit, "Serotonin Uptake Blockers and Voluntary Alcohol Consumption. A Review of Recent Studies," *Recent Developments in Alcoholism* 7 (1989): 225–248.

46. C. A. Naranjo, K. E. Kadlec, P. Sanhueza, R. D. Woodley, and E. M. Sellers, "Fluoxetine Differentially Alters Alcohol Intake and Other Consummatory Behaviors in Problem Drinkers," *Clinical Pharmacology and Therapeutics* 47 (1990): 490–498.

47. D. A. Gorelick, "Serotonin Uptake Blockers and the Treatment of Alco-holism," *Recent Developments in Alcoholism* 7 (1989): 267–281.

48. D. A. Gorelick and A. Paredes, "Effect of Fluoxetine on Alcohol Consump-tion in Male Alcoholics," *Alcoholism, Clinical and Experimental Research* 16 (1992): 261–265.

49. G. Cowley, "The Culture of Prozac," *Newsweek*, February 7, 1994, pp. 41–42.

50. Janicak, Davis, Preskorn, and Ayd, *Principles and Practice of Psycho-pharmacotherapy*, p. 243.

51. W. F. Boyer and J. P. Feighner, "An Overview of Paroxetine," *Journal of Clinical Psychiatry* 53, suppl. (February 1992): 3–6.

52. C. Bolden-Watson and E. Richelson, "Blockade by Newly-Developed Antidepressants of Biogenic Amine Uptake into Rat Brain Synaptosomes," *Life Sciences* 52 (1993): 1023–1029.

53. S. A. Montgomery, "Venlafaxine: A New Dimension in Antidepressant Pharmacotherapy," *Journal of Clinical Psychiatry* 54 (1993): 119–126.

54. B. Saletu, J. Grunberger, P. Anderer, L. Linzmayer, H. V. Semlitsch, and G. Magni, "Pharmacodynamics of Venlafaxine Evaluated by EEG Brain Mapping, Psychometry, and Psychophysiology," *British Journal of Clinical*

Pharmacology 33 (1992): 589–601.

55. D. W. Black, R. Wesner, W. Bowers, and J. Gabel, "A Comparison of Fluvoxamine, Cognitive Therapy, and Placebo in the Treatment of Panic Disorder," *Archives of General Psychiatry* 50 (1993): 44–50.

56. R. Amrien, S. R. Allen, T. W. Guentert, D. Hartmann, T. Lorscheid, M.-P. Schoerlin, and D. Vranesic, "The Pharmacology of Reversible Monoamine Oxidase Inhibitors," *British Journal of Psychiatry* 155, Suppl. 6 (1989): 66–71.

57. R. G. Priest, "Antidepressants of the Future," *British Journal of Psychiatry* 155, Suppl. 6 (1989): 7–8.

CHAPTER 9

PHARMACOTHERAPY OF MOOD DISORDERS: DRUGS FOR TREATING BIPOLAR DISORDER

Bipolar disorder (bipolar depression, manic–depressive syndrome) is characterized by the occurrence of one or more manic episodes which may be interspersed with one or more depressive episodes.[1] The disorder requires therapeutic intervention when the mood changes are severe enough to disrupt the patient's life or the lives of people associated with the patient.

There is considerable evidence for a genetic link in bipolar disorder. This suggests that persons who suffer from this disorder have a biochemical abnormality.[2] Patients who suffer from unipolar depression do not swing into bouts of mania, and little evidence exists to suggest a genetic cause for that condition. Rang and Dale state:

> There is disagreement about whether these two clinical categories represent fundamentally different disorders. One view is that unipolar depression may be either "reactive" in origin or "endogenous," the former being a non-psychotic reaction to distressing circumstances, such as bereavement or poverty, while the latter is, like bipolar depression, the result of a biochemical abnormality within the brain. There is some evidence that these two types of depressive illness respond differently to antidepressant drugs. Some patients suffering from bipolar depression also show symptoms associated with schizophrenia, whereas patients with unipolar depression often show symptoms of anxiety neurosis, so the depressive illnesses appear as a broad continuum stretching from what is probably a fundamental biochemical disturbance to psychological disturbances that are initiated by external events.[2]

A manic episode is a distinct period of behavioral hyperactivity and persistently expansive or irritable mood, during which at least three of the following seven symptoms are present:[1]

   1. inflated self-esteem or grandiosity
   2. decreased need for sleep
   3. unusual talkativeness
   4. flight of ideas or racing thoughts
   5. distractibility
   6. increase in goal-directed activity
   7. excessive involvement in pleasurable activities that have a high potential for negative consequences (buying sprees, sexual indiscretions, foolish investments)

Finally, the mood disturbance is severe enough to impair work and social functioning. When this last criterion is not met, the episode is designated as *hypomania*.

The estimated risk of developing bipolar disorder is 0.5 to 1.0 percent, and is more likely in women than in men. Ninety percent of patients who experience a single manic episode experience one or more recurrences. Thus, bipolar disorder is a chronic, disabling, and even life-threatening disorder.

When first seen, patients with bipolar disorder present in either the manic or the depressive phase; thus accurate diagnosis is important. The depression of bipolar disorder differs from the depression of depressive illness in that the former is more likely to be characterized by hypersomnia, hyperphagia, weight gain, and decreased energy.[1] Occasionally manic and depressive symptoms intermix or cycle rapidly. Underscoring the importance of adequate treatment for bipolar disorder, Janicak, Davis, Preskorn, and Ayd note:

> It is estimated that one of every four or five untreated or inadequately treated patients commit suicide during the course of their illness. Further, an increase in deaths secondary to accidents or intercurrent illnesses contributes to the greater mortality rate seen in this disorder. Unfortunately, recent epidemiological studies have indicated that only one-third of bipolar patients are in active treatment despite the availability of effective therapies.[3]

Treatment of bipolar disorder has two overall goals: the reduction of symptoms and the prevention of relapse. Since the patient can present initially with either mania or depression, reduction of presenting symptoms may require either an antidepressant (for depressive presentation) or an antipsychotic drug (for manic presentation; see Chapter 11). However, successful management of the disorder itself (aside from

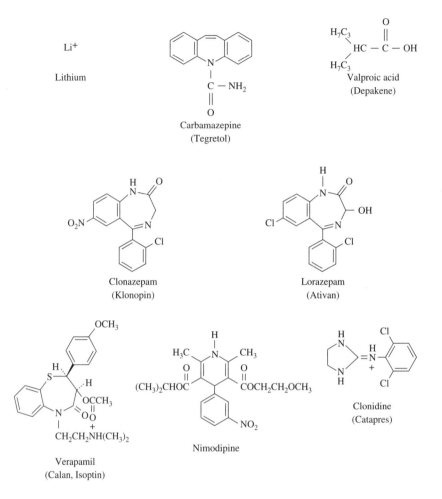

FIGURE 9.1   Drugs used in the treatment of bipolar disorder.

some of the presenting symptoms) is best accomplished by use of a mood stabilizer, especially lithium, the primary drug used to treat this disorder. In refractory cases, either of two alternative drugs (carbamazepine or valproate) can be substituted or added. Other, less-evaluated drugs include the antihypertensive drug clonidine and verapamil, a calcium channel blocker. The clinical description of bipolar disorder and the indications for drug therapy are reviewed by Janicak, Davis, Preskorn, and Ayd.[4] The chemical structures of the most used mood-stabilizing drugs are given in Figure 9.1.

Lithium

Lithium (Li⁺) is the lightest of the alkali metals (see Figure 9.1).[5] It is considered to be effective in treating 60 to 80 percent of all acute hypomanic and manic episodes.[6] Lithium is used both for treating acute mania and for maintenance therapy. Some data suggest that it is effective in treating other disorders as well, especially in augmenting antidepressant drug therapy for patients whose depression resists treatment.[7,8] Other postulated uses of lithium include treatment of obsessive-compulsive syndrome, therapy supplemental to antipsychotic medications in certain schizophrenic patients, and a possible treatment for certain types of alcoholics.[9]

History

Lithium was used in the 1920s as a sedative-hypnotic compound and as an anticonvulsant drug. During the late 1940s, lithium chloride was employed as a salt substitute for patients with heart disease. This use resulted in cases of severe toxicity and death. At about the same time, however, an Australian scientist (J. Cade) noted that when lithium was administered to guinea pigs, the animals became lethargic. Taking an intuitive leap, he administered lithium to manic patients with spectacular results. However, because of the earlier problems with lithium as a salt substitute, the medical community took longer than 20 years to accept this agent as an effective treatment for mania. It was not until the late 1960s that lithium was introduced into the United States by S. Gershon for the treatment of bipolar disorder. Today, lithium is still considered to be the standard therapy for bipolar disorder, although its limitations are recognized and alternative medications are now available.

Pharmacokinetics

Lithium is absorbed rapidly and completely when it is administered orally. Peak blood levels are reached within 1 to 3 hours, with complete absorption by 8 hours. Its therapeutic efficacy is directly correlated to its level in the blood.

Lithium crosses the blood–brain barrier slowly and incompletely; its concentration in cerebral spinal fluid only reaches about 50 percent of that in plasma. Lithium is excreted by the kidneys in two phases: About half of an oral dose is excreted within 18 to 24 hours, and the rest (which represents the amount of lithium that is taken up by cells) is excreted over the next 1 to 2 weeks. Thus, when therapy is initiated, lithium accumulates slowly over about 2 weeks until a steady state (or plateau) is reached.

The therapeutic dose of lithium is determined by closely monitoring blood levels of the drug. Indeed, lithium has a very narrow "therapeutic window," below which the drug fails to have therapeutic effect and above which side effects and toxicity dominate. Older reports and even modern textbooks[10,11] claim that a therapeutic effect is achieved at 0.8 to 1.4 milliequivalents per liter of blood, with serum toxicity at levels above 2 milliequivalents per liter. After the acute manic episode is controlled, blood levels between 0.6 and 0.8 milliequivalents per liter may be satisfactory for many patients:

> Patients who are doing well at levels of 0.8 to 1.0 mEq/L can probably stay at these levels, but if side effects are troublesome, the levels should be reduced to 0.6 to 0.8 mEq/L. Ideally, all patients should be maintained at the lowest effective blood level. Unfortunately, it is not possible to predict this level in advance. In view of these recent findings, it may make more sense to err in the direction of too high a level rather than too low.[9]

DiGregorio states that the "therapeutic serum level ranges from 0.4 to 1.0 meq per liter."[12]

Lithium, being an inorganic ion, is not metabolized in the body. Rather, it is excreted unchanged in the urine. About 80 percent of the amount of lithium filtered by the glomeruli into the renal tubules is reabsorbed back into plasma. This tends to delay excretion and accounts for the long half-life of the drug. Because lithium closely resembles normal salt (sodium chloride), when a patient lowers his or her salt intake or loses excessive amounts of salt (such as through sweating), lithium blood levels rise and intoxication may follow. Consequently, patients taking lithium should avoid marked changes in sodium intake or excretion.

Pharmacodynamics

In therapeutic concentrations, lithium has almost no discernible psychotropic effect in normal persons. It does not induce sedation, depression, or euphoria, which differentiates it from other psychoactive drugs. Indeed, it exhibits few effects on the brain aside from its specific action on mania. Its effects on memory and cognition are discussed later.

Used in patients experiencing a manic attack, lithium is effective in reducing the mania; it has little or no effect on the depressive phase. Used prophylactically, lithium prevents the recurrence of manic episodes, and it appears to modulate the cycling as well. No therapeutic effects are seen outside the central nervous system (CNS), although peripheral effects are responsible for the bothersome, and sometimes serious, side effects.

The mechanism through which lithium exerts its antimanic effect is a matter of speculation.[13] Lithium has been shown to affect nerve membranes, pre- and postsynaptic receptors, and the postsynaptic intracellular "second messenger" impulse transduction systems.[14] Here, we will attempt to summarize some of these actions.

First, lithium, as a sodiumlike ion, may increase the presynaptic reuptake of norepinephrine and serotonin, an action consistent with the biological amine theory of mania and depression (Chapter 8), since removing these neurotransmitters from the synaptic space should reduce mania and prevent its recurrence.

Second, lithium may decrease the release of both norepinephrine and serotonin; again, this action is consistent with the biological amine theory. This may occur as a result of lithium-induced attenuation of norepinephrine and serotonin autoreceptors, "possibly via alteration in presynaptic G-protein mediated mechanisms of transmitter release."[14] Manji and coworkers, however, suggest that such presynaptic mechanisms are probably not the primary sites of action of lithium.[13]

Third, lithium may decrease the number of postsynaptic norepinephrine receptors and may prevent the postsynaptic dopamine receptors from becoming supersensitive, both actions once again consistent with the biological amine theory.

Fourth, lithium may interfere with second-messenger systems in the postsynaptic neuron,* reducing the responsiveness of postsynaptic neurons to norepinephrine and serotonin.[14]

Fifth, lithium may reduce the release of thyroid hormone, reducing its behavioral stimulant action. While possible, this is not likely to be the basic mechanism of lithium's antimania action.

---

*Most models of psychoactive drug action focus on a drug's effects on the presynaptic release or the active reuptake of the chemical neurotransmitter as well as the interactions of the neurotransmitter with its receptor. Activation of a postsynaptic receptor (by either an excitatory neurotransmitter or an agonist drug) will trigger (within the postsynaptic neuron) a complex cascade of electrical and biochemical responses that result in activation of the postsynaptic neuron. This postsynaptic, intraneuronal process is called the *second-messenger system*, which translates postsynaptic receptor activation into neuronal activity (Appendix III). Increasingly, the enzymes involved in the second-messenger system are being recognized as a site of psychoactive drug action. Here, lithium may not work within the synaptic cleft, but it inhibits specific enzyme systems (phosphoinositide and/or adenyl cyclase enzymes) so that the postsynaptic neuron is down-regulated or stabilized, reducing its responsiveness to norepinephrine or serotonin.[14–17]

Sixth, lithium disrupts fluxes in transmembrane ion channels, including those of calcium ions. This may be partly responsible for the down regulation of postsynaptic, intracellular transduction mechanisms. Such blockade of the calcium channels probably occurs because of lithium-induced alterations in the second-messenger proteins, which are coupled to the calcium ion channels.

Janicak, Davis, Preskorn, and Ayd review these and other, more exotic theories of lithium's mechanisms of antimania action.[18] Risby and associates summarize as follows:

> Lithium's effects (augmentation) on adenylate cyclase activity are specific with respect to tissue and brain region and. . . lithium may interfere with guanine nucleotide binding (G) protein function. . . . lithium had significant effects on measures associated with signal transduction that might be contrasted to its more subtle effects on neuronal function (norepinephrine release). . . . Lithium's primary site of action may be on signal transduction mechanisms. These effects subsequently may be manifested in changes in neurotransmitter function that may be important to lithium's mood-stabilizing actions.[14]

Side Effects and Toxicity

Because lithium has an extremely narrow therapeutic range, blood levels of the drug must be closely monitored. The occurrence and intensity of side effects are, in most cases, directly related to plasma concentrations of lithium. When levels of lithium in plasma fall below about 0.6 milliequivalent per liter, side effects are usually minimal; they become much more bothersome at levels of 1.0 milliequivalent per liter or higher. The main toxic effects involve the gastrointestinal tract, the kidneys, the thyroid, the cardiovascular system, the skin, and the nervous system.

At plasma levels of 1.5 to 2.0 milliequivalents per liter (and sometimes at lower levels), most reactions involve the gastrointestinal tract, resulting in nausea, vomiting, diarrhea, and abdominal pain. Neurological side effects commonly seen at this level of lithium include a slight tremor, lethargy, dizziness, slurred speech, ataxia, muscle weakness, and nystagmus.

With long-term lithium therapy, the thyroid becomes enlarged in a large percentage of patients. Rashes or some other kind of skin eruption may occur. In addition, about 60 percent of patients taking lithium experience an increase in urine output, along with increased thirst and water intake. Although kidney function needs to be assessed periodically, permanent kidney damage is extremely rare.

Chronic lithium therapy may have adverse effects on memory and cognitive functioning, although these effects are hard to describe because of methodological differences in experiments.[19] Some researchers report improvements in motor performance, cognition, and creative ability after lithium withdrawal, implying detrimental effects of lithium in these areas during drug therapy.[20] Other researchers report few significant cognitive deficits associated with lithium therapy.[21,22] Richter-Leven and coworkers[23] and Manji and coworkers[24] offer some hypotheses involving neurochemical activity to explain possible cognitive, memory, and psychomotor deficits associated with lithium. Richter-Leven and coworkers point out, however, that compensatory mechanisms develop, thus preventing any severe memory impairments during lithium treatment.[23]

At plasma levels of lithium above 2.0 milliequivalents per liter, more severe side effects occur. These include fatigue, muscle weakness, slurred speech, and worsening tremors. Thyroid gland function becomes depressed, and the thyroid gland may enlarge further, resulting in goiter. Muscle fasciculations, increased reflexes, abnormal motor movements, and even seizures, psychosis, and stupor may occur. At yet higher concentrations (levels exceeding 2.5 milliequivalents per liter), toxic effects include muscle rigidity, coma, renal failure, cardiac arrhythmias, and death.

Despite this toxicity and the narrow therapeutic window, lithium can be well tolerated by patients as long as they are monitored. Its use in patients who suffer from mania and resistant depression is well established, and other uses should be discovered in coming years.

Treatment of poisoning or overdosage is nonspecific; there is no antidote to lithium. Usually drug administration is halted and sodium-containing fluids are infused immediately. If toxic signs are serious, hemodialysis, gastric lavage, diuretic therapy, antiepileptic medication, and other supports may be urgently needed. Complete recovery from intoxication may be prolonged, with full renal and neurological recovery taking weeks or months.

Fetal damage may occur when lithium is administered to a pregnant woman. The drug does appear to have teratogenic potential, especially to the heart. Therefore, lithium is contraindicated during the first trimester of pregnancy, and it should be used only if absolutely necessary during the remainder of the pregnancy. Other agents should be employed wherever possible. When a pregnant woman is on lithium therapy, the drug should be discontinued for several days before delivery, because the newborn will have difficulty excreting the drug. Other fluid and electrolyte alterations during the late stages of pregnancy can markedly alter lithium levels in the pregnant female, increasing the risk of toxicity both to the mother and to the newborn. Unfortunately, the alternatives to lithium have teratogenic potentials of their own. Therefore, the treatment of both pregnant and potentially pregnant bipolar females is difficult and must be administered with caution.

Pharmacological Alternatives to Lithium

According to a 1990 review, "heterogeneity does exist within bipolar disorder. Persons with mania differ in family history of affective illness, their age at the onset of illness, sex, and organic cause and course of the illness."[25] Therefore, it is not surprising that a substantial proportion of patients with bipolar disorder either are resistant to lithium treatment or develop side effects that limit its effectiveness.[26] Indeed, only about 60 to 70 percent of patients can be adequately controlled on lithium alone (for maintenance/prevention therapy), and the drug is even less effective in controlling episodes of acute mania. Therefore, there is a need for agents that are superior to lithium or are effective in patients for whom lithium is inadequate.

The search for alternative therapies is quite new, because lithium has been used in this country only since about 1970. I remember interviewing a famous business executive in 1972. This individual described the functional immobilization caused by intermittent attacks of "electrical explosions" in his brain. Although not epileptic in nature, these attacks responded to treatment with the antiepileptic drug phenytoin. (The man consequently spent many years unsuccessfully promoting phenytoin for nonepileptic uses.) Later that year I reported the close structural relationship between phenytoin and carbamazepine, expanding upon the newly identified antiepileptic properties of the latter drug.[27] Later, reports from Europe noted the correlation between the antiepileptic use of carbamazepine and its use as an antimanic drug. Today this use is well established.

Carbamazepine

Carbamazepine (see Figure 9.1) has been shown to be at least as effective as lithium in preventing the recurrence of mania.[28–30] In addition, some patients who do not respond adequately to either lithium or carbamazepine alone do respond when the two drugs are used together.[31] Also, carbamazepine may be superior to lithium in patients with rapid-cycling bipolar disorder, a condition for which lithium is quite ineffective.[32]

It is important to note that patients who fail to respond to carbamazepine often have taken an amount of the drug that is inadequate in plasma. Indeed, there is correlation between therapeutic effectiveness and the plasma level of the drug, with the therapeutic level of carbamazepine estimated to be between 8 and 12 milligrams per liter,[33] the same range used for antiepileptic effectiveness. Petit and coworkers reported that blood levels of the drug can be determined from a sample of saliva rather than from a blood sample, because the amount of drug in saliva correlates well with the amount of drug in blood.

Adverse effects of carbamazepine include gastrointestinal upset, sedation, ataxia, visual disturbances, and dermatological reactions. Carbamazepine may also have slight detrimental effects on cognitive functioning. However, any negative effect on higher-order cognitive functioning is rather limited[34] and is much less detrimental than effects resulting from phenytoin or the barbiturates.[35] Nevertheless, some patients may be particularly sensitive to the cognitive side effects of the drug.[35]

More serious reactions involve the blood, ranging from a relatively benign reduction in white blood cell count (leukopenia) to, on rare occasions, severe aplastic anemia. For this reason blood should be analyzed periodically.

Drug interactions involving carbamazepine are common and result from drug-induced stimulation of drug-metabolizing enzymes in the liver. As a result, tolerance to the drug develops and more drug is needed to maintain a therapeutic blood level; this tolerance also extends to other drugs metabolized by the same enzymes.

Finally, because carbamazepine is potentially teratogenic, it should not be administered during pregnancy if possible.

Valproate

As discussed in Chapter 4, valproate (see Figure 9.1) is an antiepileptic drug that acts by augmenting the postsynaptic action of GABA at its receptors. About the same time that carbamazepine was being investigated for treating mania, valproate was also being examined. Today there is increasing interest in valproate as an antimanic drug.[36–40] Valproate appears especially effective in the treatment of acute mania, mixed states, and rapid-cycling bipolar disorder. However, the drug has poor antidepressant properties.

In acute mania in treatment-resistant patients, positive response rates of up to 71 percent have been reported.[41] Valproate is also effective in some patients with schizo-affective disorder.[42] Another report suggests that the therapeutic combination of valproate and lithium may provide an effective treatment for rapid-cycling bipolar disorder.[43] Therapeutic blood levels of valproate appear to be in the range of 50 to 100 milligrams per milliliter.

Side effects associated with valproate include gastrointestinal upset, sedation, lethargy, hand tremor, alopecia (loss of hair), and some metabolic changes in the liver. Valproate may be slightly more detrimental to cognitive function than carbamazepine.[44] Very rarely valproate can be lethal, causing hepatic failure, especially in children receiving multiple drugs for the control of epileptic seizures.

Like lithium and carbamazepine, valproate can be teratogenic, and caution must be exercised in using this agent in women who might become pregnant during drug therapy.

Benzodiazepines: Clonazepam and Lorazepam

In Chapter 4 two benzodiazepines, clonazepam and lorazepam (see Figure 9.1), were discussed that have been used to treat acute mania. These two drugs seem to be most effective when combined with lithium in the treatment of lithium-resistant bipolar disorder and acute attacks of mania; in this latter application, they replace antipsychotic (neuroleptic) agents such as chlorpromazine (Chapter 11). Their antiepileptic, GABAergic effects probably contribute to their effectiveness in controlling acute mania. Gerner reviews the effectiveness of lorazepam and clonazepam in treating acute mania, referring to these drugs as "adjunctive nonspecific antimanic agents."[45]

Verapamil

The calcium channel blockers, of which verapamil (see Figure 9.1) is the prototype and most widely used, are used primarily in the treatment of cardiovascular diseases such as hypertension and angina pectoris. By modulating the influx of calcium ions across the cardiac myocytes (contractile cells of the heart), verapamil interferes with cellular function, depressing cardiac function and therefore decreasing the workload on the heart. Therapeutically, this action prevents certain cardiac arrhythmias, lowers blood pressure, decreases energy expenditure, relieves angina in patients with coronary artery disease, and reduces blood flow to cardiac muscle.

Since lithium also interferes with membrane ion function, verapamil and other calcium channel blockers have been tried in the treatment of bipolar disorder. To date, despite early reports of impressive improvements, the effectiveness of verapamil remains controversial. The numbers of patients treated have been small, and the open clinical trials have not been well controlled. Recent studies include those by Auby and coworkers,[46] Post,[47] and el-Mallakh and Jaziri.[48] Another calcium channel blocker, nimodipine (Figure 9.1), may be more effective.[49]

In patients who do not respond to lithium or the anticonvulsants, calcium channel blockers may offer some hope. Calcium channel blockers do not improve depression, but they may improve acute manic attacks. Unlike other antimanic agents, verapamil therapy does not cause cognitive deficits. Obviously, since these drugs are cardiac depressants, cardiac status (e.g., heart rate and blood pressure) must be carefully monitored, especially in the elderly.

The use of verapamil as a mood stabilizer is novel and possibly unrelated to the calcium-blocking action because verapamil also decreases the activity of several neurotransmitters. Verapamil may offer an interesting tool with which to investigate the mechanisms of bipolar disorder.

Clonidine

Clonidine (see Figure 9.1) is an antihypertensive drug that has been tried in treatment-refractory patients with bipolar disorder. Clonidine decreases the presynaptic release of norepinephrine and reduces blood pressure, hence its use in treating hypertension. Such an action should lead to a reduction in manic episodes. Indeed, positive results have been reported, although effectiveness still remains unproven.[45,50] There are no reports of any potential effectiveness of the combination of clonidine and lithium in patients who do not respond to lithium alone.

Therapy for Bipolar Disorder

A combination of drug therapy and psychotherapy is the most effective treatment modality for bipolar illness today. First, however, one must ensure that the manic state is not being caused by medications.[45] Such medications include psychiatric medicines such as antidepressants and behavioral stimulants (including illegal drugs such as cocaine), as well as nonpsychiatric medications such as corticosteroids (cortisone), anabolic steroids, caffeine, antiparkinsonian drugs, over-the-counter cough and cold preparations, and diet aids. One must also rule out diseases known to cause or exacerbate mania, most notably thyroid disease, since mania secondary to thyroid hyperactivity is common.

When the presenting phase of bipolar disorder is a manic episode, the patient may be quite agitated, out of control, or even psychotic. Here one may begin therapy with a combination of lithium and an antipsychotic medication. Once mood has been stabilized, the antipsychotic medication can be phased out. The benzodiazepines may be useful in such agitated patients. The antiepileptic-antimanic drugs car-bamazepine and valproate can be used as alternatives or as adjuncts for patients who do not tolerate or who do not respond adequately to lithium and for patients with rapid cycling or mixed bipolar states.

For initial therapy, the recommended blood level of lithium is between 1.0 and 1.2 milliequivalents per liter. Occasionally this level may approach 1.4 milliequivalents per liter for a brief period at the very beginning. Once mood is adequately stabilized, the dose can be lowered to a maintainence level of 0.8 to 1.0 milliequivalent per liter. After a period of effective maintenance therapy, the dose can be further lowered to about 0.6 to 0.8 milliequivalent per liter.

Treatment differs if the presenting phase of bipolar disorder is a depressive episode. Lithium is often ineffective in relieving depression. Thus, an antidepressant medication is given together with lithium. One risk in administering an antidepressant to a bipolar patient is that the drug may precipitate an acute shift into mania. After the depres-sive episode, lithium can be used to prevent relapse.

Psychotherapy interventions used with pharmacotherapy include cognitive-behavioral therapy and interpersonal psychotherapy. For com-plete treatment, a practitioner well versed in the pharmacological manage-ment of poorly responsive bipolar patients is necessary. Other personnel are required to monitor the effectiveness of treatment, side effects, other causative factors, and compliance with therapy. Practice guidelines for the treatment of patients with bipolar disorder have been recently published.

Study Questions

1. Describe the presenting symptoms of bipolar disorder.
2. Outline the pharmacological agents useful in treating bipolar disorder.
3. List the clinical uses of lithium.
4. Describe the correlations between the levels of lithium in plasma and the therapeutic and side effects of lithium.
5. How does lithium exert its antimania effect?
6. List the major organ systems affected by lithium. What are the drug's major side effects on each system?
7. Discuss the effects of the various antimania drugs on memory and cogni-tive behaviors.
8. Discuss the use of drug therapy in the pregnant and potentially pregnant female with bipolar disorder.
9. What antiepileptic drugs are used to treat bipolar illness, and why are they used?
10. Verapamil is a drug used to treat cardiovascular disease. Why might it be considered for the treatment of bipolar illness?
11. What medications or diseases might precipitate or worsen bipolar illness?

12. If one is not the prescribing physician, how can one contribute to the well-being of the patient with bipolar illness?

Notes

1. American Medical Association, "Drugs Used in Mood Disorders," in *Drug Evaluations, Annual 1993* (Chicago: American Medical Association, 1993), p. 278.
2. H. P. Rang and M. M. Dale, "Drugs Used in Affective Disorders," in H. P. Rang and M. M. Dale, eds., *Pharmacology*, 2nd ed. (Edinburgh: Churchill Livingstone, 1991), p. 660.
3. P. G. Janicak, J. M. Davis, S. H. Preskorn, and F. J. Ayd, Jr., *Principles and Practice of Psychopharmacotherapy* (Baltimore: Williams & Wilkins, 1993), p. 337.
4. Ibid., pp. 325–339.
5. G. J. DiGregorio, "Antipsychotic Drugs and Lithium," in J. R. DiPalma and G. J. DiGregorio, eds., *Basic Pharmacology in Medicine*, 3rd ed. (New York: McGraw-Hill, 1990), p. 263.
6. American Medical Association, "Drugs Used in Mood Disorders," p. 280.
7. J. B. Murray, "New Applications of Lithium Therapy," *Journal of Psychology* 124 (1990): 55–73.
8. H. R. Kim, N. J. Delva, and J. S. Lawson, "Prophylactic Medication for Unipolar Depressive Illness: The Place of Lithium Carbonate in Combination with Antidepressant Medication," *Canadian Journal of Psychiatry* 35 (1990): 107–114.
9. J. W. Jefferson, "Lithium: The Present and the Future," *Journal of Clinical Psychiatry* 51, suppl. (1990): 5.
10. R. J. Baldessarini, "Drugs and the Treatment of Psychiatric Disorders," in A. G. Gilman, T. W. Rall, A. S. Nies, and P. Taylor, eds., *Goodman and Gilman's The Pharmacological Basis of Therapeutics*, 8th ed. (New York: Pergamon, 1990), pp. 418–422.
11. J. A. Roth, "Antidepressants—Drugs Used in the Treatment of Mood Disorders," in C. M. Smith and A. M. Reynard, eds., *Textbook of Pharmacology* (Philadelphia: Saunders, 1992), p. 318.
12. DiGregorio, "Antipsychotic Drugs and Lithium," p. 264.
13. H. K. Manji, J. K. Hsiao, E. D. Risby, J. Oliver, M. V. Rudorfer, and W. Z. Potter, "The Mechanisms of Action of Lithium: I. Effects on Serotoninergic and Noradrenergic Systems in Normal Subjects," *Archives of General Psychiatry* 48 (1991): 505–512.
14. E. D. Risby, J. K. Hsiao, H. K. Manji, J. Bitran, F. Moses, D. F. Zhou, and W. Z. Potter, "The Mechanisms of Action of Lithium: II. Effects on Adenylate Cyclase Activity and Beta-Adrenergic Receptor Binding in Normal Subjects," *Archives of General Psychiatry* 48 (1991): 513.
15. J. M. Baraban, P. F. Worley, and S. H. Snyder, "Second Messenger Systems and Psychoactive Drug Action: Focus on the Phosphoinositide System and Lithium," *American Journal of Psychiatry* 146 (1989): 1251–1260.

16. R. H. Belmaker, A. Livne, G. Agam, D. G. Moscovich, N. Grisaru, G. Schreiber, S. Avissar, A. Danon, and O. Kofman, "Role of Inositol-1-Phosphate Inhibition in the Mechanism of Action of Lithium," *Pharmacology and Toxicology* 66, Suppl. 3 (1990): 76–83.

17. H. K. Manji, G. Chen, H. Shimon, J. K. Hsiao, W. Z. Potter, and R. H. Belmaker, "Guanine Nucleotide-binding Proteins in Bipolar Affective Disorder," *Archives of General Psychiatry* 52 (1995): 135–144.

18. Janicak, Davis, Preskorn, and Ayd, *Principles and Practice of Psychopharmacotherapy*, pp. 343–350.

19. F. Engelsmann, A. M. Ghadirian, and P. Grof, "Lithium Treatment and Memory Assessment: Methodology," *Neuropsychobiology* 26 (1992): 113–119.

20. J. H. Kocsis, E. S. Shaw, P. E. Stokes, P. Wilner, A. S. Elliot, C. Sikes, B. Myers, A. Manevitz, and M. Parides, "Neuropsychological Effects of Lithium Discontinuation," *Journal of Clinical Psychopharmacology* 13 (1993): 268–275.

21. K. Furusawa, "Drug Effects on Cognitive Function in Mice Determined by the Non-matching to Sample Task Using a 4-Arm Maze," *Japanese Journal of Pharmacology* 56 (1991): 483–493.

22. H. M. Calil, A. P. Zwicker, and S. Klepacz, "The Effects of Lithium Carbonate on Healthy Volunteers: Mood Stabilization?" *Biological Psychiatry* 27 (1990): 711–722.

23. G. Richter-Leven, H. Markram, and M. Segal, "Spontaneous Recovery of Deficits in Spatial Memory and Cholinergic Potentiation of NMDA in CA-1 Neurons during Chronic Lithium Treatment," *Hippocampus* 2 (1992): 279–286.

24. H. K. Manji, R. Etcheberrigaray, G. Chen, and J. L. Olds, "Lithium Decreases Membrane-Associated Protein Kinase C in Hippocampus: Selectivity for the Alpha Isozyme," *Journal of Neurochemistry* 61 (1993): 2303–2310.

25. B. L. Cook and G. Winokur, "Perspectives on Bipolar Illness," *Comprehensive Therapy* 16 (1990): 18–23.

26. R. T. Joffe, "Valproate in Bipolar Disorder: The Canadian Perspective," *Canadian Journal of Psychiatry* 38, Suppl. 2 (1993): S46–S50.

27. R. M. Julien and R. P. Hollister, "Carbamazepine: Mechanism of Action," in J. K. Penry and D. D. Daly, eds., *Advances in Neurology*, vol. 11 (1975), pp. 263–277.

28. N. Coxhead, T. Silverstone, and J. Cookson, "Carbamazepine versus Lithium in the Prophylaxis of Bipolar Affective Disorder," *Acta Psychiatrica Scandinavica* 85 (1992): 114–118.

29. J. G. Small, M. H. Klapper, V. Milstein, J. J. Kellams, M. J. Miller, J. D. Marhenke, and I. F. Small, "Carbamazepine Compared with Lithium in the Treatment of Mania," *Archives of General Psychiatry* 48 (1991): 915–921.

30. R. M. Lusznat, D. P. Murphy, and C. M. Nunn, "Carbamazepine vs. Lithium in the Treatment and Prophylaxis of Mania," *British Journal of Psychiatry* 153 (1988): 198–204.

31. K. G. Kramlinger and R. M. Post, "Adding Lithium Carbonate to Carbamazepine: Antimanic Efficacy in Treatment-Resistant Mania," *Acta Psychiatrica Scandinavica* 79 (1989): 378–385.

32. E. DiCostanzo and F. Schifano, "Lithium Alone or in Combination with Carbamazepine for the Treatment of Rapid-Cycling Bipolar Affective Disorder," *Acta Psychiatrica Scandinavica* 83 (1991): 456-459.

33. P. Petit, R. Lonjon, M. Cociglio, A. Sluzewska, J. P. Blayac, B. Hue, R. Alric, and P. Pouget, "Carbamazepine and Its 10,11-Epoxide Metabolite in Acute Mania: Clinical and Pharmacokinetic Correlates," *European Journal of Clinical Pharmacology* 41 (1991): 541–546.

34. A. P. Aldenkamp, W. C. J. Alpherts, G. Blennow, D. Elmwvist, J. Heijbel, H. L. Nilsson, P. Sandstedt, B. Tonnby, L. Wahlander, and E. Wosse, "Withdrawal of Antiepileptic Medication in Children—Effects on Cognitive Function: The Multicenter Holmfrid Study," *Neurology* 43 (1993): 41–50.

35. E. R. Brown, "Interictal Cognitive Changes in Epilepsy," *Seminars in Neurology* 11 (1991): 167–174.

36. J. R. Calabrese, M. J. Woyshville, S. E. Kimmel, and D. J. Rapport, "Predictors of Valproate Response in Bipolar Rapid Cycling," *Journal of Clinical Psychopharmacology* 13 (1993): 280–283.

37. J. R. Calabrese, D. J. Rapport, S. E. Kimmel, B. Reece, and M. J. Woyshville, "Rapid Cycling Bipolar Disorder and Its Treatment with Valproate," *Canadian Journal of Psychiatry* 38, Suppl. 2 (1993): S57–S61.

38. Joffe, "Valproate in Bipolar Disorder," pp. S46–S50.

39. T. W. Freeman, J. L. Clothier, P. Pazzaglia, M. D. Lesem, and A. C. Swann, "A Double-Blind Comparison of Valproate and Lithium in the Treatment of Acute Mania," *American Journal of Psychiatry* 149 (1992): 108–111.

40. H. G. Pope, Jr., S. L. McElroy, P. E. Keck, Jr., and J. I. Hudson, "Valproate in the Treatment of Acute Mania. A Placebo-Controlled Study," *Archives of General Psychiatry* 48 (1991): 62–68.

41. L. McCoy, N. A. Votolato, S. B. Schwarzkopf, and H. A. Nasrallah, "Clinical Correlates of Valproate Augmentation in Refractory Bipolar Disorder," *Annals of Clinical Psychiatry* 5 (1993): 29–33.

42. S. L. McElroy and P. E. Keck, Jr., "Treatment Guidelines for Valproate in Bipolar and Schizoaffective Disorders," *Canadian Journal of Psychiatry* 38, Suppl. 2 (1993): S62–S66.

43. V. Sharma, E. Persad, D. Mazmanian, and K. Karunaratne, "Treatment of Rapid Cycling Bipolar Disorder with Combination Therapy of Valproate and Lithium," *Canadian Journal of Psychiatry* 38 (1993): 137–139.

44. P. R. Bittencourt, M. J. Mader, M. M. Bigarella, M. P. Doro, A. M. Gorz, T. M. Marcourakis, and Z. S. Ferreira, "Cognitive Functions, Epileptic Syndromes and Antiepileptic Drugs," *Arquivos de Neuro-Psiquiatria* 50 (1992): 24–30.

45. R. H. Gerner, "Treatment of Acute Mania," *Psychiatric Clinics of North America* 16 (1993): 448.

46. P. Auby, F. Olivier, L. Schmitt, G. Peresson, and P. Moron, "Calcium Channel Blockers and Dysthymic Disorders. Recent Data," *Encephale* 18, spec. no. 1 (1992): 67–69.

47. R. M. Post, "Non-Lithium Treatment for Bipolar Disorder," *Journal of Clinical Psychiatry* 51, suppl. (1990): 9–16.

48. R. S. el-Mallakh and W. A. Jaziri, "Calcium Channel Blockers in Affective Illness: Role of Sodium-Calcium Exchange," *Journal of Clinical Psychopharmacology* 10 (1990): 203–206.

49. G. Brunet and others, "Open Trial of a Calcium Antagonist, Nimodipine, in Acute Mania," *Clinical Neuropharmacology* 13 (1990): 224–228.

50. Janicak, Davis, Preskorn, and Ayd, *Principles and Practice of Psychopharmacotherapy*, pp. 382–384.

51. American Psychiatric Association, "Practice Guideline for the Treatment of Patients with Bipolar Disorder," *American Journal of Psychiatry* 151, No. 12, suppl. (December 1994): 1–36.

CHAPTER 10

THE ANALGESICS: NARCOTIC AND NONNARCOTIC DRUGS

Pain is caused by the activation of electrical activity in small-diameter sensory (afferent) fibers of peripheral nerves. These sensory nerves originate in peripheral tissues (such as skin, muscle, and abdominal viscera) and are activated by various mechanical, thermal, chemical, and injury stimuli. Because these nerves are activated by noxious (painful) stimuli, their receptors are called *nociceptors* (Figure 10.1). The electrical discharge in these nerves is conducted to their synaptic terminals, which are located in the dorsal horn of the spinal cord, where (in its simplest concept) a chemical transmitter called *substance P* is released.

In general, there are two general classes of analgesic drugs. The first consists of "peripherally acting" drugs, such as aspirin and ibuprofen. Drugs in this class act at the site of tissue injury to reduce pain and inflammation by interfering with the synthesis of prostaglandin hormones. These drugs are discussed at the end of this chapter. The second class of analgesic drugs consists of the "centrally acting" (narcotic) analgesics, such as morphine. These drugs act on specific opioid receptors both in the spinal cord and at higher levels of

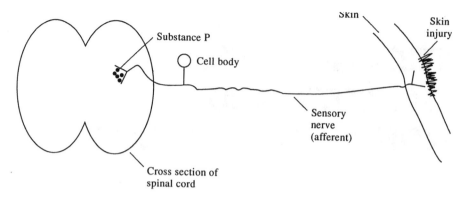

FIGURE 10.1 Activation of peripheral nociceptive (pain) fibers results in the release of substance P from nerve terminals in the dorsal horn of the spinal cord. The cell body for the nerve is located in the dorsal root ganglion.

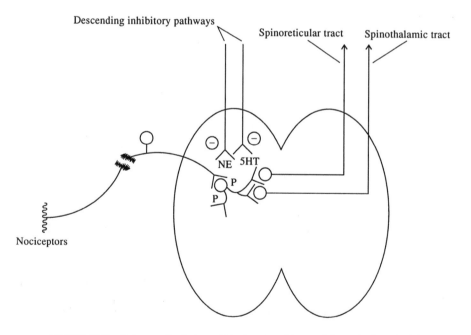

FIGURE 10.2 Release of substance P in the dorsal horn of the spinal cord with transmission of secondary relay pathways to higher centers. Descending inhibitory pathways (−) are also shown (expanded in Figure 10.3). NE, norepinephrine; 5HT, serotonin.

the central nervous system to reduce the intensity and central processing of afferent pain impulses.

Substance P, a peptide that is 11 amino acids in length, is a neurotransmitter. When it is released, it activates other neurons that transmit information about noxious stimuli to the brain by means of two specialized afferent pathways: the spinothalamic tract and the spinoreticular tract (Figure 10.2). Thus, pain is first "perceived" in the spinal cord; this perception is relayed to the brain stem and the thalamus and, eventually, to higher centers in the brain (such as the limbic system and the somatosensory cortex) for interpretation. The dorsal horn of the spinal cord, the thalamus, the brain stem, and the limbic system are all rich in opioid receptors, upon which both the opioids and naturally occurring peptides act. These centers in the brain are important sites of action for morphinelike drugs as well as for pain sensation.

Thus, pain is transmitted from the peripheral nociceptors to the brain after passing through the spinal cord. As Figure 10.3 illustrates, at least two descending pathways in the spinal cord modulate (or "gate") the transmission of pain impulses. One pathway originates in the locus coeruleus of the medulla and sends descending axons to the dorsal horn, where the neurotransmitter norepinephrine is released. There, norepinephrine inhibits the release of substance P and thus reduces nociception (that is, it is analgesic). This path is important in the mechanism for pain relief, because an injection of norepinephrine-like agonists (adrenaline or clonidine) into the spinal fluid will cause analgesia.[1,2]

The second descending analgesic pathway (see Figure 10.3) originates in the midbrain (in the periaqueductal gray matter) and in the medulla (the dorsal raphe nucleus) and sends axons down the spinal cord. These axons also synapse on the terminals of nociceptive neurons located in the dorsal horn of the spinal cord. Here, serotonin is released.[3] This pathway is an important site of action for opioid analgesics,[3] because (1) these areas of the midbrain and medulla are rich in both opioid peptides and opioid receptors, (2) electrical stimulation of these areas in the brain stem causes intense analgesia that is blocked by the narcotic antagonist naloxone,[4] and (3) serotonin induces the release of opioid peptides in the dorsal horn, inhibiting substance P release.

Thus, descending norepinephrine and serotonin pathways modulate noxious stimuli by directly or indirectly reducing the release of substance P in the spinal cord. This reduction involves the activation of opioid neurons, which release opioid peptides (mainly met-

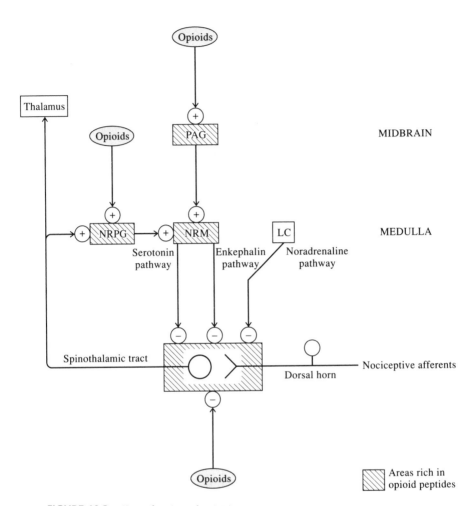

FIGURE 10.3   Sites of action of opioids on pain transmission. Opioids excite neurons in the periaqueductal gray matter (PAG) and in the midbrain and medulla. From there, serotoninergic and enkephalinergic neurons run to the dorsal horn and exert an inhibitory influence on transmission. Opioids also act directly on the dorsal horn. The locus coeruleus (LC) sends noradrenergic neurons to the dorsal horn, which also inhibits transmission. The pathways shown in this diagram represent a considerable oversimplification, but they depict the general organization of the supraspinal control mechanisms.

enkephalin and beta-endorphin), which, in turn, inhibit the release of substance P, causing an analgesic action.

Using this model, we can identify several sites of action for opioid analgesics. Drugs that potentiate serotonin cause analgesia by activating descending inhibitory pathways. Such is the case with the tricyclic antidepressants, because they are clinically effective in the treatment of chronic pain syndromes.[5] Drugs that potentiate norepinephrine produce analgesia in a similar way. Indeed, two such drugs (adrenaline and clonidine) are clinically used for this analgesic property. In addition, clonidine is useful in relieving the symptoms of opioid withdrawal in narcotic-dependent persons.[6] Finally, the substantia gelatinosa of the dorsal horn of the spinal cord and the midline structures of the medulla, midbrain, and medial thalamus are rich in opioid peptides and receptors. Morphinelike drugs exert their analgesic action by stimulating the opioid receptors in those areas.

So far, we have discussed the afferent transmission of nociceptive impulses and its modulation, which is caused by descending inhibitory influences (serotonin and norepinephrine) as well as local opioid influences. We have not addressed the *affective* component of pain—the component that determines our emotional response by reducing the distress associated with the pain. The affective component of pain may be the underlying factor in the mechanism of chronic pain states for which no objective cause can be identified.[7]

Central processing of pain involves the periaqueductal gray area, the nucleus accumbens, the amygdala, the habenula, and other structures of the mesolimbic system. Ma and Han state that

> these nuclei possibly act through a "mesolimbic neural loop" to exert an analgesic effect, in which met-enkephalin and beta-endorphin have been implicated as the 2 major opioid peptides involved in antinociception. . . . [These structures] are connected in a network served by a positive feedback circuitry.[8]

This pathway appears to involve both dopaminergic and serotonergic pathways.[9,10]

Chronic pain states may arise from deficits in this central processing of nociceptive afferent actions, whereby input that might be innocuous in some persons debilitates others. In such persons, treatment with opioids is not effective (and sometimes even harmful because dependence can develop). Thus, for these persons, treatment is focused on behavior modification, cognitive-behavioral therapy, or self-management approaches that include biopsychosocial models of therapy.

OPIOID ANALGESICS

The opioid analgesics are a group of naturally occurring and synthetic drugs* that exert actions on the body that are similar to those induced by morphine, the major pain-relieving agent that is obtained from opium. Opium has been used for thousands of years to produce euphoria, analgesia, sleep, and relief from diarrhea. The earliest descriptions of the effects of opium were written about 300 B.C., although references have been found dating to about 3000 B.C. Opium was used in early Egyptian, Greek, and Arabic cultures primarily for its constipating effect in the treatment of diarrhea. Later, opium's sleep-inducing properties were noted by writers such as Homer, Virgil, and Ovid. Opium was used to treat a variety of medical problems, including snakebite, asthma, cough, epilepsy, colic, urinary complaints, headache, and deafness. Recreational abuse of opium was also quite common. Addiction to opium was common, even among the high-standing military and political figures of Rome.

From the early Greek and Roman days through the sixteenth and seventeenth centuries, the medicinal and recreational uses of opium were well established throughout Europe. Because much of the opium came from the Near East and the Orient, a bustling trade in opium existed between the East and the West. Indeed, control of opium was a central issue during the wars in China in 1839.

Until the nineteenth century, the opioids that were used medicinally and recreationally consisted of crude opium, which is the extract of the exudate from the opium poppy, *Papaver somniferum*. It was not until the early 1800s that morphine was isolated from opium. The purification of morphine revolutionized the use of opioids, and since then morphine (rather than crude opium) has been used throughout the world as the premier agent for treating severe pain.

In the United States, morphine and opium were widely used during the nineteenth century. Opium and morphine were freely available from physicians, drugstores, and general stores; by mail order; and in patent medicines sold through a variety of channels. It was not until

---

*Naturally occurring opioids are derived from either of two sources: (1) drugs (morphine and codeine) obtained from the opium poppy and (2) endogenous morphinelike compounds (e.g., the endorphins) found in the brain. Synthetic drugs include the semisynthetic modifications of morphine (e.g., heroin) and totally synthetic drugs (e.g., meperidine).

after the Civil War (when opioid addiction was referred to as the "soldier's disease") and the invention of the hypodermic needle (in 1856) that a new type of drug user appeared in the United States—one who administered opioids to himself by injection.

By the early part of the twentieth century, the use of opium was widespread, and concern began to mount about the dangers of opioids and the dependence that they could induce. By 1914, the Harrison Narcotic Act was passed, and the use of most opioid products was strictly controlled. Nonmedical uses of opioids were banned.

The use of opioids is deeply entrenched in society; it is widespread and impossible to stop. The pharmacology of the opioids should be discussed like that of any other class of psychoactive drugs that have pleasurable effects, produce tolerance and physiological dependence, and have a potential for compulsive misuse. Emotional reactions and extensive legal efforts will probably fail to eradicate the recreational use of these drugs. Also, the opioids will continue to be used in medicine because they are irreplaceable as pain-relieving agents. In addition, the profound effects of opioids on the central nervous system (CNS) induce an enormous potential for compulsive abuse—a liability that is likely to resist any efforts at total control. Goldstein writes of the opioids, "they dramatically relieve emotional as well as physical pain. This property contributes to making them extremely seductive for self-administration."[11]

Opioid Receptors and Classification of Opioid Analgesics

Opioid receptors are widely distributed throughout the gray matter of the brain and the spinal cord, with limbic and limbic-associated areas tending to have the highest concentration. These receptors are not all identical; distinct types exist, with different affinities for binding with different opioid analgesics.[12-14] The major categories of receptors have been identified and are designated as *mu, kappa,* and *delta* receptors. Subtypes of some of these receptors have also been identified (for example, mu-1 and mu-2).

Despite some overlap, mu, delta, and kappa receptors are concentrated in different areas of the body. Mu receptors are located mostly at supraspinal sites, which are responsible both for morphine-induced analgesia as well as the emotional quieting and reinforcing properties of morphine and other opioids. Such areas include the medial thalamus and brain stem areas (locus coeruleus, periaqueductal gray matter of the midbrain, and the nucleus raphe magnus of the medulla). Activation of mu receptors in these areas seems to underlie the analgesic, respiratory depressant, miotic (pinpoint pupils), euphoric, and physical dependence properties of morphine and its related drugs.

It is thought that the mu-1 subtype modulates analgesia and euphoria primarily, while the mu-2 subtype modulates respiratory depression. Because no analgesics specific to the mu-1 receptors are clinically available at present, analgesia cannot be separated from respiratory depression in patients who are taking opioids. In addition, the intense analgesia that is caused by opioids has not been separated from the euphoria that is induced. All analgesics that stimulate mu receptors induce euphoria, have potent behavior-reinforcing properties, and thus are capable of causing drug dependence. Some mu receptors are also located in the spinal cord, and these receptors may modulate at least part of the spinal analgesia that is induced by morphine. There are several candidates for endogenous transmitters at mu receptors. These include beta-endorphin and possibly even naturally occurring morphine.

Kappa receptors are located principally within the dorsal horn of the spinal cord. Thus, kappa receptors produce analgesia by depressing the initial relay site of pain transmission. Other kappa receptors are located in the brain stem (medullary reticular formation) and in supraspinal structures. Kappa-specific drugs produce miosis and sedation but not euphoria, physical dependence, or respiratory depression. Indeed, drugs that stimulate kappa receptors produce aversive effects in animals and dysphoria (rather than euphoria) in humans,[15] probably because they also inhibit mu opioid activity.[16]

Delta receptors are poorly delineated as yet, but they may be involved at brain stem and spinal levels in analgesic effects and in some of the positive reinforcing properties of morphine.

Using this knowledge of opioid receptors, we can classify the opioid analgesics. First, we can tabulate the activity of each drug at each type of receptor and indicate whether it activates (agonistic action) or inhibits (antagonistic action) receptor function. We can thus categorize each drug as a *pure agonist,* a *pure antagonist,* or a *mixed agonist/antagonist* (Table 10.1). Pure agonists include most of the morphinelike drugs.

Pure agonists exhibit a high binding affinity for (and exert high activity with) mu receptors, and they also have affinity for kappa receptors. Pure antagonists bind to opioid receptors with varying affinity, but they do not exert agonist activity at any receptor. Finally, the mixed agonist/antagonists exhibit modest morphinelike activity at some receptors, but they can also antagonize the effects of mor-

TABLE 10.1 Classification of opioid analgesics by analgesic properties.

Pure agonists	Mixed agonist/Antagonists	Pure antagonists
Morphine	Nalbuphine (Nubain)	Naloxone (Narcan)
Codeine	Butorphanol (Stadol)	Naltrexone (Trexan)
Heroin	Pentazocine (Talwin)	
Meperidine (Demerol)	Buprenorphine (Buprenex)	
Methadone (Dolophine)	Dezocine (Dalgan)	
Oymorphone (Numorphan)		
Hydromorphone (Dilaudid)		
Fentanyl (Sublimaze)		

phine at some, or all, of the receptors. Several such agents are available clinically. Table 10.2 lists some opioids and their actions at opioid receptors.

Some opioid receptors are located outside the CNS. Here we refer primarily to receptors located in the gastrointestinal tract and in other parts of the autonomic nervous system. Such peripheral receptors are involved in the production of some of the bothersome side effects of opioids.

TABLE 10.2 Classification of opioid analgesics by actions at opioid receptors.

Compound	Receptor types[a]		
	Mu	Kappa	Delta
Morphine	+++	+	+
Naloxone	−	−	−
Pentazocine	+/0	+	NA
Butorphanol	+/0	+	NA
Nalbuphine	−	+	NA
Buprenorphine	+	−	NA
Fentanyl	+++	+	+
Dezocine	+	+	+

[a]The mu receptor is thought to mediate supraspinal analgesia, respiratory depression, euphoria, and physical dependence; the kappa receptor, spinal analgesia, miosis, and sedation. Categorizations are based on best inferences about actions in humans. See text for further explanation. Agonists are indicated by one or more plus signs, antagonists by one or more minus signs, and agents that have no significant action at the receptor by zero. NA, data not available.

Morphine

Opium contains two pharmacologically active analgesic drugs, morphine and codeine. Morphine, the more effective pain-relieving drug, represents approximately 10 percent of the crude exudate. Codeine is closely related to morphine structurally, but it is much less potent and constitutes only 0.5 percent of the crude exudate.

Despite decades of research, no other drug has been found that exceeds morphine's effectiveness as an analgesic. Indeed, morphine and codeine remain vital weapons in the armamentarium of the physician in the struggle against pain.

Pharmacokinetics

Morphine may be administered orally, rectally, or by injection. In general, absorption of morphine from the gastrointestinal tract (oral or rectal) is slow and incomplete compared to absorption following injection: Blood levels reach only about half of that achieved when the drug is administered by injection. Absorption through the rectum is adequate, and several opioids (morphine, hydromorphone, and oxymorphone) are available in suppository form. Such preparations might be indicated in patients suffering from muscle-wasting diseases (such as in patients with terminal cancer) who cannot tolerate other routes of administration.

Highly fat-soluble opioids (such as fentanyl, discussed later) are readily absorbed from the oral mucosa, and this route of administration is being investigated as a possible way to treat postsurgical pain in children. Also, fentanyl has recently become available in a skin patch. In this instance, the fentanyl diffuses slowly across the skin into plasma, providing a steady and reasonably consistent blood level over a period of about 24 hours. Such a preparation is useful for patients with chronic pain who desire to avoid the peaks and valleys associated with intermittent administration of drug.

Finally, morphine and certain other opioids can be administered directly into the spinal canal (through small catheters) to control the pain of obstetric labor and delivery, to treat postoperative pain, and (for long-term use) to relieve the pain associated with terminal cancer. Indeed, such technology is revolutionizing the treatment of terminally ill patients who are suffering from severe pain: No individual today should have to suffer severe, unremitting pain as his or her life ends.[17] The drugs and the technology exist to alleviate such pain, allowing death with dignity.

Morphine is usually administered by intramuscular, subcutaneous, or intravenous injection. The problems and limitations of the injection of drugs (Chapter 1) include accidental overdose, rapid onset of adverse drug reactions, the necessity of using sterile techniques, and the inability to retrieve the drug if too much is administered. However, administering the specific pharmacological antagonist naloxone (Narcan) antagonizes the effects of morphine.

As is well-known from the history of opium smoking in Asian cultures, the opioids may be administered by inhalation, most commonly by inhaling the smoke from burning crude opium. The rapidity of onset of drug action rivals that following intravenous injection.

Opioids achieve significant levels in the brain within seconds to minutes after an intravenous injection. The more water-soluble (lipid-insoluble) opioids, such as morphine, penetrate the blood–brain barrier somewhat more slowly than do the more lipid-soluble opioids. Thus, morphine exists in the bloodstream in a relatively lipid-insoluble form, which does not cross the blood–brain barrier easily. Only small amounts of morphine (20 percent) ever penetrate the brain. In contrast, heroin (discussed later in this chapter) crosses the blood–brain barrier easily. This difference may explain why the "flash" or "rush" following intravenous injection of heroin is so much more intense than that perceived after injecting morphine. The opioids also reach all body tissues, including the fetus; infants born of addicted mothers are physically dependent on opioids and exhibit withdrawal symptoms that require intensive therapy.

Morphine is metabolized by the liver, and its metabolites are excreted by the kidneys. Morphine is metabolized rapidly, and its duration of action is about 4 to 5 hours. This factor is critically important to drug-dependent persons, because they must continually seek and administer the drug at intervals that are as short as 3 to 5 hours. Morphine's half-life is about 2 hours.

Urine-screening tests to determine whether a person has used narcotics detect codeine and morphine as well as their metabolites. Because heroin is metabolized to morphine, and because street heroin also contains acetylcodeine (which is metabolized to codeine), heroin use is suspected when both morphine and codeine are present in a patient's urine. However, such tests cannot accurately determine which specific drug (heroin, codeine, or morphine) has been used. Furthermore, codeine is widely available in cough syrups and analgesic preparations, and even poppy seeds contain small amounts of morphine.[18] Thus, depending on the drug that was taken, morphine and codeine may be detected in a patient's urine for 2 to 4 days after he or she has taken the opioid.

Pharmacological Effects

Morphine, the prototype of a pure opioid agonist, exerts its major effects primarily by stimulating opioid receptors. As a result, morphine produces a syndrome that consists of analgesia, relaxed euphoria, sedation, a sense of tranquility, reduced apprehension and concern, respiratory depression, suppression of the cough reflex, and pupillary constriction.

Analgesia   Morphine produces intense analgesia and indifference to pain, reducing the intensity of pain and thus reducing the associated distress by altering the central processing of pain (at the level of the thalamus, limbic system, and cerebral cortex).[19] Thus, morphine is analgesic because it stimulates opioid receptors (of the mu type) in the brain stem, spinal cord, and brain. Analgesia can be produced in animals by injecting morphine directly into the periaqueductal gray matter, the nucleus raphe magnus, or the dorsal horn of the spinal cord. An injection of naloxone (Narcan) or the surgical interruption of the descending inhibitory opioid pathways will block the analgesia induced by morphine.[19]

Euphoria   Morphine produces a pleasant euphoric state, which includes a strong feeling of contentment, well-being, and lack of concern. Indeed, this is part of the affective, or reinforcing, response of the drug.

> Opioids, like cocaine, are used for their positive effects. Use of exogenous opioids gives the addict access to the reinforcement system . . . in the locus coeruleus and elsewhere. This positive reward system, normally reserved to reward the performance of species-specific survival behaviors, once reached by exogenous self-administration of drugs of abuse, provides the user with an experience that the brain equates with profoundly important events like eating, drinking, and sex. Opioid use becomes an acquired drive state that permeates all aspects of human life. Withdrawal from opioid use is mediated by separate neural pathways that cause withdrawal events to be perceived as life-threatening, and the subsequent physiologic reactions often lead to renewed opioid consumption.[6]

Regular users and those who are psychologically attracted to morphine describe the effects of intravenous injection in ecstatic and often sexual terms. However, the euphoric effect becomes progressively less intense after repeated use. At this point, users inject the drug for one or more of several possible reasons: to try to reexperience the extreme euphoria experienced after the first few injections, to maintain a state of pleasure and well-being, to prevent mental discomfort that may be associated with reality, or to prevent withdrawal symptoms.

Perhaps part of the psychological attraction to morphine is its ability to alter a person's perception of pain by inducing a lack of concern for it. Medical practitioners and researchers often tend to describe pain resulting from physical causes (such as cancer or a broken leg). However, pain also occurs that is emotional or psychological in origin, having no evident organic cause. Thus, some persons who are attracted to the opioids may be attempting to dull psychological pain, which may partly account for the profound psychological effects and the feeling of well-being that have been reported following the use of opioid drugs.

Because morphine exerts powerful effects on pain and emotion by stimulating receptors that bind with naturally occurring opioid peptides, we might ask what role these peptides play in our bodies. Are they natural analgesics or natural euphoriants? The answer is not clear, especially since the pure narcotic antagonist naloxone, when it is injected intravenously into a normal person, does not induce pain or dysphoria. In marathon runners, however, endorphin levels in plasma increase fourfold;[20,21] these natural analgesics reduce depression and provide an overall feeling of well-being (a "runner's high"). Endorphins appear to be part of a natural euphoric reward system and a determinant of our mood.

The mechanism of morphine's positive reinforcing and euphoria-producing action probably involves more than one system. Indeed, Di Chiara and North argue that both dopaminergic and nondopaminergic systems are involved in opioid reward.[22] Opioids are known to activate opioid receptors within the mesolimbic dopamine reward system by means of the same pathway involved in the rewarding effects of cocaine, the benzodiazepines, and alcohol.[23–27] Indeed, opioid receptors in or near the ventral tegmental area are the likely sites where opioids activate the mesolimbic dopamine system expressed through the nucleus accumbens.[27] Di Chiara and North summarize the complexity of this action:

> Opioids excite dopamine neurons in the ventral tegmental area, but this is indirect. Local GABA-releasing interneurons have mu-opioid receptors, via which opioids cause hyperpolarization by increasing the K^+ (potassium ion) conductance; as a result, GABA release onto the dopamine cells is reduced and the firing rate (of the dopamine cells) increases.[22]

This receptor action is illustrated in Figure 10.4.

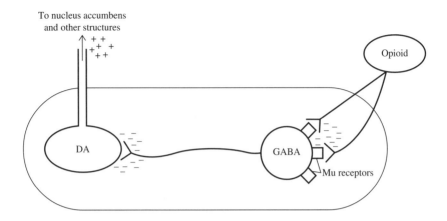

FIGURE 10.4 Schematic illustration of how dopamine-secreting neurons in the ventral tegmental area are excited by opioids. Dopamine-containing neurons are hyperpolarized by GABA acting at $GABA_A$ receptors. GABA-containing neurons are hyperpolarized by opioids acting at mu receptors. Thus, opioids reduce the inhibition exerted by GABA on dopamine neurons. DA, dopamine.

The nondopaminergic substrate of opioid-induced reward is the endogenous opioid system itself.[22] Beta-endorphin, which underlies the maintenance of our normal state of affect (i.e., our mood), is probably the primary endogenous opioid involved.

Finally, environmental cues repeatedly paired with drug-induced reward (the primary incentive) acquire their own motivational properties and become powerful secondary incentives for goal-directed behavior.[22] Such secondary incentives can increase self-administration (one mechanism of tolerance) and can provide powerful incentives for relapse and the maintenance of opioid addiction.

Sedation and Anxiolysis Morphine produces anxiolysis, sedation, and drowsiness, but the level of sedation is not as deep as that produced by the CNS depressants. Although persons who are taking morphine will doze, they can usually be readily awakened. During this state, "mental clouding" is prominent, which is accompanied by a lack of concentration, apathy, complacency, lethargy, reduced mentation, and a sense of tranquility. These anxiolytic actions of opioids likely follow from mu receptor inhibition of neuronal activity in the locus coeruleus, the principal clustering of norepinephrine neurons in the brain.[15]

Depression of Respiration Morphine causes a profound depression of respiration by decreasing the respiratory center's sensitivity to higher levels of carbon dioxide in the blood. The respiratory rate is reduced even at therapeutic doses; at higher doses the rate slows even further, respiratory volume decreases, breathing patterns become shallow and irregular, and, at sufficiently high levels, breathing ceases. Respiratory depression is the major acute side effect of morphine, and it is the cause of death when a person takes an acute drug overdose.

Suppression of Cough   Opioids suppress the "cough center," which is also located in the brain stem. Thus, opioid narcotics have historically been used as cough suppressants, codeine being particularly popular for this purpose. Today, however, less addicting drugs are used as cough suppressants; opioids are inappropriate choices for treating persistent cough.

Pupillary Constriction   Morphine (as well as other mu and kappa agonists) causes pupillary constriction (miosis). Indeed, pupillary constriction in the presence of analgesia is characteristic of narcotic ingestion.

Nausea and Vomiting   Morphine stimulates receptors in an area of the medulla that is called the *chemoreceptor trigger zone.* Stimulation of this area produces nausea and vomiting, which are the most characteristic and unpleasant side effects of morphine and other opioids.

Gastrointestinal Symptoms   Morphine and the other opioids relieve diarrhea as a result of their direct actions on the intestine. They cause intestinal tone to increase, motility to decrease, feces to dehydrate, and intestinal spasm (and cramping) to occur. This combination of a decreased propulsion, an increased intestinal tone, a decrease in the rate of movement of food, and dehydration hardens the stool and further retards the advance of fecal material. All these effects contribute to the constipating effect of opioids. Because tolerance to the constipating effects of the opioids does not develop, drug-dependent individuals have long-term problems with constipation. Similarly, drug withdrawal is characterized by severe abdominal cramping and diarrhea, as intestinal tone returns to normal.

Nothing more effective than the opioids has yet been developed for treating severe diarrhea. In recent years two opioids have been developed that only very minimally cross the blood–brain barrier into the CNS. The first is *diphenoxylate* (the primary active ingredient in Lomotil) and *loperamide* (Imodium). These drugs are exceedingly effective opioid antidiarrheals but are not analgesics, nor are they prone to compulsive abuse, since their distribution and their action is restricted to areas outside the CNS (such as the intestine).

Other Effects   Morphine can release histamine from its storage sites in mast cells in the blood but to a much lesser extent than other opioids. This can result in localized itching or more severe allergic reactions, including bronchoconstriction (an asthmalike constriction of the bronchi of the lungs). Opioids also affect white blood cell function, perhaps producing alterations in the immune system that are as yet poorly defined. The science of psychoneuroimmunology (PNI) has been actively investigating this area of opioid action.

Tolerance and Dependence

Tolerance to morphine and to the other opioid narcotics varies according to the patient's physiological response, the dose, and the frequency of administration. Tolerance to the respiratory depressant, analgesic, euphoric, and sedative effects develops as a result of using any opioid.

The rate at which tolerance develops varies widely. When morphine or other opioid narcotics are used only intermittently, little, if any, tolerance develops. Thus, when a person's sprees of drug use are separated by prolonged periods without using drugs, the opioids retain their initial efficacy. For example, if a person uses an opioid for recreational purposes only occasionally, low doses may continue to be effective and may not have to be increased markedly (unless, of course, a greater or more intense effect is desired). As drug use is increased, greater dependence and greater tolerance occur. When administration is repeated, tolerance may become so marked that massive doses have to be administered to either maintain a degree of euphoria or prevent withdrawal discomfort (avoidance of discomfort is more common). The degree of tolerance is illustrated by the fact that the dose of morphine can be increased from clinical doses (i.e., 50 to 60 milligrams per day) to 500 milligrams per day over as short a period as 10 days.[15]

Tolerance to opioids develops from any of three mechanisms. First is the induction of hepatic drug-metabolizing enzymes; as a result, more opioid is needed to maintain the same level of opioid in blood (i.e., drug is metabolized more quickly). Second, opioid receptors in the CNS may down-regulate, or lose their sensitivity to the presence of opioids; consequently, a higher blood level of opioid is necessary to stimulate the receptors. Third, environmental conditioning and behavioral sensitization produce conditioned and extinguishable tolerance to the effects of opioids.[29–31] The behavioral sensitization to opioids is modeled by injection of morphine into the ventral tegmental area but not into the nucleus accumbens.[32–33] Thus, this sensitization is related to an increased activation of dopamine neurons in the ventral tegmental area.[34]

Tolerance to one opioid leads to cross tolerance to all other natural and synthetic opioids, even if they are chemically dissimilar. Cross tolerance, however, does not develop between the opioids and the sedative hypnotics. In other words, a person who has developed a tolerance for morphine will also have a tolerance for heroin but not for alcohol or barbiturates. This point is extremely important, because accidental death may result from the additive effects of using a sedative and an opioid together. For example, if a person takes moderate doses of opioids and then drinks alcohol or takes a sedative, respiration will be further depressed, potentially leading to coma or death. Deaths from the combined effects of opioids and general depressants are common.

In Chapter 1, we described physical dependence as an altered state of biology induced by a drug whereby withdrawal of a drug is followed by a complex set of biological events typical for that class of drugs. Acute withdrawal from opioids has been well studied, since it can be easily precipitated in drug-dependent individuals by injecting the opioid antagonist naloxone (Narcan). Withdrawal results in a profound reduction in the release of dopamine in the nucleus accumbens,[22] a reduction in the level of dynorphin in the nucleus accumbens,[35] and a large (300 percent) increase in the release of norepinephrine in various structures including the hippocampus,[36] nucleus accumbens,[37] and locus coeruleus.[38]

Immediate symptoms of withdrawal include restlessness, drug craving, sweating, extreme anxiety, depression, irritability, dysphoria, fever, chills, violent retching and vomiting, increased respiratory rate (panting), cramping, insomnia, explosive diarrhea, and intense aches and pains. The magnitude of these acute withdrawal symptoms depends on the dose of opioid, the frequency of previous drug administration, and the duration of drug dependence. Acute opioid withdrawal is not considered to be life-threatening, although it can seem unbearable to the person experiencing it.

More recently recognized is a *protracted abstinence syndrome.*[15] This syndrome begins when the acute phase of opioid withdrawal ends, persisting for up to 6 months. Symptoms of this syndrome include depression, abnormal responses to stressful situations, drug hunger, decreased self-esteem, anxiety, and other psychological disturbances. Complicating the diagnosis of prolonged abstinence syndrome is the high prevalence of other psychiatric disorders (e.g., affective and personality disorders) in opioid-dependent individuals. Thus, recurrence or expression of underlying personality problems that drug use may have masked should be expected, diagnosed, and treated appropriately.

Several behavioral theories have been posited to account for continued opioid use:[15,39]

1. Continued use avoids the distress and dysphoria associated with withdrawal.

2. The euphoria (a positive reinforcing effect) produced by the opioids leads to their continued use.

3. Preexisting dysphoric or painful affective states are alleviated.

4. The euphoric response is an atypical response to opioids that occurs in individuals with preexistent psychopathology.

5. Preexisting psychopathology may be the basis for initial experimentation and euphoria, but repeated use is prompted by the desire to avoid withdrawal.

6. Some individuals have deficient endorphin systems that are corrected by the use of opioids.

7. Repeated use of opioids leads to permanent dysfunction in the endorphin system such that normal function requires the continued use of exogenous opioids.

8. Drug effects and drug withdrawal can become linked through environmental cues and internal mood states. Here, emotions and external cues recall the distress of withdrawal or the memory of opioid euphoria or opioid reduction of dysphoria or painful affective states.

To varying degrees, all of these theories are probably involved in a given individual's use of opioids. The propensity toward opioid dependence lies not merely in a few predisposed individuals, because dependence can develop in anyone who uses the drugs repeatedly; all users (even short-term users) experience some withdrawal when drug use is ended. The listed behavioral theories may be of value in identifying individuals who may be more susceptible to relapse during or after prolonged abstinence syndrome.

Other Pure Agonist Opioids

Morphine is the prototype of a pure opioid agonist. Several similar opioids are also available.

Heroin (diacetylmorphine) is produced from morphine by a slight modification of chemical structure (Figure 10.5). Heroin is about three times as potent as morphine. Its increased lipid solubility leads to faster penetration of the blood–brain barrier, producing an intense rush when it is either smoked or injected intravenously. Heroin is metabolized to morphine, which is eventually metabolized and excreted. Heroin is legally available in Great Britain, where it is used clinically. The drug is not legal in the United States. The trend toward the smoking of heroin tends to reduce some of the risks of injection (exposure to hepatitis and AIDS). When heroin is smoked together with crack cocaine, euphoria is intensified, the anxiety and paranoia associated with cocaine are tempered, and the depression that follows

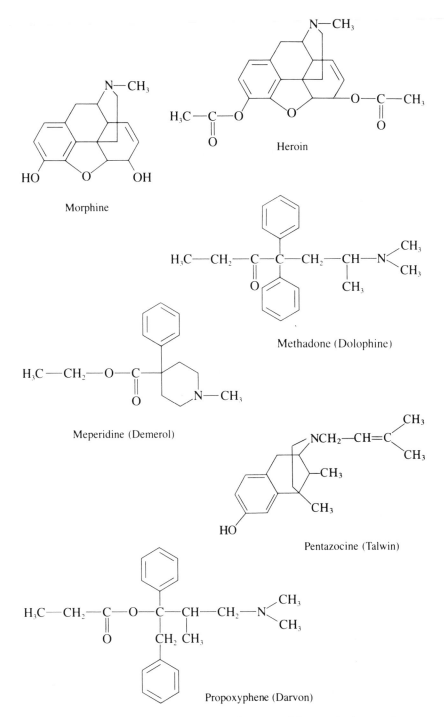

FIGURE 10.5   Structural formulas of morphine, heroin, and four synthetic narcotic analgesics.

after the effects of cocaine wear off is reduced. Unfortunately, this combination creates a polydrug addiction that is extremely difficult to treat.

Codeine, along with morphine, occurs naturally in opium. It is only about one-tenth as potent as morphine, but it is absorbed better than morphine when taken orally. Codeine is often combined with aspirin or acetaminophen (Tylenol) in oral tablets for use as a moderately effective analgesic combination.

Hydromorphone (Dilaudid) and *oxymorphone* (Numorphan) are both structurally related to morphine. Both of these drugs are effective mu receptor stimulants that are about 6 to 10 times as potent as morphine.

Meperidine (Demerol) is a synthetic opioid whose structure differs from that of morphine (see Figure 10.5). Originally meperidine was thought to be free of many of the undesirable properties associated with the use of opioids that are structurally related to morphine. However, meperidine is now considered addictive and can be substituted for morphine or heroin in addicts. Meperidine is widely prescribed medically. It is one-tenth as potent as morphine, produces a similar type of euphoria, and is equally likely to cause dependence. Meperidine's side effects differ from morphine's and include tremors, delirium, hyperreflexia, and convulsions. These effects are produced by a metabolite of meperidine (normeperidine) that has no analgesic action but can cause CNS excitation. Meperidine can accumulate in individuals who have kidney dysfunction or who use only meperidine for their opioid addiction.

Methadone (Dolophine) is a synthetic opioid, the pharmacological activity of which is very similar to that of morphine.

> The outstanding properties of methadone are its effective analgesic activity, its efficacy by the oral route, its extended duration of action in suppressing withdrawal symptoms in physically dependent individuals, and its tendency to show persistent effects with repeated administration.[40]

To control opioid withdrawal, methadone, an orally absorbed opioid, is substituted for the injected opioid to which the patient is addicted. Later the dependent individual can be withdrawn slowly from the methadone or the methadone can be continued indefinitely.

LAAM (levo-alpha-acetylmethadol) is an oral opioid analgesic approved in mid-1993 (after many years of delay) for the clinical management of opioid dependence. Similar in many respects to methadone, LAAM is well absorbed from the gastrointestinal tract. It has a slow onset and a long duration of action. It is metabolized to compounds that are also active as opioid agonists. Its primary advantage over methadone is its long duration of action; in maintenance therapy it is administered by mouth three times a week. Its use in the treatment of opioid dependence is discussed later in this chapter.

Propoxyphene (Darvon) is an analgesic compound that is structurally similar to methadone (see Figure 10.5). As an analgesic, it is less potent than codeine but more potent than aspirin in therapeutic doses. When propoxyphene is taken in large doses, opioidlike effects are seen; when it is used intravenously, it is recognized by addicts as a narcotic. Taken orally, propoxyphene does not have much potential for abuse. Some cases of drug dependence have been reported, but to date they have not been of major concern. Because commercial intravenous preparations of propoxyphene are not available, intravenous abuse is encountered only when persons attempt to inject solutions of the powder that is contained in capsules, which are intended for oral use.

Fentanyl (Sublimaze) and two related compounds, *sufentanil* (Sufenta) and *alfentanil* (Alfenta), are short-acting, intravenously administered, agonist opioids that are structurally related to meperidine. These compounds are intended to be used during and after surgery to relieve surgical pain. As discussed earlier, fentanyl is now available in a skin patch, with the transdermal route of drug delivery offering prolonged, rather steady levels of drug in blood. The drug is used to treat chronic, intractable pain. A fentanyl "lollypop" was made available in selected hospitals in late 1994 for the treatment of post-operative pain in children.

Fentanyl and its derivatives are 80 to 500 times as potent as morphine as analgesics, have rather short durations of action, and profoundly depress respiration. Death from these agents is invariably caused by respiratory failure. In illicit use, fentanyl is known as "China white." Numerous derivatives (such as methylfentanyl) can be manufactured illegally; they emerge periodically and have been responsible for multiple fatalities.*

---

*To control the manufacture and distribution of illicit derivatives of fentanyl, the Federal Drug Enforcement Agency (DEA) has been authorized to declare any drug a Schedule I narcotic substance if it poses an immediate public health hazard. Within the past 10 years, dozens of analogue drugs have been placed under Schedule I control, including MMDA (Chapter 12) and certain meperidine (Demerol) derivatives, especially MPPP and MPTP. Both MPPP and MPTP are neurotoxic by-products of meperidine, and both induce a severe, irreversible, and progressive parkinsonian disease state. Such control was first invoked for the fentanyl analogue 3-methylfentanyl in 1985. Since then many other fentanyl analogues have been placed under control. Newer legislation makes it illegal to engage in any drug activities using these illicit analogues, regardless of whether the drug has been duly scheduled under the DEA's Controlled Substance Act.

Buprenorphine (Buprenex) is a newer opioid whose action is characterized by a limited stimulation (partial agonist action) of mu receptors, which is responsible for its analgesic properties. However, as a partial agonist, there is a ceiling to its analgesic effectiveness as well as to its potential for inducing euphoria and respiratory depression. It has a very long duration of action, presumably because of its strong binding to mu receptors. Such binding, however, occasionally limits its reversibility by naloxone when a reversal is considered necessary.

At low doses, buprenorphine can substitute for morphine (in morphine-dependent individuals) and it is analgesic (in nontolerant individuals). However, higher doses do not substitute well for morphine, and they can precipitate withdrawal symptoms.

Buprenorphine is being evaluated as an alternative, or subsequent step, to methadone for narcotic detoxification and maintenance programs. It may provide an easier transition from methadone to a pure narcotic antagonist such as naltrexone.[41] Gold[6] reviews the literature relevant to this use.

Opioids with Mixed Actions

Four drugs that all bind with varying affinity to the mu and kappa receptors are pentazocine (Talwin), butorphanol (Stadol), nalbuphine (Nubain), and dezocine (Dalgan) (Figure 10.6). These drugs, in general, are weak mu agonists, with most of their analgesic effectiveness (which is quite limited) resulting from their stimulation of kappa receptors (see Table 10.2). Low doses cause moderate analgesia; higher doses produce little additional analgesia. In opioid-dependent individuals, these drugs can precipitate withdrawal, likely by inhibiting mu-agonist-induced activation of the mesolimbic dopamine pathway.[16]

Pentazocine and *butorphanol* are prototypical mixed agonist/antagonists, being both weak mu agonists and stronger kappa agonists of limited analgesic effectiveness. Neither of these drugs has much potential for producing respiratory depression or physical dependence.

In November 1993 butorphanol, previously available only for use by injection, became available as a nasal spray.[42] The spray is indicated for use against any type of pain for which an opioid analgesic is appropriate. After spraying into the nostrils, peak plasma levels (and maximal effect) are achieved in about 1 hour, with a duration of 4 to 5 hours. Few studies are available that document the effectiveness of this route. If effective, convenience will be a positive factor. Whether the abuse potential of butorphanol will increase with this preparation is as yet unclear.

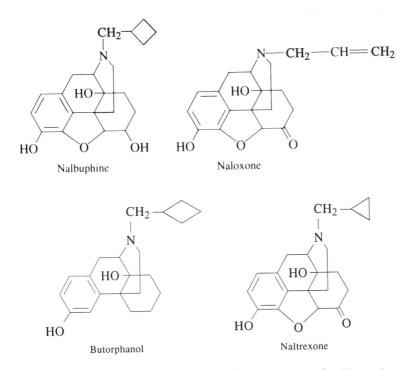

FIGURE 10.6 Structural formulas of four morphine analogues. Nalbuphine and butorphanol have mixed agonistic/antagonistic properties, while naloxone and naltrexone are pure antagonists.

In recent years abuse of pentazocine has been increasing, particularly in combination with tripelennamine, an antihistamine. This combination of drugs, called "Ts and blues," has caused serious medical complications, including seizures, psychotic episodes, skin ulcerations, abscesses, and muscle wasting. (The latter three effects are caused by the repeated injections rather than by the drugs themselves.)

Nalbuphine is primarily a kappa agonist of limited analgesic effectiveness. Because it is also a mu antagonist, it is not likely to produce either respiratory depression or patterns of abuse. Structurally nalbuphine is closely related to naloxone (Narcan; see Figure 10.6), which is a pure narcotic antagonist (discussed in the following section).

Dezocine, the newest of the mixed agonist/antagonist opioids, was introduced in 1990. As a moderate mu agonist and a weak delta and kappa agonist, dezocine can substitute for morphine. Its clinical efficacy and potential for abuse appear limited.

Opioid Antagonists

Two clinically available drugs, naloxone (Narcan) and naltrexone (Trexan), have affinity for opioid receptors (especially mu receptors), but after binding they exert no agonist effects of their own. Therefore, they completely antagonize the effects of agonist opioids at all their receptors. These drugs are termed *pure opioid antagonists,* just as flumazenil was called a pure benzodiazepine antagonist (Chapter 4).

Naloxone has little or no effect when injected into non-opioid-dependent persons, but it rapidly precipitates withdrawal when injected into opioid-dependent persons. Because it is a pure opioid antagonist, naloxone is neither analgesic nor subject to abuse, and it antagonizes the actions of morphine at all its receptors, with mu receptors being 10 times more sensitive to naloxone than kappa receptors. Because naloxone is not absorbed from the gastrointestinal tract, it must be given by injection. Furthermore, its duration of action is very brief, in the range of 15 to 30 minutes. Thus, for continued opioid antagonism, it must be reinjected at short intervals to avoid "renarcotization."

Naloxone is used to reverse the respiratory depression that follows acute narcotic intoxication (overdoses) and to reverse narcotic-induced respiratory depression in newborns of opioid-dependent mothers. The limitations of naloxone include its short duration of action and its parenteral route of administration. Administered to anyone in pain who has received opioids as pain relievers, naloxone will displace the opioid and precipitate the perception of pain.

Naltrexone became clinically available in 1985 as the first orally absorbed, pure narcotic antagonist. Its actions resemble those of naloxone, but naltrexone is well absorbed orally and has a long duration of action, necessitating only a single daily dose of about 40 to 80 milligrams. It is useful in narcotic treatment programs when it is desirable to maintain a person on chronic therapy with a narcotic antagonist. In persons who take naltrexone daily, any injection of a pure opioid agonist will be ineffective. The primary clinical use of naltrexone is to treat opioid-dependent individuals who realize that they have more to gain by being drugfree than by being drug dependent. The major problem with long-term naloxone therapy is that it must be taken daily to render any opioids ineffective.

Treatment of Opioid Dependence

Hypotheses to account for continued opioid use despite its life-threatening consequences are listed on pages 249–250. As with all behavior-reinforcing drug addictions, an opioid-dependent individual goes for therapy for any of a number of reasons. These range from referral for negative legal, family, social, or job consequences to a personal desire to be free of opioid use and the drug-oriented life-style.

As with the abuse of stimulants (Chapter 6), therapy is aimed at clearing the offending drug from the body, managing withdrawal, diagnosing coexisting psychopathology, treating any psychpathological disorders, and preventing relapse. With the opioids, however, the situation has an important difference.

First, cocaine and the amphetamines are "power drugs," while opioids promote a state of tranquility, analgesia, and sedation. Power-drug users while intoxicated tend to display aggressive, hostile behavior with thought processes that can lead to a state of manic paranoia. Violent acts of aggression and crimes while the drug user is intoxicated are not unusual. With intoxication by opioids, behavior is calm, with mental quieting and tranquility. Crime associated with opioid use usually results from trying to obtain money to buy more drugs and is usually performed when the user is not intoxicated or is in withdrawal. If adequate drug is supplied (usually at little cost), violent acts and crime are usually not a problem.

Total abstinence from all opioids need not be an objective for all addicts. Goals, however, should include prevention of relapse to the use of illicitly obtained, injectable opioids (such as heroin). Continuing, medically managed opioid therapy may be necessary for many addicts, and such an approach follows medical models of illness.[43] For example, a diabetic may require insulin for the remainder of his or her life, a patient with high blood pressure may require antihypertensive medication for a lifetime, and a patient with bipolar disorder might require long-term lithium therapy for mood stabilization. Similarly, a narcotic addict may require ongoing opioid therapy, perhaps for a lifetime. Nevertheless, such therapy requires the elimination both of the parenteral route of drug administration and the need to seek expensive, illicit sources of drugs.

We must carefully distinguish between *physical dependence* and *addiction*. The former implies drug intake to block a set of biological reactions that occur when the drug is not taken. The latter includes not only dependence but a total life-style oriented to obtaining and using a drug in the face of severe adverse consequences. A patient with terminal cancer may have pain that can be relieved only by the use of opioids. This person is likely to become physically dependent on the opioid and experience withdrawal if the drug is withheld. Concern over whether the patient is addicted (physically dependent) becomes secondary to the humane management of pain in the terminally ill patient. The pain associated with terminal illness requires aggressive management, and worry about a developing "addiction" is a minor concern. In contrast, the drug dependence that develops as a result of using opioids for nonmedical use has been treated very differently. Until very recently, the objective has been medically managed withdrawal, with the following sequence of goals:

1. cessation of illicit opioid use

2. transition to orally administered methadone

3. maintenance on methadone for a few days or weeks

4. methadone withdrawal with clonidine administered to make the withdrawal syndrome more tolerable

5. assisted living to help adjust to a drugfree state, usually with the addition of naltrexone to block any effects of any opioid that the individual might take

6. return to the community

Such a sequence of withdrawal with naltrexone maintenance is most successful in patients who are highly motivated to remain totally opioid-free. Examples include addicted physicians and other medical personnel whose continued licensure to practice their profession is contingent on completely abstaining from opioids. The supervised ingestion of naltrexone (about 3 to 4 times per week) implies that any other opioid will be ineffective.

As an alternative to switching from the illicit opioid to methadone, some addicts can be switched from the opioid to buprenorphine,[44] the partial mu agonist discussed above. "Patients transferred to buprenorphine experience little or no withdrawal and craving is generally suppressed. Buprenorphine can then be discontinued or naltrexone treatment can be initiated."[15] Currently, however, most opioid addicts are withdrawn from narcotic use by being switched to methadone and then either being eventually withdrawn from methadone or put on long-term methadone maintenance.

The process of acute withdrawal using methadone is not too difficult and can be achieved in only a few days. However, this process does not treat protracted abstinence syndrome and is almost universally followed by relapse to former patterns of drug use (i.e., treatment failure).

Until recently it was generally believed that an opioid addict must sooner or later be returned to a totally drugfree state. The goal of therapy, therefore, was to eliminate opioid intake from the addict's life. Even recent reviews state that, regardless of the various pharmacological options and the psychological and social support techniques, opioids must be withdrawn from opioid-dependent individuals.[6,15]

If one takes opioids for a prolonged period of time, long-lasting neuronal adaptive changes can be induced that require continued administration of opioids to maintain normal mood states and normal responses to stress. Long-term opioid craving might result from a pre-existing or an opioid-dependency-induced hypofunction of the endoge-nous endorphin system. Therefore, to rehabilitate these addicts and keep them in a functional state, low levels of opioid may be necessary.

With methadone maintenance, addicts are stabilized on metha-done and remain productive members of their communities without withdrawing from the orally administered opioid. After one or two years, many former heroin addicts can be withdrawn from the metha-done over a period of several weeks. The withdrawal discomforts are relatively minor, and some patients can complete the withdrawal process and not relapse to the use of heroin or other illicit opioid. Others later return to using heroin. Still others discontinue the with-drawal process and remain on methadone maintenance. The opioid, however, must be combined with intensive psychological counseling, and the patient must adopt a productive life-style.

It is not enough to switch addicts from heroin to an oral opioid and then return them to the street. When an addict is simply returned to the street, he or she often compulsively abuses the methadone or returns to the use of heroin. Addicts must be helped to find a new life-style and positive reinforcements to replace the motivation to use opi-oids. Certainly, it is better to maintain an opioid addict on methadone than to return him or her to the street and to former habits of drug acquisition and use, with its negative consequences.

Goldstein reviews over 20 years of administering methadone main-tenance therapy to 1000 heroin addicts in New Mexico.[45] Over half of the patients were traced and analyzed. Of these, over one-third are now dead; causes include violence, overdosage, and alcoholism. About one-quarter are still enmeshed in the criminal justice system. About one-quarter go on and off methadone maintenance, indicating that opioid dependence, whether on heroin or on methadone, is a lifelong condition for a considerable fraction of the addict population. With one-half of the treated population of 1000 addicts unaccounted for, the data are obviously incomplete. Likely many of these unaccounted-for former addicts are either drugfree or are stabilized on an opioid and remain functional in their communities. Indeed, the successful gradu-ates of therapy are the most difficult to track, usually preferring to re-main anonymous in their communities.

Regardless, treatment of opioid dependence leads to a productive life-style in only a minority of cases. The most interesting data now support lifelong opioid maintenance as a treatment possibility, with withdrawal (and perhaps naltrexone treatment) as necessary primarily for those addicts who have much to gain by being drugfree or who desire to be drugfree. When drugfree individuals relapse, they must be readmitted to methadone (or LAAM) maintenance immediately. Unfortunately, many people still see physical dependence on an opioid as "bad" in and of itself. These attitudes must be changed before widespread attempts at long-term opioid maintenance can be fully evaluated.

NONNARCOTIC ANALGESIC AND ANTI-INFLAMMATORY DRUGS

The nonnarcotic analgesics are a group of chemically unrelated drugs (Figure 10.7) that produce both analgesic and anti-inflammatory effects. They block the generation of peripheral pain impulses by inhibiting the synthesis and release of prostaglandins.*,[46],[47] These drugs do not bind to opioid receptors. Their effects include (1) reduction of inflammation (anti-inflammatory effect), (2) reduction in body temperature when the patient has a fever (antipyretic effect), (3) reduction in pain without sedation (analgesic effect), and (4) inhibition of platelet aggregation (anticoagulant effect).

Numerous drugs are classified as nonnarcotic analgesics, including aspirin and other salicylates, ibuprofen, acetaminophen, indomethacin, phenylbutazone, ketorolac, and naproxen. Many of these drugs are used to reduce both the inflammation and the pain associated with arthritis. Gastric irritation limits their long-term usefulness.

Aspirin

In the United States, about 10 to 20 thousand tons of aspirin are consumed each year; it is our most popular and most effective analgesic, antipyretic, and anti-inflammatory drug. It is most effective for low-

---

*Prostaglandins are autacoids (Chapter 7) that induce local inflammatory responses. Aspirinlike drugs inhibit the enzyme cyclooxygenase (prostaglandin synthetase), which is responsible for the biosynthesis of certain prostaglandins. In addition, recent studies suggest that the inhibition of prostaglandin synthesis is only part of aspirin's action;[48] the local anti-inflammatory action also results from aspirin's ability to disrupt white blood cell responsiveness to tissue injury, thus preventing the cellular release of tissue-disruptive enzymes.

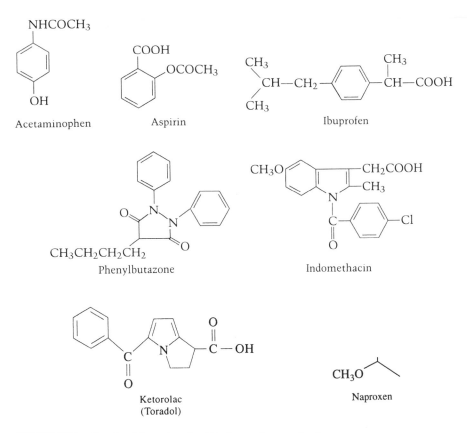

FIGURE 10.7   Structural formulas of anti-inflammatory analgesics.

intensity pain. The analgesic and anti-inflammatory effects follow peripheral inhibition of both prostaglandin synthesis and white blood cell responsiveness to injury. Its antipyretic effect follows the inhibition of prostaglandin synthesis in the hypothalamus, a structure in the brain that modulates body temperature. However, one caution is necessary regarding the use of aspirin to reduce fever. An association exists between the use of aspirin for the fever that accompanies varicella (chicken pox) or influenza and the subsequent development of Reye's syndrome, including severe liver and brain damage and even death.[49]

Aspirin increases oxygen consumption by the body, which increases the production of carbon dioxide, an effect that stimulates respiration. Therefore, an overdose with aspirin is often characterized by a marked increase in respiratory rate, which causes the overdosed person to appear to pant. This occurrence results in other, severe metabolic consequences that are beyond this discussion.

Aspirin has important effects on blood coagulation.[48] For blood to coagulate, platelets must first be able to aggregate, an action requiring the presence of prostaglandins. (Platelets are small components of the blood that adhere to vascular membranes after injury to a vessel. They form an initial plug, over which a blood clot eventually forms to limit bleeding from a lacerated blood vessel.) Aspirin can inhibit the aggregation of platelets and therefore reduce the formation of intravascular clots. Low doses of aspirin (for example, one tablet daily) are now widely used for preventing strokes and heart attacks, which can be caused by atherosclerosis, intravascular clotting, or the formation of emboli on either artificial or damaged heart valves.

Side effects of aspirin are common. Gastric upset occurs most frequently. In addition, poisoning by aspirin occurs thousands of times each year and can be fatal. Mild intoxication can produce ringing in the ears, auditory and visual difficulties, mental confusion, thirst, and hyperventilation.

Acetaminophen, Ibuprofen, and Related Drugs

Acetaminophen (Tylenol) is an effective alternative to aspirin as an analgesic and antipyretic agent. However, its anti-inflammatory effect is minor, and it is not clinically useful in treating acute inflammation or arthritis. Because acetaminophen does not inhibit platelet aggregation, it is not useful for preventing vascular clotting or for prophylaxis against heart attacks or stroke. No reports have associated acetaminophen with Reye's syndrome. It should be noted that an acute overdose (either accidental or intentional) may produce severe or even fatal liver damage.

Acetaminophen generally has fewer side effects than aspirin; the drug produces less gastric distress and less ringing in the ears. Alcoholics appear to be especially susceptible to the hepatotoxic effects of even moderate doses of acetaminophen.[50] Indeed, alcoholics should avoid acetaminophen while they persist in heavy consumption of alcohol.

Acetaminophen has been proven to be a reasonable substitute for aspirin when analgesic or antipyretic effectiveness is desired, especially in children and in patients who cannot tolerate aspirin. Candidates for acetaminophen might include patients with peptic ulcer disease or gastric distress or anyone in whom aspirin is poorly tolerated.

Ibuprofen (Advil, Motrin, Nuprin, and Medipren) is an aspirinlike analgesic, antipyretic, and anti-inflammatory agent. Compounds that are similar to ibuprofen include *naproxen* (Aleve, Naprosyn, and Anaprox) and *fenoprofen* (Nalfon).

All three compounds are effective analgesic, anti-inflammatory, and antipyretic agents. Their effectiveness is comparable to or greater than that of acetaminophen, aspirin, codeine, aspirin with codeine, and propoxyphene (Darvon).[47] Their actions presumably occur as a result of drug-induced inhibition of prostaglandin synthesis. The incidence and severity of side effects produced by these agents are somewhat lower than those of aspirin, but gastric distress and the formation of peptic ulcers have been reported. Like aspirin but unlike acetaminophen, these compounds inhibit platelet aggregation and therefore interfere with the clotting process. These drugs should be used with caution in patients who suffer from peptic ulcer disease or bleeding abnormalities. At the present time, ibuprofen and naproxen are not recommended for use by pregnant women. They are not secreted in breast milk.

Phenylbutazone (Butazolidin) is an older, effective anti-inflammatory agent that was once widely used to relieve the inflammation associated with rheumatoid arthritis. However, significant side effects have limited its long-term usefulness. Unlike most of the other anti-inflammatory drugs, its half-life is quite long (about 2 days).

Most patients who take phenylbutazone experience some side effects, usually in the form of gastric distress and skin rashes. More severe problems include ulcer formation, allergies, liver and renal dysfunction, and a variety of severe abnormalities in various types of blood cells. At present, phenylbutazone is considered to be a secondary choice for treating the symptoms of rheumatoid arthritis and similar disorders.

Indomethacin (Indocin) is an effective anti-inflammatory drug that is used primarily for treating rheumatoid arthritis and similar disorders. Like phenylbutazone, its use is limited because of its toxicity. Indomethacin is an analgesic, antipyretic, and anti-inflammatory agent. Indeed, its clinical effects closely resemble those of aspirin. Side effects occur in about 50 percent of the patients who take indomethacin, with gastric dysfunction being most prominent. Paradoxically, drug-induced headache limits its use in many patients. Other side effects are rare but potentially serious.

Ketorolac (Toradol) is a new analgesic and anti-inflammatory agent; it is the first of these agents to be available in injectable form for use in the treatment of pain after an operation. Administered intramuscularly, it is quite effective in the short-term postoperative treatment of moderate to severe pain.[51,52] Like the analgesics already discussed, it indirectly inhibits prostaglandin synthesis. Its analgesic potency is comparable to that of low doses of morphine administered intramuscularly, and it appears to offer greater anti-inflammatory action. Its half-life is about 4 to 6 hours in most persons, but it is longer in the elderly. Ketorolac is not recommended for use in obstetrics (because it and all other inhibitors of prostaglandin synthesis can adversely affect uterine contraction and fetal circulation).[51]

Study Questions

1. Describe the location of opioid receptors in the brain and the spinal cord.
2. How are pain impulses modulated as they enter the spinal cord?
3. What is substance P and how is it influenced by narcotic analgesics?
4. What is an opioid agonist? What is an opioid antagonist? What is a mixed agonist/antagonist? Give an example of each.
5. What might lead a person to misuse or abuse opioid narcotics?
6. Differentiate between naloxone and naltrexone. How might each of these drugs be used?
7. Describe the various ways that opioid dependence might be handled or treated.
8. Why are tricyclic antidepressants analgesic? (Answer from your knowledge of descending spinal cord analgesic pathways.)
9. Differentiate between the opioid modulation of afferent pain impulses and the affective component of pain.
10. Give evidence for and against the existence of endogenous opioid peptides (e.g., endorphins) that serve as "natural opioids."
11. Explain how the actions of aspirin differ from those of the opioids.
12. Why is aspirin anti-inflammatory and morphine not?

Notes

1. Y. Kuraishi and others, "Noradrenergic Inhibition of the Release of Substance P from the Primary Afferents in the Rabbit Spinal Dorsal Horn," *Brain Research* 359 (1985): 177–182.
2. J. C. Eisenach, D. M. Dewan, J. C. Ruse, and J. M. Angelo, "Epidural Clonidine Produces Antinociception, But Not Hypotension, in Sheep," *Anesthesiology* 66 (1987): 496–501.
3. M. E. S. Alojado, Y. Ohta, T. Yamamura, and O. Kemmotsu, "The Effect of Fentanyl and Morphine on Neurons in the Dorsal Raphe Nucleus in the Rat: An *In Vitro* Study," *Anesthesia and Analgesia* 78 (1994): 726–732.

4. K. H. Gwirtz, "Intraspinal Narcotics in the Management of Postoperative Pain," *Anesthesiology Review* 17 (1990): 16–28.
5. D. Coquoz, H. C. Porchet, and P. Dayer, "Central Analgesic Effects of Desipramine, Fluvoxamine, and Moclobemide after Single Oral Dosing: A Study in Healthy Volunteers," *Clinical Pharmacology and Therapeutics* 54 (1994): 339–344.
6. M. S. Gold, "Opiate Addiction and the Locus Coeruleus: The Clinical Utility of Clonidine, Naltrexone, Methadone, and Buprenorphine," *Psychiatric Clinics of North America* 16 (1993): 65.
7. R. W. Hansen and K. E. Gerber, *Coping with Chronic Pain: A Guide to Patient Management* (New York: Guilford, 1990).
8. Q. P. Ma and J. S. Han, "Neurochemical Studies on the Mesolimbic Circuitry of Antinociception," *Brain Research* 566 (1991): 95–102.
9. Q. P. Ma and J. S. Han, "Neurochemical and Morphological Evidence of an Antinociceptive Neural Pathway from Nucleus Raphe Dorsalis to Nucleus Accumbens in the Rabbit," *Brain Research Bulletin* 28 (1992): 931–936.
10. Q. Pei, T. Zetterstrom, R. A. Leslie, and D. G. Grahame-Smith, "5-HT$_3$ Receptor Antagonists Inhibit Morphine-Induced Stimulation of Mesolimbic Dopamine Release and Function in the Rat," *European Journal of Pharmacology* 230 (1993): 63–68.
11. A. Goldstein, *Addiction: From Biology to Drug Policy* (New York: W. H. Freeman and Company, 1994), p. 138.
12. J. H. Jaffe and W. R. Martin, "Opioid Analgesics and Antagonists," in A. G. Gilman, T. W. Rall, A. S. Nies, and P. Taylor, eds., *Goodman and Gilman's The Pharmacological Basis of Therapeutics*, 8th ed. (New York: Pergamon, 1990), pp. 485–489.
13. R. M. Brown, D. H. Clouet, and D. Friedman, eds., *Opiate Receptor Subtypes and Brain Function*, National Institute on Drug Abuse, Monograph No. 71, Department of Health and Human Services Publication No. ADM 86-1462 (Washington, D.C.: U.S. Government Printing Office, 1986).
14. E. J. Simon, "Opiates: Neurobiology," in J. H. Lowinson, P. Ruiz, R. B. Millman, and J. G. Langrod, eds., *Substance Abuse: A Comprehensive Textbook*, 2nd ed. (Baltimore: Williams & Wilkins, 1993), p. 192.
15. J. H. Jaffe, "Opiates: Clinical Aspects," in J. H. Lowinson, P. Ruiz, R. B. Millman, and J. G. Langrod, eds., *Substance Abuse: A Comprehensive Textbook*, 2nd ed. (Baltimore: Williams & Wilkins, 1993), pp. 186–194.
16. M. Narita, T. Suzuki, M. Funada, M. Misawa, and H. Nagase, "Blockade of the Morphine-Induced Increase in Turnover of Dopamine on the Mesolimbic Dopaminergic System by Kappa-Opioid Receptor Activation in Mice," *Life Sciences* 52 (1993): 397–404.
17. A. Jacox et al., *Management of Cancer Pain*, Clinical Practice Guideline No. 9, AHCPR Publication No. 94-0592 (Rockville, Md.: Agency for Health Care Policy and Research, U.S. Department of Health and Human Services, Public Health Service, March 1994).
18. K. Verebey, "Diagnostic Laboratory: Screening for Drug Abuse," in J. H. Lowinson, P. Ruiz, R. B. Millman, and J. G. Langrod, eds., *Substance

Abuse: A Comprehensive Textbook, 2nd ed. (Baltimore: Williams & Wilkins, 1993), pp. 425–437.

19. Q. P. Ma, Y. S. Shi, and J. S. Han, "Further Studies of Interactions between Periaqueductal Gray, Nucleus Accumbens and Habenula in Antinociception," *Brain Research* 583 (1992): 292–295.

20. D. A. Mahler, L. N. Cunningham, G. S. Skrinar, W. J. Kraemer, and G. L. Colice, "Beta-Endorphin Activity and Hypercapnic Ventilatory Responsiveness after Marathon Running," *Journal of Applied Physiology* 66 (1989): 2431–2436.

21. G. A. Sforzo, "Opioids and Exercise. An Update," *Sports Medicine* 7 (1989): 109–124.

22. G. Di Chiara and R. A. North, "Neurobiology of Opiate Abuse," *Trends in Pharmacological Sciences* 13 (1992): 187.

23. T. S. Shippenberg, R. Bals-Kubik, and A. Herz, "Examination of the Neurochemical Substrates Mediating the Motivational Effects of Opioids: Role of the Mesolimbic Dopamine System and D-1 vs. D-2 Dopamine Receptors," *Journal of Pharmacology and Experimental Therapeutics* 265 (1993): 53–59.

24. X. R. Yuan, S. Madamba, and G. R. Siggins, "Opioid Peptides Reduce Synaptic Transmission in the Nucleus Accumbens," *Neuroscience Letters* 134 (1992): 223–228.

25. C. Kornetsky and L. J. Porrino, "Brain Mechanisms of Drug-Induced Reinforcement," *Research Publications—Association for Research in Nervous and Mental Disease* 70 (1992): 59–77.

26. S. T. Cunningham and A. E. Kelley, "Evidence for Opiate-Dopamine Cross-Sensitization in Nucleus Accumbens: Studies of Conditioned Reward," *Brain Research Bulletin* 29 (1992): 675–680.

27. S. D. Glick, C. Merski, S. Steindorf, S. Wank, R. W. Keller, and J. N. Carlson, "Neurochemical Predisposition to Self-Administer Morphine in Rats," *Brain Research* 578 (1992): 215–220.

28. P. Leone, D. Pocock, and R. A. Wise, "Morphine-Dopamine Interaction: Ventral Tegmental Morphine Increases Nucleus Accumbens Dopamine Release," *Pharmacology, Biochemistry & Behavior* 39 (1991): 469–472.

29. S. T. Tiffany and P. M. Maude-Griffin, "Tolerance to Morphine in the Rat: Associative and Nonassociative Effects," *Behavioral Neuroscience* 102 (1988): 534–543.

30. J. Moring and J. Strang, "Cue Exposure as an Assessment Technique in the Management of a Heroin Addict: Case Report," *Drug and Alcohol Dependence* 24 (1989): 161–167.

31. S. Siegel, "Heroin 'Overdose' Death: Contribution of Drug-Associated Environmental Cues," *Science* 216 (1982): 436–437.

32. M. Gaiardi, M. Bartoletti, A. Bacchi, C. Gubellini, M. Costa, and M. Babbini, "Role of Repeated Exposure to Morphine in Determining Its Affective Properties: Place and Taste Conditioning Studies in Rats," *Psychopharmacology* 103 (1991): 183–186.

33. P. Vezina and J. Stewart, "Amphetamine Administered to the Ventral

Tegmental Area But Not to the Nucleus Accumbens Sensitizes Rats to Systemic Morphine: Lack of Conditioned Effects," *Brain Research* 516 (1990): 99–106.

34. P. W. Kalivas and P. Duffy, "Sensitization to Repeated Morphine Injection in the Rat: Possible Involvement of A10 Dopamine Neurons," *Journal of Pharmacology and Experimental Therapeutics* 241 (1987): 204–212.

35. R. Y. Yukhananov, Q. Z. Zhai, S. Persson, C. Post, and F. Nyberg, "Chronic Administration of Morphine Decreases Level of Dynorphin A in the Rat Nucleus Accumbens," *Neuropharmacology* 32 (1993): 703–709.

36. P. H. Silverstone, C. Done, and T. Sharp, "In Vivo Monoamine Release during Naloxone-Precipitated Morphine Withdrawal," *Neuroreport* 4 (1993): 1043–1045.

37. E. Acquas and G. Di Chiara, "Depression of Mesolimbic Dopamine Transmission and Sensitization to Morphine during Opiate Abstinence," *Journal of Neurochemistry* 58 (1992): 1620–1625.

38. R. Maldonado, L. Stinus, L. H. Gold, and G. F. Koob, "Role of Different Brain Structures in the Expression of the Physical Morphine Withdrawal Syndrome," *Journal of Pharmacology & Experimental Therapeutics* 261 (1992): 660–677.

39. J. H. Jaffe and F. K. Jaffe, *Historical Perspectives on the Use of Subjective Effects Measures in Assessing the Abuse Potential of Drugs,* Research Monograph 92 (Washington, D.C.: National Institute on Drug Abuse, 1989), pp. 43–72.

40. J. H. Jaffe and W. R. Martin, "Opioid Analgesics and Antagonists," in A. G. Gilman, T. W. Rall, A. S. Nies, and P. Taylor, eds., *Goodman and Gilman's The Pharmacological Basis of Therapeutics,* 13th ed. (New York: Pergamon, 1990), p. 508.

41. E. C. Strain and others, "Comparison of Buprenorphine and Methadone in the Treatment of Opioid Dependence," *American Journal of Psychiatry* 151 (1994): 1025–1030.

42. "Butorphanol Nasal Spray for Pain," *The Medical Letter* 35 (12 November 1993): 105–106.

43. A. Goldstein, "Heroin Addiction: Neurobiology, Pharmacology, and Policy," *Journal of Psychoactive Drugs* 23 (1991): 123–133.

44. R. A. Rawson and W. Ling, "Opioid Addiction Treatment Modalities and Some Guidelines to Their Optimal Use," *Journal of Psychoactive Drugs* 23 (1991): 151–163.

45. A. Goldstein, *Addiction,* pp. 142–154.

46. P. A. Insel, "Analgesic-Antipyretics and Anti-Inflammatory Agents: Drugs Employed in the Treatment of Rheumatoid Arthritis and Gout," in A. G. Gilman, T. W. Rall, A. S. Nies, and P. Taylor, eds., *Goodman and Gilman's The Pharmacological Basis of Therapeutics,* 8th ed. (New York: Pergamon, 1990), pp. 638–681.

47. "Analgesics," in *Drug Evaluations Annual 1994* (Milwaukee, Wis.: American Medical Association, 1993), pp. 114–131.

48. G. Weissmann, "Aspirin," *Scientific American* 264 (1991): 84–90.

49. P. Pinsky, E. S. Hurwitz, L. B. Schonberger, and W. J. Gunn, "Reye's Syndrome and Aspirin. Evidence for a Dose–Response Effect," *Journal of the American Medical Association* 260 (1988): 657–661.

50. L. B. Seeff, B. A. Cuccherini, H. J. Zimmerman, E. Adler, and S. B. Benjamin, "Acetaminophen Hepatotoxicity in Alcoholics. A Therapeutic Misadventure," *Annals of Internal Medicine* 104 (1986): 399–404.

51. "Ketorolac Tromethamine," *The Medical Letter on Drugs and Therapeutics* 32 (1990): 79–81.

52. M. M.-T. Buckley and R. N. Brogden, "Ketorolac: Review of Its Pharmacodynamic and Pharmacokinetic Properties, and Therapeutic Potential," *Drugs* 39 (1990): 86–109.1

CHAPTER 11

ANTIPSYCHOTIC (NEUROLEPTIC) AND ANTIPARKINSONIAN DRUGS

At first glance, considering drugs used to treat schizophrenia and Parkinson's disease (parkinsonism) in the same chapter seems unusual. However, both classes of drugs act upon similar receptor systems. Furthermore, the drugs used to treat schizophrenia produce side effects that closely resemble the symptoms of idiopathic parkinsonism. Similarly, the drugs used to treat the side effects of antischizophrenia therapy are the same drugs used to treat parkinsonism. Indeed, schizophrenia has long been associated with dysfunction of a subclass of dopamine receptors, while parkinsonism follows from a deficiency in the number and function of certain dopamine-secreting neurons. Most of this chapter is devoted to the drugs used to treat schizophrenia; the chapter ends with a brief discussion of antiparkinsonism drugs.

ANTIPSYCHOTIC (NEUROLEPTIC) DRUGS

Schizophrenia has long been recognized as one of the most severe and debilitating of psychiatric illnesses.[1] It is also a common disorder, with approximately 1 in every 100 persons developing it during his or her lifetime.[2] Approximately 1.2 million people have schizophrenia in the United States at the present time.[3] A majority of affected individuals are unemployed, and family costs (e.g., lost work time and treatment expenses) may range from $410 to $15,000 per year per patient.[2] The national costs are equally staggering.

Schizophrenia typically has an onset in individuals in their late teens and early twenties, with young males having the worst prognoses. Like the affective disorders, schizophrenia is associated with an increased risk of suicide: Approximately 10 to 15 percent of individuals with schizophrenia take their own lives, usually within the first 10 years of developing the disorder. The present state of treatment for schizophrenia is summarized in a recent congressional report:

> Currently, there is no way to prevent or cure schizophrenia: however, treatments that control some of its symptoms are available. The optimal treatment generally integrates antipsychotic drugs and supportive psychosocial treatment. Individuals acutely ill with schizophrenia may require hospitalization. Furthermore, rehabilitation is generally necessary to enhance social and occupational outcomes.[3]

The first part of this chapter focuses on the pharmacology of drugs used to treat schizophrenia. Psychosocial treatment cannot be overlooked, however. Supportive psychotherapy is aimed at helping patients understand their illness, reduce stress, enhance coping abilities, secure the patient's cooperation in treatment, and perhaps reduce the amount of medication required to prevent relapse.[4,5] Educating the family, as well as providing them with the tools to deal with stress, is also vital. Finally, a wide range of social and vocational rehabilitation programs are important adjuncts—but not alternatives—to antipsychotic medication and supportive psychotherapy.[4]

It was formerly thought that schizophrenia was a single disease process of which the primary pathology was a dissociation of thoughts, emotion, and behavior. Today, however, schizophrenia is generally considered a clinical syndrome encompassing a continuum ranging from mild attenuated personality traits resembling schizophrenia to severe, unremitting psychosis.[6] Indeed, schizotypical personality disorder is a prototype of the schizophrenia-related personality disorders and is a diagnosis related to classical schizophrenia.[6]

The schizophrenias are characterized by disturbances of thought and cognition. The components of thought may become dissociated or fragmented, with the flow of thought interrupted. "Schizophrenia typically impairs the ability to integrate information, to reason, to concentrate, or to focus attention or purpose. The consequence is often an observed vagueness, illogicality, and bizarreness of thinking that, when severe, restricts interpersonal communication."[3]

Persons who suffer from schizophrenia display an impaired capacity to recognize reality, communicate, or associate with others to such a degree that they cannot deal with the ordinary demands of life. Affected persons can exhibit abnormal behavior as well as a serious inability to think coherently, to comprehend reality, or to gain insight into their abnormality. These conditions often include delusions and hallucinations (usually auditory).

Classically, the symptoms of schizophrenia have been classified as "positive" and "negative." The positive symptoms are those typical of psychosis and include delusions and hallucinations, bizarre behaviors, dissociated or fragmented thoughts, incoherence, and illogicality. The negative symptoms include blunted affect, impaired emotional responsiveness, apathy, loss of motivation and interest, and social withdrawal. This differentiation of symptomatology is of importance in the pharmacology of antipsychotic drugs since the classic agents affect primarily the positive symptoms, while the "new generation," or "atypical," antipsychotic drugs relieve the negative symptoms.

Etiology of Schizophrenia

There is no doubt that there is a genetic component to schizophrenia.[7,8] Figure 11.1 illustrates the risk that relatives of affected individuals will develop schizophrenia. In addition, the schizoaffective and

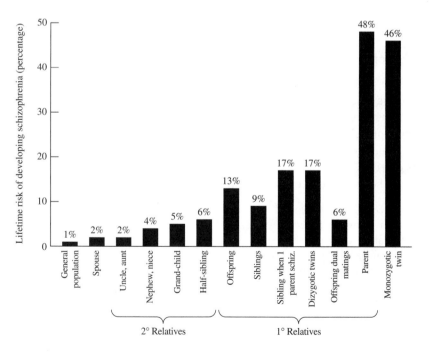

FIGURE 11.1   Lifetime risks of developing schizophrenia among relatives of an affected individual. Data from about 40 European family and twin studies conducted between 1920 and 1987. [From Gottesman, *Schizophrenia Genesis* (New York: W. H. Freeman and Company, 1991); with permission.]

schizotypal personality disorders also have a genetic component.[7] However, nongenetic factors also play important roles, and the exact genetic factor remains unknown. Indeed, interplay between genetic and environmental factors seems to be important in the pathogenesis of schizophrenia.

Until recently, scientific evidence favored a dopamine theory of schizophrenia,[9] according to which the disorder arises from dysregulation in certain brain regions of the dopamine system.[10] This theory was based on several facts:

1. The standard antipsychotic (neuroleptic) drugs are all potent and effective blockers of a certain subclass of dopamine receptors (the dopamine$_2$ receptor).

2. Blockage of the dopamine$_2$ receptors by binding assay linearly correlates with clinical potency as antipsychotic agents (Figure 11.2).

3. Drugs such as cocaine, which potentiate the activity of dopamine (Chapter 6), can precipitate or aggravate schizophrenia-like psychosis.

4. The atypical antipsychotic drug clozapine is a blocker of a different subclass of dopamine receptors, the dopamine$_4$ receptors.

5. The new, atypical neuroleptic, risperidone, is a blocker of both dopamine$_2$ and serotonin$_2$ receptors.

6. Some studies have shown increased densities of dopamine receptors in the brains of deceased schizophrenics.

Despite this evidence, there is only a correlation between schizophrenia and increased dopamine activity; causation has never been demonstrated. In addition, while a hyperdopaminergic theory of schizophrenia may partially explain psychosis, it does not account for the complex and multidimensional nature of the disease, including its diversity of clinical expression (especially the negative symptoms).

Other hallmarks of schizophrenia are the following:

1. correlation of frontal lobe deficits with negative and disorganized symptoms in schizophrenia; 2. abnormalities in the hippocampus relating to symptoms such as memory disturbance; and 3. compromised activity in the left relative to the right hemisphere as a common finding in the disorder.[2]

More recently disturbances of brain development during the prenatal period in genetically predisposed individuals have been examined as causative factors of schizophrenia.[11,12] This has led to the neurodevelopmental theory of schizophrenia. In support of this hypothesis, Akbarian and coworkers identified disturbances in normal patterns of cellular development and migration, which are thought

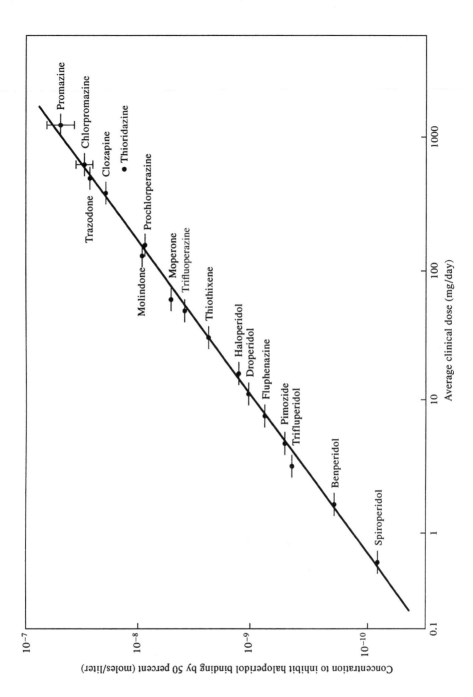

FIGURE 11.2 Correlation between the clinical potency and receptor-binding activities of neuroleptic drugs. Clinical potency is expressed as the daily dose used in treating schizophrenia, and binding activity is expressed as the concentration needed to produce 50 percent inhibition of haloperidol binding. Haloperidol binds to dopamine$_2$ receptors; other antipsychotic drugs compete for the same receptors. Thus, measuring the competitive inhibition of haloperidol binding correlates with potency as an antipsychotic drug.

to occur during the second trimester of pregnancy;[13,14] these altered cellular patterns have serious consequences for the establishment of a normal pattern of cortical connections leading to a potential break-down of frontal lobe function in schizophrenics.[13] Their similar findings in the hippocampus indicate that there may be a more global developmental defect that leads to both the positive (limbic system) and the negative (prefrontal cortex) symptoms of schizophrenia. The authors postulate that "viral infection during the second trimester [of pregnancy] elevates the risk of schizophrenia in susceptible offspring ... in line with this theory."[14] Thus, there may be a "two-hit" etiology of schizophrenia, in which individuals at risk because of genetic factors, having been exposed as fetuses to viral infections of the mother (e.g., influenza) in the second trimester of pregnancy, show an increased incidence of the disease.[15]

Bloom[12] challenges whether a virus is necessary to cause this developmental etiology, suggesting that other mechanisms might alter neuronal development, such as "premature switching off of genes responsible for trophic factors or their receptors in response to fever or famine rather than a viral pestilence."[16] Alternatively, the "genome of a given family tree might 'simply' fail to maintain the expression of one or the other of the genes required to complete the process of cortical neuronal migration."[16] Whatever the etiology, these data provide exciting new insights into the pathogenesis of schizophrenia and may eventually lead to new, more effective treatments and medications.

Overview of Antipsychotic Drugs

Since the mid-1950s, neuroleptic drugs have been the primary treatment for both chronic and acute schizophrenia. They effectively relieve the signs and symptoms of acute schizophrenia and prevent relapse in stabilized patients.[17] As positive as this sounds, these drugs are extremely limited and limiting. First, antipsychotic drugs do not cure the disease; they treat only the clinical symptoms. Even this statement must be qualified, because the drugs are more effective in controlling the positive symptoms of schizophrenia than the negative symptoms.[18] Second, some patients fail to respond to these drugs; approximately 30 percent of schizophrenics have little response to drug treatment of acute symptomatology.[19,20] Third, these drugs have severe side effects. Thus, clinicians "are forced to balance clinical effectiveness (which is less than ideal) against uncomfortable and sometimes disabling side effects."[17]

Today there is hope that newer compounds (such as clozapine, risperidone, and remoxipride) will be more effective in relieving negative symptoms and have fewer side effects, including those that manifest during treatment and those that persist after therapy is discontinued.[21] Finally, if an intrauterine-viral etiology in genetically susceptible individuals is confirmed, treatment of viral influenza during pregnancy may actually prevent schizophrenia rather than merely treat its symptoms.

Historical Background

Clinical descriptions of schizophrenic patients date back at least to 1400 B.C. Until the 1930s isolation of and caring for these patients was the only known therapy. Some schizophrenics were effectively treated with care that resembles today's group and social therapy. However, when huge mental hospitals were introduced in the twentieth century, the personal approach disappeared; the therapeutic gains that were made with such individualized attention were no longer seen.

In 1933 Sakel introduced insulin coma as a form of therapeutic treatment. In this method, insulin was injected until the patient became hypoglycemic enough to lose consciousness, perhaps convulse, and lapse into a coma. A series of several of these treatments was reported to help schizophrenic patients. Shortly thereafter drug-induced convulsions and electroconvulsive therapy (ECT) were introduced. A series of these treatments frequently brought relief to patients experiencing acute psychotic episodes. Today such therapies have been abandoned (although ECT is no longer used to treat schizophrenia, it is still used to treat major depression).

Thus, prior to 1950, effective drugs for treating psychotic patients were virtually nonexistent, and such patients were usually permanently or semipermanently hospitalized. By 1955 more than half a million psychotic persons in the United States were residing in mental hospitals. However, in 1956 a dramatic and steady reversal in this trend began (Figure 11.3). By 1983 fewer than 220,000 were institutionalized. This decline has occurred despite a doubling in the numbers of admissions to state hospitals. We now stabilize schizophrenics on medication and discharge them from institutions quite rapidly.*

---

*Although we have a high discharge rate of schizophrenics from institutions, we must be concerned about the ultimate functioning of these persons in society. Many of these patients fail to continue their medication and function poorly as a result. It has been estimated that about 50 percent of our adult homeless population may suffer from inadequately controlled schizophrenia.

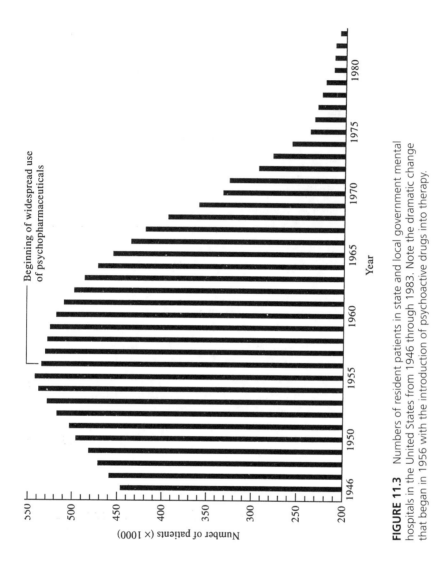

FIGURE 11.3 Numbers of resident patients in state and local government mental hospitals in the United States from 1946 through 1983. Note the dramatic change that began in 1956 with the introduction of psychoactive drugs into therapy.

What accounts for such a dramatic shift in treatment? The answer lies in the history of a class of drugs called the *phenothiazines*.

In 1952 Laborit used promethazine (the first of the phenothiazines) to deepen anesthesia. Later that year, other French researchers studied a second phenothiazine, chlorpromazine (Thorazine). This drug was administered in a "cocktail" to patients the night before surgery to allay their fears and anxieties. Chlorpromazine (Figure 11.4) was found to lower the amount of anesthetic drugs that a patient needed without making the patient unconscious; instead, treatment with chlorpromazine produced a state characterized by calmness, conscious sedation, and disinterest in and detachment from external stimuli. This condition was termed a *neuroleptic state,* and chlorpromazine was the first neuroleptic drug.

Because of these behavioral effects, chlorpromazine was tried in the treatment of schizophrenic episodes and found to be remarkably

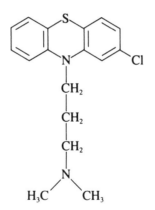

Chlorpromazine (Thorazine)

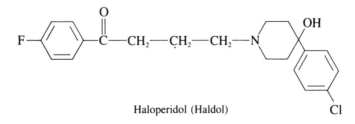

Haloperidol (Haldol)

FIGURE 11.4 Structural formulas of a phenothiazine (chlorpromazine) and a butyrophenone (haloperidol).

effective. Thus, for the first time, a drug had been found that altered the clinical manifestations of the psychotic process itself. Although chlorpromazine did not provide a permanent cure, its use in conjunction with supportive therapy allowed thousands of patients who otherwise would have been hospitalized permanently to return to their communities.

In the continuing search for more effective and less bothersome drugs, alternatives to the phenothiazines have been (and are continuing to be) developed. Reserpine (Serpasil) was an early alternative, but significant side effects have today rendered the drug obsolete. The second class of alternative agents was the *butyrophenones,* developed in Belgium in the mid-1960s. Two butyrophenones are currently available: haloperidol (Haldol; see Figure 11.4) and droperidol (Inapsine). Neither drug seems to have significant advantages over the phenothiazines, but haloperidol is occasionally used for patients who cannot tolerate the phenothiazines.

During the 1970s and 1980s, other agents became available. These include *loxapine* (Loxitane) and *molindone* (Moban), both of which have significant side effects (parkinsonian, involuntary, extrapyramidal motor movements).

In the 1990s, we are in a new era of treatment goals for the schizophrenic patient. Management of only the positive symptoms of schizophrenia may make the patient more manageable, but it begs an important question: How do these changes actually benefit the person with schizophrenia?[2] Previously peripheral concerns, such as quality of life, are now being addressed.[2] The advent of the atypical neuroleptics, clozapine and risperidone, are providing the means to address these vital issues. In addition, they are providing tools with which researchers can explore the mechanisms underlying the genesis of the illness. Finally, these atypical drugs have vast implications for how health care is delivered to these patients.

Mechanism of Action

The standard antipsychotic drugs antagonize the neurotransmitter actions of dopamine by competitively blocking dopamine$_2$ receptors.[2] This action is responsible for most of their clinical effects, correlates strongly with antipsychotic potency, and is responsible for many of their side effects.[22] By extension, schizophrenia has been explained in terms of dopamine hyperactivity in the mesolimbic area of the brain,[2] but this is certainly an overly simplistic view of the disorder.[23]

Dopamine receptors have been classified into at least six subtypes;[24] the most important in the study of schizophrenia are the dopamine$_2$ and the dopamine$_4$ receptors. Hallucinations and positive symptomatology of schizophrenia are blunted when about 70 percent of the dopamine$_2$ receptors are blocked by neuroleptic drugs.[25] The dopamine$_4$ receptor, located in both the mesolimbic system and the frontal cortex, is blocked by clozapine, which binds strongly to this receptor,[25] although it also binds to other receptors as well.[26]

Dopamine$_2$ and dopamine$_4$ receptors are located at several sites within the brain:

1. mesolimbic (nucleus accumbens, amygdala, hippocampus) and frontal cortical areas of the brain (Activation of these receptors is thought to be responsible for the therapeutic action of the drugs.)

2. extrapyramidal system (the caudate nucleus and the putamen of the basal ganglia) (Activation of these receptors results in the motor dysfunctions that are produced by the drugs.)

3. hypothalamic–pituitary axis (Activation of these receptors correlates with the hormonal alterations that are induced by these agents.)

4. certain centers of the brain stem, especially the chemoreceptor trigger zone of the medulla (Activation of these receptors correlates with the antivomiting [antiemetic] effect of these drugs.)

Much of the molecular biology of these dopamine receptors remains to be elucidated.

In addition to the dopamine receptors, the serotonin$_2$ receptor (also found in the frontal cortex) may be important in the pharmacological treatment of schizophrenia, especially the negative symptoms. The newly released drug risperidone has marked affinity for both the dopamine$_2$ and the serotonin$_2$ receptors and is effective in treating both positive and negative symptoms, further supporting a multireceptor theory of schizophrenia.[27]

Major versus Minor Tranquilizers

The benzodiazepine sedatives, or tranquilizers (Chapter 4), reduce anxiety states and neurotic behavior. They are generally not considered to be effective in managing schizophrenic patients; however, one benzodiazepine, clonazepam, has been utilized in the initial treatment of agitated psychotic patients with manic symptoms who are in need of rapid tranquilization.[28]

In contrast, the antipsychotic tranquilizers discussed in this chapter are the drugs of choice in treating schizophrenic persons, reducing both the acute episodes and the frequency of relapses. The terms *major tranquilizer, neuroleptic, antipsychotic,* and *antischizophrenic* refer to drugs that can relieve the symptoms of schizophrenia. Major tranquilizers, therefore, induce the neuroleptic state described above: psycho-motor slowing, emotional quieting, and an indifference to external stimuli.

Note that the word *tranquilizer* implies an agent that induces a peaceful, tranquil, calm, or pleasant state. Such a state can, indeed, be produced by a minor tranquilizer such as a benzodiazepine. However, the psychological effects produced by the major tranquilizers—the antipsychotic drugs—are seldom pleasant or euphoric. Indeed, they may cause unpleasant or dysphoric feelings, especially when admin-istered to nonpsychotic persons. Hence, these drugs do not cause posi-tive behavioral reinforcement and are seldom encountered as drugs of abuse.

Classification

Antipsychotic drugs have been broadly classified into two groups: (1) standard, or traditional, agents and (2) atypical, or new-generation, agents. The phenothiazines are the prototypical agents of the first class, while clozapine and risperidone are the most popular atypical agents of the second class in the United States.

With the standard agents, it has not been possible to separate the therapeutic effects on the positive symptoms from their prominent side effects involving the extrapyramidal motor system. These side effects closely resemble the motor alterations observed in patients who have Parkinson's disease, consisting of rigidity, tremor, slowed move-ments, and restlessness. Some of these symptoms disappear when the medication is discontinued, but persistent or permanent motor dis-orders (e.g., tardive dyskinesia) also occur.

The atypical agents have two advantages: (1) They may be thera-peutically effective without causing this neuroleptic syndrome, and (2) they help relieve the negative symptoms.

Phenothiazine Derivatives

The phenothiazines are the most widely used neuroleptic antipsychotic drugs. However, they are also used extensively for other purposes, for example, to treat nausea and vomiting, to sedate patients before anes-thesia, to delay ejaculation, to relieve severe itching, to treat alcoholic hallucinosis, and to manage the hallucinations caused by psychedelic agents (Chapter 12).

Table 11.1 lists 10 phenothiazine derivatives available for clinical use. Our discussion focuses on the prototypical agent of this class, chlorpromazine (Thorazine).

TABLE 11.1 Antipsychotic drugs.

Chemical classification	Drug name: Generic (Trade)	Dose equivalent (mg)	Sedation	Autonomic side effects[a]	Involuntary movement
Phenothiazine	Chlorpromazine (Thorazine)	100	High	High	Moderate
	Prochlorperazine (Compazine)	15	Moderate	Low	High
	Fluphenazine (Prolixin)	2	Low	Low	High
	Trifluoperazine (Stelazine)	5	Moderate	Low	High
	Perphenazine (Trilafon)	8	Low	Low	High
	Acetophenazine (Tindal)	20	Moderate	Low	High
	Carphenazine (Proketazine)	25	Moderate	Low	High
	Triflupromazine (Vesprin)	25	High	Moderate	Moderate
	Mesoridazine (Serentil)	50	High	Moderate	Low
	Thioridazine (Mellaril)	100	High	Moderate	Low
Thioxanthene	Thiothixene (Navane)	4	Low	Low	High
	Chlorprothixene (Taractan)	100	High	High	Moderate
Butyrophenone	Haloperidol (Haldol)	2	Low	Low	High
	Droperidol (Inapsine)	NA[b]	Low	Low	High
Miscellaneous	Loxapine (Loxitane)	10	Moderate	Low	Moderate
	Molindone (Moban)	10	Moderate	Moderate	Moderate

[a]Autonomic side effects include dry mouth, blurred vision, constipation, urinary retention, and reduced blood pressure.   [b]Not available.

Pharmacokinetics

The phenothiazines are absorbed erratically and unpredictably from the gastrointestinal tract. However, because patients usually take these drugs for long periods of time (even for a lifetime), the oral route of administration is still effective and commonly used. Intramuscular injection of phenothiazines is also quite effective; it increases the effectiveness of the drug to about 4 to 10 times that achieved with oral administration. Once these drugs are in the bloodstream, they are rapidly distributed throughout the body. The levels of phenothiazines that are found in the brain are low compared with the levels found in other body tissues; the highest concentrations are found in the lungs, liver, adrenal glands, and spleen.

The phenothiazines have half-lives of 24 to 48 hours, and they are slowly metabolized in the liver. The clinical effects of a single dose persist for at least 24 hours. Thus, taking the daily dose at bedtime will often minimize certain side effects (such as excessive sedation). The phenothiazines become extensively bound to body tissues, which partially accounts for their slow rate of elimination. Indeed, metabolites of some of the phenothiazines can be detected for as long as several months after the drug has been discontinued. Such slow elimination may also contribute to the slow rate of recurrence of psychotic episodes following the cessation of drug therapy.

To date, therapeutic drug monitoring and correlation of plasma levels of neuroleptics with clinical response and toxicity have not been widely utilized; most dosage decisions are made on a trial-and-error basis.[17] Studies have shown, however, that the plasma concentrations vary widely among patients given similar amounts of orally administered neuroleptics.[29] These differences probably result from large variations in drug absorption and metabolism. Of the antipsychotics, haloperidol (Haldol) and fluphenazine have been the most studied in this regard.

Marder and coworkers summarize the usefulness of plasma level monitoring in those circumstances where

> (1) patients fail to respond to what is usually an adequate dose; (2) when it is difficult . . . to discriminate drug side effects . . . from symptoms of schizophrenia; (3) when antipsychotic drugs are combined with other drugs . . . which may affect the antipsychotic's pharmacokinetics; (4) in the very young, the elderly, and the medically compromised, in whom the pharmacokinetics of neuroleptics may be altered . . . ; and (5) if noncompliance or poor compliance is suspected.[17]

Pharmacological Effects

In addition to blocking the dopamine$_2$ receptors, the phenothiazines also block acetylcholine, serotonin, histamine, and norepinephrine receptors. Blockade of acetylcholine receptors results in dry mouth, dilated pupils, blurred vision, constipation, urinary retention, and tachycardia. Blockade of norepinephrine receptors can result in hypotension and sedation. Haloperidol (a nonphenothiazine neuroleptic) produces a lower incidence of these effects, because it does not block norepinephrine receptors as well. Blockade of histamine receptors has sedating as well as antiemetic effects. Indeed, these drugs are widely used in medicine for their antinausea effect.

The consequences of blocking serotonin receptors by neuroleptic drugs are unclear. Certainly, the blockade of serotonin$_2$ receptors may be involved in therapeutic efficacy.[27,30] Such action might also explain why antipsychotic drugs partially ameliorate the hallucinogenic effects of LSD, a psychedelic drug that acts by stimulating serotonin receptors (Chapter 12). It is also thought that the blockade of serotonin receptors may be linked to a disinhibition of dopamine function and "lead to enhanced dopamine function in the frontal lobes (the putative neuroanatomic locus of negative symptoms)."[31]

Limbic System   Dopamine-secreting neurons located in the central midbrain portion of the brain stem send axonal projections to those parts of the limbic system that regulate emotional expression as well as to the limbic forebrain areas, where thought and emotions are integrated. Indeed, an increased sensitivity of dopamine receptors in those areas may be responsible for the positive symptomatology of schizophrenia. Thus, chlorpromazine decreases paranoia, fear, hostility, and agitation; it also reduces the intensity of schizophrenic delusions and hallucinations. In addition, chlorpromazine dramatically relieves the agitation, restlessness, and hyperactivity associated with an acute schizophrenic attack. The delusions and hallucinations are particularly sensitive to treatment.

Brain Stem   Through actions on the brain stem, phenothiazines suppress the centers involved in behavioral arousal (the ascending reticular activating center) and vomiting (the chemoreceptor trigger zone). By suppressing activity in the reticular formation, the phenothiazines induce an indifference to external stimuli, reducing the inflow of sensory stimuli that would otherwise reach higher brain centers.

Basal Ganglia Neuroleptic drugs produce two main kinds of motor disturbances, which comprise both the most bothersome and the most serious side effects associated with the use of these agents.[32] The two syndromes are (1) acute extrapyramidal reactions, which develop early in treatment in up to 90 percent of patients, and (2) tardive (late) dyskinesia, which occurs much later, during and even after cessation of chronic neuroleptic therapy.

The acute extrapyramidal side effects are threefold: (1) akathesia, which is a syndrome of the subjective feeling of anxiety, accompanied by restlessness, pacing, constant rocking back and forth, and other repetitive, purposeless actions; (2) dystonia, which is characterized by involuntary muscle spasms and sustained abnormal, bizarre postures of the limbs, trunk, face, and tongue; and (3) neuroleptic-induced parkinsonism, which resembles idiopathic (of unknown etiology) Parkinson's disease. This is characterized by tremor at rest, rigidity of the limbs, and slowing of movement with a reduction in spontaneous activity. In idiopathic parkinsonism, these latter symptoms occur when the concentration of dopamine in the nuclei of the basal ganglia (caudate nucleus, putamen, and globus pallidus) decreases to about 20 percent of normal. Here neuroleptic drug-induced blockade of dopamine receptors produces the parkinsonismlike symptoms. The side effects are closely related to the dose that is used; they develop quite rapidly and are reversed when the neuroleptic drug is discontinued.

Tardive dyskinesia is a much more puzzling and serious form of movement disorder. Victims exhibit involuntary hyperkinetic movements, often of the face and tongue but also of the trunk and limbs, which can be severely disabling. More characteristic are sucking and smacking of the lips, lateral jaw movements, and darting, pushing, or twisting of the tongue. Choreiform movements of the extremities are frequent. The syndrome appears a few months to several years after the beginning of neuroleptic treatment (hence the description *tardive*) and is often irreversible. The incidence of tardive dyskinesia has been estimated at more than 10 percent of patients who are treated with neuroleptic drugs, but this side effect depends greatly on the dosage, the age of the patient (it is most common in patients older than 50) and the particular drug used. Adequately controlling dyskinesia may necessitate restarting the neuroleptic medication or increasing the dosage, which is a problem if parkinsonian side effects are troublesome. Casey[32] and Baldessarini[33] review these effects at length.

Hypothalamus–Pituitary Pathways of dopamine-secreting neurons extend from the hypothalamus to the pituitary gland. The hypothalamus is intimately involved in the emotions, eating and drinking, sexual behavior, and the secretion of some pituitary hormones. By suppressing the function of the hypothalamus, phenothiazines interrupt these functions. By suppressing the appetite, food intake may be reduced. By suppressing the temperature-regulating centers of the hypothalamus, body temperature will fall in a cold room and rise in a hot room (poikilothermy). In addition, several body hormones are affected. Dopamine is likely the hormone that inhibits the release of prolactin in the hypothalamus. Thus, when dopamine receptors are blocked, the hormone prolactin is released, which often causes breast enlargement in males and lactation in females. Phenothiazines also reduce the release of hormones from the pituitary gland, which regulate the secretions of sex hormones (Chapter 14). Thus, in men, ejaculation may be blocked, and in women, libido may be decreased, ovulation may be blocked, and normal menstrual cycles may be suppressed, resulting in infertility.

Side Effects and Toxicity

The therapeutic use of the phenothiazines invariably leads to many side effects (see Table 11.1). Indeed, much of the art of managing patients with schizophrenia is in the diagnosis and management of the side effects of the neuroleptics.[34] One chooses one drug over another not so much because of differences in therapeutic efficacy but because of the relative intensities of their side effects. In general, the "high potency" phenothiazines (e.g., fluphenazine, trifluoperazine, and perphenazine; see Table 11.1), cause less sedation, fewer anticholinergic side effects, less postural hypotension, and more extrapyramidal side effects than the "low potency" phenothiazines (e.g., chlorpromazine and thioridazine). Where sedation is desirable, either a low-potency phenothiazine used alone or a high-potency drug combined with a benzodiazepine will have the desired therapeutic effect. Where the anticholinergic side effects limit drug compliance, a high-potency drug is desirable, and the drug-induced movement disorders can often be controlled with other medications (anticholinergic, antihistaminic, anti-adrenergic, or antiparkinsonian drugs), which will not be elaborated upon here. In patients at risk for developing extrapyramidal side effects and who cannot tolerate the low-potency phenothiazines, two options are available: (1) They can be prophylactically medicated with anticholinergic, antiparkinsonian, or anti-adrenergic drugs, or (2) they can receive a trial of clozapine or risperidone (discussed below) as replacements for the phenothiazine. Casey describes a treatment algorithm for managing drug-induced motor syndromes.[32]

Other potentially serious but much less common side effects of phenothiazines include altered pigmentation of the skin, pigment deposits in the retina, permanently impaired vision, decreased pituitary function, menstrual disorders, and allergic (or hypersensitivity) reactions, which include liver dysfunction and blood disorders.

Cognitive disturbances indisputably exist in schizophrenic patients,[35] and neuroleptic drugs intensify these disturbances, with the newer agents possibly disturbing cognition somewhat less.[35]

Any of these side effects can cause significant clinical problems, because nonhospitalized patients tend to stop taking medicine that causes them and inevitably suffer a return of psychotic symptoms. Thus, patient compliance is a significant problem. However, these drugs are relatively nonlethal, even when a massive overdose is taken.

Tolerance and Dependence

One of the positive attributes of the phenothiazines is that they are not behaviorally reinforcing and so are not prone to abuse. They do not produce tolerance, physical dependence, or psychological dependence. Psychotic patients may take phenothiazines for years without increasing their dose because of tolerance; if a dose is increased, it is usually done to increase the control of psychotic episodes. Discontinuation of a phenothiazine is not followed by symptoms of withdrawal, possibly because it may take many months for the drug and its metabolites to be excreted completely.

Haloperidol

In 1967, haloperidol (see Figure 11.4) was introduced to the United States as the first of the *butyrophenone derivatives*. A second compound, droperidol, has subsequently been introduced. Haloperidol is used primarily for its antipsychotic effects, while droperidol is used primarily for its antinausea and antiemetic properties.

Pharmacologically haloperidol is remarkably similar to the phenothiazines. Haloperidol produces sedation and an indifference to external stimuli; it reduces initiative, anxiety, and activity. It is well absorbed orally and has a moderately slow rate of metabolism and excretion. Indeed, stable blood levels can be seen for up to 3 days following discontinuation of the drug. It takes approximately 5 days for 40 percent of a single dose to be excreted by the kidneys.[36]

The mechanism of the antipsychotic action of haloperidol is like that of the phenothiazines—it blocks dopamine$_2$ receptors. Haloperidol does not produce many of the serious side effects occasionally observed in patients who are taking phenothiazines (jaundice, blood abnormalities, and so on), but it causes parkinsonian motor movements that are of the same or greater intensity as those induced by the high-potency phenothiazines. Prophylactic antiparkinsonian medication may be needed. Sedation is unusual. In general, however, haloperidol is an effective drug for treating psychotic patients, offering an alternative for patients who do not respond to the phenothiazines.

Atypical Antipsychotic Drugs

Until recently most attempts at finding alternative agents to the phenothiazines have met with little success. However, four such alternatives, the atypical antipsychotic drugs,[37] are currently available for clinical use, with two of them (clozapine and risperidone) currently attracting much interest.

Molindone

Molindone (Moban) is structurally unique as an antipsychotic medication, resembling the neurotransmitter serotonin. Whether such structural resemblance is related to its antipsychotic action is unknown. Molindone resembles other antipsychotic drugs in therapeutic efficacy, occupancy of dopamine receptors, and side effects. It produces moderate sedation, increased motor activity, and possibly euphoria. It can also lead to abnormal motor movements that resemble those observed in patients taking phenothiazines. Molindone is rapidly absorbed when it is taken orally, and it is metabolized before it is excreted. Clinical effects following a single dose of molindone persist for about 24 to 36 hours. Interestingly, it is also a blocker of the enzyme monoamine oxidase (Chapter 8), and its use is infrequently associated with tardive dyskinesia.[38]

Loxapine

Loxapine (Loxitane) is an antipsychotic drug with a unique structure (Figure 11.5). It resembles somewhat the tricyclic antidepressants, especially amoxapine (Asendin; see Chapter 8). However, its actions differ little from those of the older antipsychotic drugs. It has antipsychotic, antiemetic, and sedative properties and causes abnormal motor movements. It lowers convulsive thresholds somewhat more than do the phenothiazines. Taken orally, loxapine is well absorbed, and it is metabolized and excreted within about 24 hours.

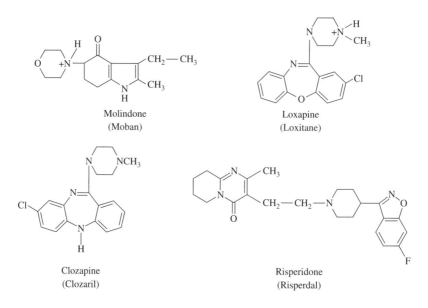

FIGURE 11.5   Structural formulas of atypical antipsychotic drugs.

Clozapine

Clozapine (Clozaril) is an antipsychotic drug whose structure is closely related to that of loxapine (Figure 11.5). Clozapine is useful in treating treatment-resistant schizophrenics, relieves much of the negative symptomatology of schizophrenia, and lacks many of the extrapyramidal side effects associated with the standard neuroleptics. Extensive discussion of clozapine may be found in several recent publications.[17,21,34,37,39,40]

Background   Although of intense interest only lately, clozapine is not a new drug. Synthesized in 1959, clozapine was introduced into clinical practice in Europe in the early 1970s. Its lack of extrapyramidal side effects was appreciated immediately. However, in 1975 several schizophrenic patients in Finland died of severe infectious diseases after developing *agranulocytosis* (loss of white cells in the blood) while taking clozapine.[17,21] As a result, clinical testing ceased and the drug was withdrawn from unrestricted use in Europe. Later, clozapine was reexamined for two major reasons: (1) The agranulocytosis was found to be reversible when the drug was discontinued, and (2) the drug was found to be therapeutically beneficial in schizophrenic patients who failed to respond to the traditional neuroleptic compounds. In 1986 a large, multicenter trial of the drug in the United States found a 30 percent improvement among 318 severely psychotic schizophrenics who were unresponsive to other drugs; only 1 to 2 percent developed agranulocytosis. More recent studies show that the rate of improvement may approach 60 percent with longer therapy.[41]

> In some cases, the improvements in both positive and negative symptoms will result in striking changes with patients who appeared hopelessly lost in a psychotic world, emerging as individuals who can be discharged from hospitals or participate meaningfully in rehabilitation programs. Other clozapine "responders" may not improve substantially in their positive symptoms, but will report that their mood and sense of well-being are much improved. For these individuals, the deficits associated with schizophrenia may not improve, but the quality of life is better.[17]

Meltzer states that clozapine is also particularly effective against a third type of psychotic symptomatology (besides the positive and negative symptoms), which he calls *disorganization*.[21] This set of symptoms consists of loose association, inappropriate affect, incoherence, and reduction in rational thought processes.

Thus, while agranulocytosis limits the drug's use in patients adequately controlled by traditional neuroleptics, clozapine is indicated for use in treatment-resistant schizophrenics and patients who suffer severe extrapyramidal side effects with conventional drugs, who have severe negative symptoms, and perhaps who have severe tardive dyskinesia.

Pharmacokinetics The pharmacokinetics of clozapine varies significantly among patients.[42] Plasma levels of the drug peak in about 1 to 4 hours, and its distribution in the body appears to vary, with some patients sequestering significant quantities of drug. Clozapine is metabolized in the liver into two major metabolites, desmethyl-clozapine and clozapine-N-oxide. These metabolites plus small amounts of unchanged clozapine are excreted in the urine. The reported metabolic half-life of clozapine is 9 to 17 hours in one study[42] and 6 to 33 hours in another.[17]

Jann and coworkers addressed the relationship between plasma levels of clozapine and therapeutic effectiveness. They estimated that in the treatment of patients with refractory schizophrenia, a minimum concentration of 350 micrograms per liter was needed.[42]

Pharmacodynamics   The mechanisms of the antipsychotic action of clozapine remain elusive.[26,42,43,44] Coward states that

> binding studies show that clozapine's highest affinities (for binding to receptors in the brain) to be for dopamine$_4$, seotonin$_{1C}$ (a subgroup of serotonin receptors), serotonin$_2$, alpha-1 (an adrenergic receptor), muscarinic (an acetylcholine receptor), and histamine-1 receptors, but moderate affinity is also seen for many other receptor subtypes.[40]

Although most researchers agree that binding to the dopamine$_4$ receptor is important, Meltzer stresses the critical importance of drug binding to the serotonin receptors.[30] Regardless of the pharmacodynamics, clozapine and its derivatives provide researchers with important new tools for investigating the cellular mechanisms of the schizophrenias.

Side Effects and Toxicity   The most common side effect of clozapine is sedation, which can limit the amount of drug administered. Other bothersome side effects include hypotension, tachycardia, fever (including a rare *neuroleptic malignant syndrome*), increased salivation, dizziness, and weight gain.

As discussed already, the major concern with clozapine is the 1 to 2 percent risk of developing severe, life-threatening (though reversible) agranulocytosis. White blood cell counts must be monitored at least weekly for the first 4 to 5 months of therapy and monthly thereafter, with more frequent monitoring if the white blood cell count is decreasing. Other drugs that can cause reductions in white blood cell count (most notably carbamazepine) should not be taken concomitantly.

The etiology of clozapine-induced agranulocytosis remains unknown. Most likely is a cellular-toxic mechanism.[45,46] In support of this concept, Uetrecht reported that clozapine can be metabolized not only in the liver but also by the *neutrophils* (a specialized type of white blood cell) themselves![47] An intermediate compound in this latter metabolic process is reactive and is postulated to be toxic to the cell, possibly killing the cell that formed it either directly or through an immunological mechanism. If this is true, it should not be too difficult to develop a derivative of clozapine that is as therapeutically effective but is not metabolized by white blood cells to a toxic metabolite.

Cost Concerns   Clozapine is much more expensive than other antipsychotic drugs because of its limited market—only 40,000 of the 2,000,000 schizophrenic patients in the United States. It also has special requirements that include blood monitoring, a national registry of users, and education for prescribing physicians.[48] Currently, the annual cost of taking clozapine (including the costs of weekly blood monitoring) totals about $10,000. Meltzer places this expense in perspective by comparing it with the expense of psychiatric hospitalization.[21] He concludes that "large savings are possible with clozapine treatment for treatment-resistant schizophrenics who have had frequent hospitalizations." He estimates that there are 300,000 to 600,000 schizophrenics who do not respond to other neuroleptics or who cannot tolerate their side effects.[48] These people form a large potential market for clozapine, but the high costs make mental health workers reluctant to prescribe the drug more.

Risperidone

Risperidone (Risperdal), introduced in the United States in March 1994, is the newest of the atypical antipsychotic drugs. The drug was first administered to schizophrenic patients in 1986; since then it has been used in Europe and its pharmacology extensively studied.

Risperidone acts as a potent inhibitor of both dopamine$_2$ and serotonin$_2$ receptors, with the drug having greater affinity for the serotonin receptors.[27,49] This observation has provoked reevaluation of schizophrenia as purely a disorder of hyperdopaminergic dopamine$_2$ activity.[50] Indeed, serotonin antagonists can improve psychotic symptoms and alleviate preexisting neuroleptic-induced extrapyramidal side effects.[27] According to one review, "High concentrations of serotonin$_2$ receptors are found in the neocortex, and serotoninergic efferent fibers originating in the raphe magnus project into the midbrain, where they can inhibit the release of dopamine."[27] Thus, some of the therapeutic benefit of risperidone (and of clozapine) can follow from drug-induced release of dopaminergic neurons from tonic serotoninergic inhibition.

There is also some suggestion that the negative symptoms of schizophrenia are associated with elevated densities of serotonin$_2$ receptors; thus blockade of these receptors would reduce the negative symptoms and diminish extrapyramidal side effects.

> Risperidone's therapeutic effect in schizophrenia is the result of its clinically effective blockade of both cortical serotonin$_2$ and limbic dopamine$_2$ systems. More dopamine is released in cortical regions as a result of relatively selective serotonin$_2$ blockade in these areas, ameliorating the core negative symptoms of schizophrenia as well as neurophysiologic/cognitive deficits. From the distribution of serotonin$_2$ receptors, one would expect dopaminergic transmission to be enhanced in the basal ganglia as well, resulting in diminished extrapyramidal symptoms. . . . Improved frontal cortical function

results in the normalization of descending GABA and NMDA neuronal function . . . systems also implicated in the pathogenesis of positive and negative symptoms.[27]

The pharmacokinetics of risperidone have been well studied.[51,52] The drug is well absorbed when administered orally and is highly bound to plasma proteins. It is metabolized to an active intermediate (9-hydroxy-risperidone), but the rate of metabolism varies because of genetic differences (genetic polymorphism). The metabolic half-life in rapid metabolizers is about 3 hours, 10 hours in intermediate metabolizers, and 21 hours in slow metabolizers. The half-life of the active intermediate is about 20 hours in all groups. Whether these various rates of hepatic metabolism have important clinical consequences in unclear.

Risperidone improves both positive and negative symptoms and has a low incidence of extrapyramidal motor side effects.[53,54,55] Common side effects include agitation, anxiety, insomnia, headache, extrapyramidal effects, and nausea. According to Remington, risperidone can be considered as a first-line agent in treating schizophrenia because of its efficacy and safety profile.[50]

Remoxipride

Remoxipride is another atypical antipsychotic agent whose availability in the United States is currently under active consideration. Pharmacologically, remoxipride is a weak but relatively selective antagonist of central dopamine$_2$ receptors, possibly with a preferential affinity for extrastriatal dopamine$_2$ receptors.[56] Why remoxipride has a lower incidence of extrapyramidal side effects despite its dopamine$_2$-blocking action is not clear, although some researchers speculate that remoxipride, unlike haloperidol, can discriminate among different types of dopamine-mediated functions, probably by having a preferential action on subpopulations of functionally coupled dopamine$_2$ receptors.[57] The symposium edited by Sedvall discusses the pharmacology of remoxipride at length.[58]

ANTIPARKINSONIAN DRUGS

As discussed, neuroleptic drugs produce side effects that closely resemble the movement disorders seen in idiopathic parkinsonism. Therefore, the drugs used to treat the side effects of neuroleptics are the same drugs used to treat Parkinson's disease. For this reason, these drugs will be briefly described.

Parkinson's disease is a neurodegenerative disease that occurs in about 1 percent of all adults over the age of 65 years. Although the cause of parkinsonism remains unknown, its symptoms clearly follow from a deficiency in the numbers and function of dopamine-secreting neurons located in the basal ganglia of the brain. In outline, functional activity of the basal ganglia is determined by a balance of dopamine-secreting (inhibitory) neurons and acetylcholine-secreting (excitatory) neurons. The clinical disease emerges when dopamine is depleted to about 20 percent of normal; as noted above, neuroleptic drugs produce parkinsonian side effects at a similar level of dopamine depletion. Thus, therapy is aimed at either resupplying the dopamine that is absent or else blocking the unopposed acetylcholine system.

Levodopa

Because a loss of dopamine is the primary problem in patients who have Parkinson's disease, replacement of the dopamine ameliorates the symptoms of the disease. However, when dopamine is present in plasma, it does not cross the blood–brain barrier into the brain. Therefore, dopamine itself is therapeutically ineffective. However, levodopa (dihydroxyphenylalanine), which is the immediate metabolic precursor of dopamine, does cross the blood–brain barrier, and in the CNS it is metabolized into dopamine by the enzyme dopa decarboxylase.

Administered orally, levodopa is rapidly absorbed into the bloodstream, where most of it (about 95 percent) is converted to dopamine in the plasma. Although only a small amount (about 5 percent) of levodopa crosses the blood–brain barrier and is converted to dopamine in the brain, it is enough to alleviate the symptoms of parkinsonism. However, the remaining high levels of dopamine in the systemic circulation produce bothersome side effects. Thus, such therapy, though effective, is obviously not optimal. A method is needed to reduce the high levels of dopamine in the systemic circulation while maintaining sufficient quantities in the brain.

To invent such a drug, one must examine the biosynthetic pathway that leads to dopamine. Since the enzyme dopa decarboxylase is responsible for converting dopa to dopamine, by inhibiting this enzyme in the systemic circulation but not in the brain, systemic biotransformation of the drug should be reduced, with a concomitant reduction in blood levels of dopamine and therefore in side effects. An example of such a peripherally restricted dopa decarboxylase inhibitor is the drug *carbidopa,* which is available in combination with levodopa

(Sinemet). By combining carbidopa with levodopa, the effective dose of levodopa is reduced by 75 percent, with a concomitant reduction in side effects and no loss of CNS therapeutic effect. Thus, the current treatment of parkinsonism relies heavily on this combination of levodopa and carbidopa. This is not a useful method for treating neuroleptic drug-induced parkinsonism, because the dopamine receptors are blocked and any resupplied dopamine cannot reach the receptors.

Anticholinergic Drugs

Anticholinergic drugs are effective for treating both the symptoms of parkinsonism and the motor side effects caused by neuroleptic drugs. These drugs exert their effect by blocking the excitatory cholinergic (acetylcholine) neurons that persist in the basal ganglia after the inhibitory dopamine neurons have either degenerated or been pharmacologically "blocked." Representative agents include trihexyphenidyl (Artane), procyclidine (Kemadrin), and biperiden (Akineton). Significant side effects include blurred vision, constipation, urinary retention, mental confusion, and delirium. Today these agents are used primarily in the early stages of the disease. They are also used when levodopa therapy has failed or been suboptimal and when patients experience the extrapyramidal side effects of the neuroleptics.

Amantadine (Symmetrel)

Amantadine is an antiviral agent that, through an unknown mechanism, relieves the symptoms of parkinsonism. It is likely that amantadine releases dopamine from whatever dopamine neurons remain in the patient's basal ganglia. Amantadine also appears to potentiate the therapeutic effects of levodopa, although such potentiation is not consistent. Thus, amantadine is much less effective than levodopa for long-term relief of the symptoms of parkinsonism. Adverse effects include slurred speech, ataxia, gastric distress, hallucinations, confusion, and nightmares.

Dopamine Receptor Stimulants (Agonists)

About 1 to 5 years after the start of levodopa therapy, most patients gradually become less responsive. This development may be related to a progressive inability of dopamine neurons to synthesize and store dopamine. To alleviate this problem, attempts have been made to identify drugs that will directly stimulate postsynaptic dopamine receptors in the basal ganglia. To date, two such agents are available: bromocrip-

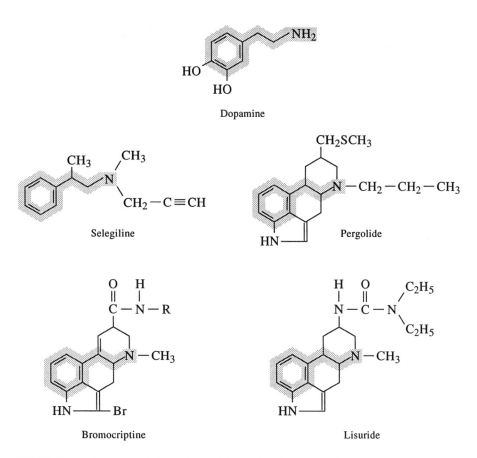

FIGURE 11.6 Structures of dopamine and dopaminergic agonists that are used to treat parkinsonism. The shaded portions, which are shared by all these structures, resemble dopamine.

tine (Parlodel) and pergolide (Permax). Both of these drugs are derived from the ergot alkaloid lysergic acid (Chapter 12), and both have structures that closely resemble that of dopamine (Figure 11.6). A third lysergic acid derivative, lisuride, is being studied.

Bromocriptine is a potent agonist (stimulant) of dopamine$_2$ receptors. It is used as an adjunct to levodopa in patients whose disease is not adequately controlled with levodopa. This combination improves the patient's therapeutic response to a reduced dose of levodopa and thus reduces the side effects of therapy. Because the efficacy of bromocriptine is often not sustained, its therapeutic usefulness is limited. Patient responsiveness also varies widely. Bromocriptine is incompletely absorbed when it is taken orally and has a plasma half-life of about 3 hours. Side effects include nausea, vomiting, hypotension, and mental disturbances.

Pergolide closely resembles bromocriptine but is more potent and has a longer half-life. Pergolide may be effective following a loss of responsiveness to bromocriptine. Thus, a patient's failure to respond to one dopaminergic agonist may not necessarily rule out a response to another.

Selegiline (Eldepryl) is also used to treat parkinsonism. In Chapter 8, we discussed two types of the enzyme monoamine oxidase (MAO) and the emerging use of selective MAO-A inhibitors as clinical antidepressants. In contrast to MAO-A (which is more closely involved with norepinephrine and serotonin nerve terminals), MAO-B has preferential affinity for dopamine neurons. MAO-B is selectively inhibited by selegiline. Selegiline also inhibits the local breakdown of dopamine, thus preserving the small amounts of dopamine that are present. Both actions enhance the therapeutic effect of levodopa. Selegiline is being used increasingly in the treatment of newly diagnosed, younger patients who have Parkinson's disease, because it appears to slow down the early progression of the disease and delays the need for initiating levodopa therapy. Interestingly, selegiline is metabolized to several by-products, including amphetamine and methamphetamine. Thus, metabolism of this drug provides a third mechanism that helps to alleviate the dopamine deficiency. In summary, selegiline may contribute to therapy for parkinsonism through any of three mechanisms: (1) inhibition of MAO-B, (2) inhibition of the breakdown of dopamine, and (3) metabolism into the active intermediates amphetamine and methamphetamine.

Study Questions

1. How are neuroleptics and antipsychotics alike? How do they differ?
2. What is a nonneuroleptic antipsychotic drug? How might such an agent differ from a traditional antipsychotic drug?
3. Describe the overall appearance of a schizophrenic person before and after treatment with chlorpromazine.
4. Discuss the meaning of the term *tranquilizer*.
5. What is the difference between a major tranquilizer and a sedative-hypnotic antianxiety agent?
6. The major tranquilizers have been called "chemical straitjackets." Do you agree or disagree?
7. Discuss the mechanism of action of neuroleptic antipsychotic drugs.
8. Discuss the major side effects of phenothiazines.

9. Discuss the consequences of reducing the numbers of institutionalized schizophrenic patients.
10. Compare and contrast clozapine and chlorpromazine.
11. Compare and contrast clozapine and risperidone.
12. What is meant by the term *atypical antipsychotic drug?*

Notes

1. P. Powchik and S. C. Schulz II, "Preface," *Psychiatric Clinics of North America* 16, no. 2 (June 1993): xi–xii.
2. B. Jones, "Schizophrenia: Into the Next Millennium," *The Canadian Journal of Psychiatry* 38, Suppl. 3 (September 1993): S67–S69.
3. U.S. Congress, Office of Technology Assessment, *The Biology of Mental Disorders* (Washington, D.C.: U.S. Government Printing Office, September 1992), p. 7.
4. Ibid., p. 53.
5. N. R. Schooler and S. J. Keith, "Role of Medication in Psychosocial Treatment," *Handbook of Schizophrenia, Psychosocial Treatment of Schizophrenia,* vol. 4 (New York: Elsevier, 1990).
6. L. J. Siever, O. F. Kalus, and R. S. E. Keefe, "The Boundaries of Schizophrenia," *Psychiatric Clinics of North America* 16, no. 2 (June 1993): 217–244.
7. C. A. Prescott and I. I. Gottesman, "Genetically Mediated Vulnerability to Schizophrenia," *Psychiatric Clinics of North America* 16, no. 2 (June 1993): 245–267.
8. U.S. Congress, Office of Technology Assessment, *Biology of Mental Disorders,* pp. 106–107.
9. G. Sedvall, "Monoamines and Schizophrenia," *Acta Psychiatrica Scandinavica* 82, Suppl. 358 (1990): 7–13.
10. Y. Su, J. Burke, A. O'Neil, B. Murphy, L. Nie, B. Kipps, J. Bray, R. Shinkwin, M. N. Nuallain, C. J. MacLean, D. Walsh, S. R. Diehl, and K. S. Kendler, "Exclusion of Linkage Between Schizophrenia and the D_2 Dopamine Receptor Gene Region of Chromosome 11q in 112 Irish Multiplex Families," *Archives of General Psychiatry* 50 (1993): 205–211.
11. H. A. Nasrallah, "Neurodevelopmental Pathogenesis of Schizophrenia," *Psychiatric Clinics of North America* 16, no. 2 (June 1993): 269–293.
12. F. E. Bloom, "Advancing a Neurodevelopmental Origin for Schizophrenia," *Archives of General Psychiatry* 50 (1993): 224–227.
13. S. Akbarian, W. E. Bunney, Jr., S. C. Potkin, S. B. Wigal, J. O. Hagman, C. A. Sandman, and E. G. Jones, "Altered Distribution of Nicotinamide-Adenine Dinucleotide Phosphate-Diaphorase Cells in Frontal Lobe of Schizophrenics Implies Disturbances of Cortical Development," *Archives of General Psychiatry* 50 (1993): 169–177.
14. S. Akbarian, A. Vinuela, J. J. Kim, S. C. Potkin, W. E. Bunney, Jr., and E. G. Jones, "Distorted Distribution of Nicotinamide-Adenine Dinucleotide Phosphate-Diaphorase Neurons in Temporal Lobe of Schizophrenics Implies Anomalous Cortical Development," *Archives of General Psychiatry* 50 (1993): 178–187.

15. S. A. Mednick and T. D. Cannon, "Fetal Development, Birth, and the Syndromes of Adult Schizophrenia," in S. A. Mednick, T. D. Cannon, C. E. Barr, and M. Lyon, eds., *Fetal Neural Development and Adult Schizophrenia* (New York: Cambridge University Press, 1991), pp. 3–13.

16. F. E. Bloom, "Advancing a Neurodevelopmental Origin for Schizophrenia," *Archives of General Psychology* 50 (1993): 226.

17. S. R. Marder, D. Ames, W. C. Wirshing, and T. VanPutten, "Schizophrenia," *Psychiatric Clinics of North America* 16, no. 3 (September 1993): 568–570.

18. U.S. Congress, Office of Technology Assessment, *Biology of Mental Disorders*, pp. 50–51.

19. J. Kane, "The Current Status of Neuroleptics," *Journal of Clinical Psychiatry* 50 (1989): 322–328.

20. J. A. Lieberman, D. Jody, S. Geisler, J. Alvir, A. Loebel, S. Szymanski, M. Woerner, and M. Borenstein, "Time Course and Biological Correlates of Treatment Response in First-Episode Schizophrenia," *Archives of General Psychiatry* 50 (1993): 369–376.

21. H. Y. Meltzer, "New Drugs for the Treatment of Schizophrenia," *Psychiatric Clinics of North America* 16, no. 2 (June 1993): 365–385.

22. P. Seeman, "Dopamine Receptors and the Dopamine Hypothesis of Schizophrenia," *Synapse* 1 (1987): 133–152.

23. P. Seeman, "Atypical Neuroleptics: Role of Multiple Receptors, Endogenous Dopamine, and Receptor Linkage," *Acta Psychiatrica Scandinavica* 82, Suppl. 358 (1990): 14–20.

24. U.S. Congress, Office of Technology Assessment, *Biology of Mental Disorders*, p. 75.

25. P. Seeman, "Dopamine Receptor Sequences. Therapeutic Levels of Neuroleptics Occupy D2 Receptors, Clozapine Occupies D4," *Neuropsychopharmacology* 7 (1992): 261–284.

26. H. Y. Meltzer and C. A. Stockmeier, "In Vitro Occupancy of Dopamine Receptors by Antipsychotic Drugs," *Archives of General Psychiatry* 49 (1992): 588–589.

27. L. Ereshefsky and S. Lacombe, "Pharmacological Profile of Risperidone," *Canadian Journal of Psychiatry* 38, Suppl. 3 (1993): S81–S83.

28. G. Chouinard, L. Annable, L. Turnier, N. Holobow, and N. Szkrumelak, "A Double-Blind Randomized Trial of Rapid Tranquilization with I. M. Clonazepam and I. M. Haloperidol in Agitated Psychotic Patients with Manic Symptoms," *Canadian Journal of Psychiatry* 38, Suppl. 4 (1993): S114–S121.

29. S. H. Preskorn, M. J. Burke, and G. A. Fast, "Therapeutic Drug Monitoring," *Psychiatric Clinics of North America* 16, no. 3 (September 1993): 611–641.

30. H. Y. Meltzer, "The Importance of Serotonin–Dopamine Interactions in the Action of Clozapine," *British Journal of Psychiatry* 17, suppl. (May 1992): 22–29.

31. Marder, Ames, Wirshing, and VanPutten, "Schizophrenia," p. 577.

32. D. E. Casey, "Neuroleptic-Induced Acute Extrapyramidal Syndromes and Tardive Dyskinesia," *Psychiatric Clinics of North America* 16, no. 3 (September 1993): 589–610.

33. R. J. Baldessarini, "Drugs and the Treatment of Psychiatric Disorders," in A. G. Gilman, T. W. Rall, A. S. Nies, and P. Taylor, eds., *Goodman and Gilman's The Pharmacological Basis of Therapeutics*, 8th ed. (New York: Pergamon, 1990), pp. 395–400.

34. A. Rifkin, "Pharmacologic Strategies in the Management of Schizophrenia," *Psychiatric Clinics of North America* 16, no. 2 (June 1993): 359.

35. W. H. Strauss and E. Klieser, "Cognitive Disturbances in Neuroleptic Therapy," *Acta Psychiatrica Scandinavica* 82, Suppl. 358 (1990): 56–57.

36. B. K. Colasanti, "Antipsychotic Drugs," in C. R. Craig and R. E. Stitzel, eds., *Modern Pharmacology*, 3rd ed. (Boston: Little, Brown, 1990), pp. 461–472.

37. Scientific Update Meeting, "Clozapine (Leponex/Clozaril)," *Psychopharmacology* 99, suppl. (1990).

38. R. R. Owen, Jr., and J. O. Cole, "Molindone Hydrochloride: A Review of Laboratory and Clinical Findings," *Journal of Clinical Psychopharmacology* 9 (1989): 268–276.

39. J. A. Lieberman and A. Z. Safferman, "Clinical Profile of Clozapine: Adverse Reactions and Agranulocytosis," *Psychiatric Quarterly* 63 (1992): 51–70.

40. D. M. Coward, "General Pharmacology of Clozapine," *British Journal of Psychiatry* 17, suppl. (May 1992): 5–11.

41. A. Breier, R. W. Buchanan, D. Irish, and W. T. Carpenter, Jr., "Clozapine Treatment of Outpatients with Schizophrenia: Outcome and Long-term Response Patterns," *Hospital and Community Psychiatry* 44 (1993): 1145–1149.

42. M. W. Jann, S. R. Grimsley, E. C. Gray, and W. H. Chang, "Pharmacokinetics and Pharmacodynamics of Clozapine," *Clinical Pharmacokinetics* 24 (1993): 161–176.

43. R. J. Baldessarini, D. Huston-Lyons, A. Campbell, E. M. Marsh, and B. M. Cohen, "Do Central Antiadrenergic Actions Contribute to the Atypical Properties of Clozapine?" *British Journal of Psychiatry* 17, suppl. (May 1992): 12–16.

44. B. S. Bunney, "Clozapine: A Hypothesized Mechanism for Its Unique Clinical Profile," *British Journal of Psychiatry* 17, suppl. (May 1992): 17–21.

45. S. L. Gerson and H. Meltzer, "Mechanisms of Clozapine-Induced Agranulocytosis," *Drug Safety* 7, Suppl. 1 (1992): 17–25.

46. A. V. Pisciotta, S. A. Konings, L. L. Ciesemier, C. E. Cronkite, and J. A. Lieberman, "On the Possible Mechanisms and Predictability of Clozapine-Induced Agranulocytosis," *Drug Safety* 7, Suppl. 1 (1992): 33–44.

47. J. P. Eutrecht, "Metabolism of Clozapine by Neutrophils. Possible Implications for Clozapine-Induced Agranulocytosis," *Drug Safety* 7, Suppl. 1 (1992): 51–56.

48. H. Y. Meltzer, "Clozapine: A Major Advance in the Treatment of Schizophrenia," *The Harvard Mental Health Letter* 10 (August 1993): 4–6.

49. R. W. Kerwin, G. F. Busatto, and L. S. Pilowsky, "Dopamine D_2 Receptor Occupancy *in Vivo* and Response to the New Antipsychotic Risperidone," *British Journal of Psychiatry* 163 (1993): 833–834.

50. G. J. Remington, "Clinical Considerations in the Use of Risperidone," *Canadian Journal of Psychiatry* 38, Suppl. 3 (1993): S96–S100.

51. G. Mannens, M.-L. Huang, W. Meuldermans, J. Hendrickx, R. Woesten-borghs, and J. Heykants, "Absorption, Metabolism, and Excretion of Risperidone in Humans," *Drug Metabolism and Disposition* 21 (1993): 1134–1141.

52. M. Huang, A. Van Peer, R. Woestenborghs, R. De Coster, J. Heykants, A. A. I. Jansen, Z. Zylicz, H. W. Visscher, and J. H. G. Jonkman, "Pharmacokinetics of the Novel Antipsychotic Agent Risperidone and the Prolactin Response in Healthy Subjects," *Clinical Pharmacology and Therapeutics* 54 (1993): 257–268.

53. G. Chouinard and W. Arnott, "Clinical Review of Risperidone," *Canadian Journal of Psychiatry* 38, Suppl. 3 (1993): S89–S95.

54. K. Heinrich, E. Klieser, E. Lehmann, E. Kinzler, and H. Hruschka, "Risperidone versus Clozapine in the Treatment of Schizophrenic Patients with Acute Symptoms: A Double Blind, Randomized Trial," *Progress in Neuro-Psychopharmacology and Biological Psychiatry* 18 (1994): 129–137.

55. M. G. Livingston, "Risperidone," *Lancet* 343 (1994): 457–460.

56. A. N. Wadworth and R. C. Heel, "Remoxipride: A Review of Its Pharmacodynamic and Pharmacokinetic Properties and Therapeutic Potential in Schizophrenia," *Drugs* 40 (1990): 863–879.

57. S.-O. Ogren, L. Florvall, H. Hall, O. Magnusson, and K. Angeby-Moller, "Neuropharmacological and Behavioral Properties of Remoxipride in the Rat," *Acta Psychiatrica Scandinavica* 82, Suppl. 358 (1990): 21–26.

58. G. Sedvall, "Development of a New Antipsychotic, Remoxipride," *Acta Psychiatrica Scandinavica* 82, Suppl. 358 (1990).

CHAPTER 12

PSYCHEDELIC DRUGS: MESCALINE, LSD, AND OTHER "MIND EXPANDING" HALLUCINOGENS

Psychedelic drugs comprise a group of heterogeneous compounds that induce visual and auditory hallucinations, separating the persons who use them from reality. These agents may disturb cognition and perception and, in some instances, produce behavior that is similar to that observed in psychotic patients. Because of this wide range of psychological effects, it has long been debated as to what single term might best be used to classify these agents.[1]

The term *hallucinogen* has been widely used for psychedelic drugs, because most of these agents can induce hallucinations in high enough doses. However, that term appears to be somewhat inappropriate because hallucinations are unusual at normally encountered doses, at which illusory phenomena and perceptual distortions are more common. Thus, the term *illusionogenic* has been used. The term *psychotomimetic* has also been assigned to these compounds because of their alleged ability to mimic psychoses or induce psychotic states. However, the effects of these drugs do not produce the same behavioral patterns that are observed in persons who experience psychotic episodes. Because no one of these terms characterizes the pharmacology of these drugs, we must rely on a descriptive term, such as *phantasticum* (proposed by Lewin in 1924) or *psychedelic* (proposed by Osmond in 1957), to imply that these agents all have the ability to alter sensory perception and therefore to be "mind expanding."

Many psychedelic agents occur in nature; other, newer psyche-delics are synthetically produced in laboratories, many of which are clandestine. Naturally occurring psychedelic drugs have been used for thousands of years primarily for their effects on sensory perception. To some individuals, these drugs have magical or mystical properties. Prior to the 1960s, the compounds were restricted primarily to relig-ious rituals, and most persons were barely aware of their existence. During the late 1960s and 1970s, however, the psychedelic agents were "discovered"; some people advocated their use to enhance perception, expand reality, promote personal awareness, and stimulate or induce comprehension of the spiritual or supernatural.

> There is heightened awareness of sensory input, often accompanied by an enhanced sense of clarity, but a diminished control over what is experienced. Frequently there is a feeling that one part of the self seems to be a passive observer (a "spectator ego") rather than an active organizing and directing force, while another part of the self participates and receives the vivid and unusual sensory experiences. The attention of the user is turned inward, preempted by the seeming clarity and portentous quality of his own thinking processes. In this state the slightest sensation may take on profound meaning. Commonly, there is a diminished capacity to differentiate the bound-aries of one object from another and of the self from the environ-ment. Associated with the loss of boundaries there may be a sense of union with "mankind" or the "cosmos."[2]

Because psychedelic drugs differ widely in chemical structure, they are difficult to classify on that basis. However, their structures do resemble those of certain neurotransmitters, and so they can be classi-fied according to the transmitters that they most closely resemble (Table 12.1). The transmitters that the psychedelic drugs resemble are acetylcholine, two catecholamines (norepinephrine and dopamine), and serotonin. These structural similarities lead to three classes for categorizing psychedelic drugs: *anticholinergic, catecholamine-like,* or *serotonin-like.* Also included in Table 12.1 is a fourth class of psyche-delic drugs, the psychedelic anesthetics.

The psychedelic drugs produce their effects through several mechanisms. The anticholinergic psychedelics produce intoxication, amnesia, and delirium by blocking postsynaptic acetylcholine recep-tors. The catecholamine-like and serotonin-like psychedelics act by influencing a subset of serotonin receptors. Finally, the psychedelic anesthetic drugs produce a unique spectrum of psychedelic actions by blocking the passage of calcium ions through a specific receptor for the excitatory amino acid glutamate. Each of these will be discussed in turn.

TABLE 12.1 Classification of psychedelic drugs.

ANTICHOLINERGIC PSYCHEDELIC DRUGS

Atropine

Scopolamine

CATECHOLAMINE-LIKE PSYCHEDELIC DRUGS

Mescaline

DOM (STP), MDA, MMDA, TMA, DMA, MDMA

Myristin, elemicin

SEROTONIN-LIKE PSYCHEDELIC DRUGS

Lysergic acid diethylamide (LSD)

Dimethyltryptamine (DMT)

Psilocybin, psilocin, bufotenine

Ololiuqui (morning glory seeds)

Harmine

PSYCHEDELIC ANESTHETIC DRUGS

Phencyclidine (Sernyl)

Ketamine (Ketalar)

Anticholinergic Psychedelic Drugs

Scopolamine, which attaches to and occupies acetylcholine receptor sites, is the classic example of an anticholinergic psychedelic drug (Figure 12.1). Having no intrinsic activity, scopolamine does not activate these receptors; it merely blocks the access of acetylcholine to them.

Historical Background   The history of scopolamine is long and colorful. The drug is distributed widely in nature; it is found, along with another anticholinergic compound called *atropine,* in especially high concentrations in the plant *Atropa belladonna* (known as belladonna or deadly nightshade), as well as in *Datura stramonium* (Jamestown weed, jimsonweed, stinkweed, thorn apple, or devil's apple) and *Mandragora officinarum* (mandrake). Both professional and amateur poisoners of the Middle Ages frequently used deadly nightshade as a source of poison. In fact, the plant's name, *Atropa belladonna,* is derived from *Atropos,* the name of the Greek goddess who supposedly cuts the thread of life. *Belladonna* means "beautiful

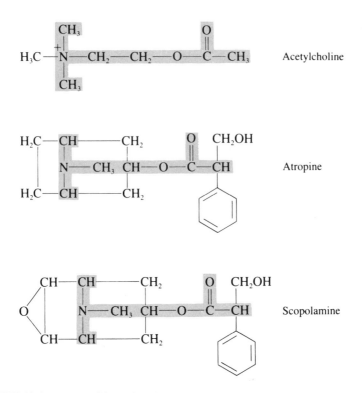

FIGURE 12.1 Structural formulas of acetylcholine (a chemical transmitter) and the anticholinergic psychedelic drugs atropine and scopolamine. Atropine and scopolamine act by blocking acetylcholine receptors. The shaded portion of each molecule illustrates structural similarities, which presumably contribute to receptor "fit."

woman," which refers to its ability to dilate the pupils when it is applied topically to the eyes (eyes with widely dilated pupils were presumably a mark of beauty).

Plants that contain atropine and scopolamine have been used and misused for centuries. For example, the delirium caused by these substances may have persuaded certain persons that they could fly—that they were witches. Marijuana and opium preparations from the Far East were once fortified with material from *Datura stramonium*. Today cigarettes made from the leaves of *Datura stramonium* and *Atropa belladonna* are smoked occasionally to induce intoxication. Such cigarettes were sold in pharmacies until the 1970s to treat asthma. Throughout the world, leaves of plants that contain atropine or scopolamine are still used to prepare intoxicating beverages.

Pharmacological Effects   Atropine and scopolamine act on the peripheral nervous system to depress salivation (causing dry mouth), reduce sweating, increase body temperature, dilate the pupils, blur vision, and markedly increase heart rate. Because these drugs inhibit the secretion of acid into the stomach, they have been used in the medical treatment of ulcers. However, their effectiveness is limited, and better drugs have been developed for this purpose.

Atropine only very poorly crosses the blood–brain barrier. Therefore, of the two drugs, scopolamine is the primary CNS-active intoxicant. Within the CNS, low doses of scopolamine produce drowsiness, mild euphoria, profound amnesia, fatigue, delirium, mental confusion, dreamless sleep, and loss of attention. Rather than expanding consciousness, awareness, and insight, scopolamine clouds consciousness and produces amnesia; it does not expand sensory perception.

In higher doses, a behavioral state that resembles a toxic psychosis occurs. Delirium, mental confusion, sedation, and amnesia dominate CNS effects; superimposed on these effects are peripheral actions such as tachycardia, blurred vision, urinary retention, and dry mouth. All these effects can convey a sense of excitement and loss of control to the user. However, the clouding of consciousness and the absence of any memory of the episode render scopolamine unattractive as a psychedelic drug. Indeed, it would be more appropriate to refer to it as a somewhat dangerous intoxicant, amnestic, and deliriant.

Catecholamine-like Psychedelic Drugs

Norepinephrine and dopamine synapses are important sites of action for a large group of psychedelic drugs that are structurally similar to both catecholamine neurotransmitters, as well as to cocaine and the amphetamines (Figure 12.2). Structurally, the catecholamine psychedelics differ from norepinephrine, dopamine, cocaine, and amphetamine by the addition of one or more methoxy (OCH$_3$) groups to the carboxy ring structure. Such modification increases the psychedelic properties of the drug, while behavior is stimulated to varying degrees. Such methoxylated amphetamine derivatives include mescaline, DOM (also called STP), TMA, MDA, MDMA ("ecstasy"), MMDA, DMA, and certain drugs that are obtained from nutmeg (myristin and elemicin). Compared to the amphetamines and cocaine, these compounds have more intense psychedelic action and less intense behavioral stimulant action.[3] Thus, they produce significant adrenaline-like peripheral effects, as well as strong behavior-reinforcing effects, similar to the effects obtained with cocaine and the amphetamines (Chapter 6).

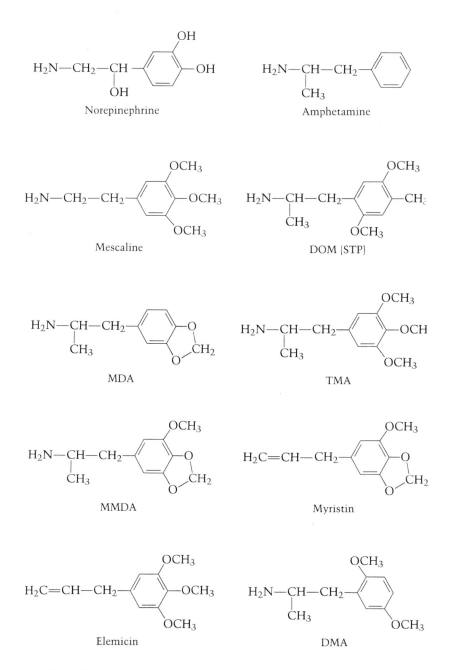

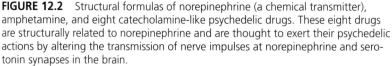

FIGURE 12.2 Structural formulas of norepinephrine (a chemical transmitter), amphetamine, and eight catecholamine-like psychedelic drugs. These eight drugs are structurally related to norepinephrine and are thought to exert their psychedelic actions by altering the transmission of nerve impulses at norepinephrine and serotonin synapses in the brain.

Despite these catecholamine-like actions, however, their psychedelic actions are likely exerted by changes in the neurotransmission of serotonin, which results in LSD-like effects.[4] Thus, we should first expand upon the mechanism of action of these drugs, which the serotonin psychedelic drugs, discussed later, also share.

As early as the late 1960s, most psychedelics were known to produce a remarkably similar set of effects.[5] These included sensory-perceptual (time) distortion; altered perceptions of colors, sounds, and shapes; complex hallucinations and synesthesia; dreamlike feelings; depersonalization; altered affect (depression or elation); and somatic effects (tingling skin, weakness, tremor, and so on). As further indication of their common action, many of these drugs demonstrate cross tolerance with each other.*

It was then discovered that psychedelic drugs produce marked alterations in brain serotonin.

> Once a drug acts upon the brain serotonin system, it sets in motion a cascade of events involving much of the enormous complexity of the brain and many of its constituent neurochemical systems. Thus, the brain serotonin system acts as a trigger for a multitude of changes whose elaboration generates the hallucinatory experience.[6]

Indeed, these drugs appear to act on postsynaptic (rather than presynaptic) receptors of the serotonin$_2$ subtype.[7] However, whether these drugs act as agonists or antagonists at these receptors remained quite unclear until recently.[8] Now it is generally accepted that the psychedelics act as *high-affinity serotonin$_2$ partial agonists*.[9] Ungerleider and Pechnick[1] and Teitler and coworkers[10] recently reviewed the interactions of psychedelic drugs with serotonin$_2$ receptors.

Mescaline

Peyote (*Lophophora williamsii*) is a common plant in the southwestern United States and Mexico. It is a spineless cactus that has a small crown, or "button," and a long root. When the plant is used for psychedelic purposes, the crown is cut from the cactus and dried into a hard brown disc. This disc, which is frequently referred to as a mescal

---

*Of note, phencyclidine (discussed later in this chapter) and marijuana (Chapter 13) do not demonstrate cross tolerance with either the catecholamine-like or the serotonin-like psychedelics,[5] suggesting that phencyclidine and marijuana interact with different sets of receptors—a supposition that we will see is quite true.

button, may later be softened in a person's mouth and swallowed. The psychedelic chemical in the button is mescaline.

Historical Background The use of peyote extends back to pre-Columbian times, when the cactus was used in the religious rites of the Aztecs and other Mexican Indians. Currently, peyote is legally available for use in the religious practice of the Native American Church of North America—an organization that claims some 250,000 members from Indian tribes throughout North America. Members of the Native American church regard peyote as sacramental, much the same way that members of Christian churches regard bread and wine as sacramentals. The use of peyote for religious purposes is not considered to be abuse. Indeed, peyote is seldom abused by members of the Native American church. Today the federal government and 23 states permit the sacramental use of peyote. However, the U.S. Supreme Court, which had earlier ruled that no federal control should interfere with freedom of religion, ruled that states may ban even religious uses of peyote without violating the constitutional right of free religious exercise. Thus, the controversy over the nonmedical use of psychoactive drugs continues.

Pharmacological Effects The initial research on the active ingredients of the peyote cactus was carried out near the end of the nineteenth century by German pharmacologists. In 1896 mescaline was identified as the active ingredient in peyote. After the chemical structure of mescaline was elucidated in 1918, the compound was produced synthetically. Because of its structural resemblance to norepinephrine, a wide variety of synthetic mescaline derivatives have now been synthesized, and all have methoxy (OCH_3) groups or similar additions on their benzene rings (see Figure 12.2). Why methoxylation of the benzene ring adds psychedelic properties to the drug is not clear, but it is thought that at higher doses (for example, at doses higher than those that exert amphetamine-like behavioral stimulation), these molecules "fit" the presynaptic serotonin receptors better and thus exert LSD-like psychedelic effects (discussed below).

When taken orally, mescaline is rapidly and completely absorbed, and significant concentrations are usually achieved in the brain within 30 to 90 minutes. The effects of a single dose of mescaline persist for approximately 10 hours. The drug does not appear to be metabolized before it is excreted.

As would be predicted by its resemblance to norepinephrine, low doses of mescaline (2 to 3 milligrams per kilogram of body weight) produce amphetamine-like behavioral effects that are characteristic of the fight/flight/fright syndrome. These effects include dilatation of the pupils, increased blood pressure and heart rate, an increase in body temperature, EEG and behavioral stimulation, and other excitatory symptoms. However, such actions are not the primary effects that are sought by persons who use mescaline.

> Interest in mescaline centers on the fact that it causes unusual psychic effects and visual hallucinations. The usual oral dose (5 mg/kg) in the average normal subject causes anxiety, sympathomimetic effects, hyperreflexia of the limbs, static tremors, and vivid hallucinations that are usually visual and consist of brightly colored lights, geometric designs, animals and occasionally people; color and space perception is often concomitantly impaired, but otherwise the sensorium is normal and insight is retained.[11]

Synthetic Amphetamine Derivatives

DOM, MDA, TMA, MDMA, MMDA, and DMA are structurally related to mescaline and methamphetamine and, as might be expected, produce similar effects. They have moderate amphetaminelike effects at low doses, but LSD-like serotonin-mediated effects dominate as doses increase. These derivatives are considerably more potent and more toxic than mescaline.

DOM (also known as STP for "serenity, tranquility, and peace") has effects that are similar to those of mescaline; doses of 1 to 6 milligrams produce euphoria, which is followed by a 6- to 8-hour period of hallucinations. DOM is 100 times more potent than mescaline but much less potent than LSD. The use of DOM is associated with a high incidence of overdose (because it is potent and street doses are poorly controlled). Acute toxic reactions are common; they consist of tremors that may eventually lead to convulsive movements and prostration, which may be followed by death. Because these effects are common, the use of DOM is not widespread.

MDA, MMDA, TMA, and numerous other structural variations are encountered occasionally as designer drugs. Producers of these drugs attempt to circumvent legal regulations by producing compounds that have modest structural differences from FDA-regulated compounds. In general, the pharmacological effects of these drugs resemble those of mescaline and LSD; they reflect the mix of catecholamine and serotonin interactions.

MDMA ("ecstasy") resembles MDA in structure but may be less hallucinogenic, with a less extreme sense of disembodiment and visual distortion.[12] The amphetamine-like feelings of elation may be greater than those obtained with mescaline. In experiments, MDMA has been shown to release serotonin and cause acute depletion of serotonin from most axon terminals in the forebrain, as well as to produce irreversible destruction of serotonin neurons in laboratory animals.[13,14] Ricaurte and coworkers argue for a similar toxic action in humans.[15] Thus, MDMA is potentially too dangerous for human use. The neurotoxicity may be due to MDMA itself or to a by-product of its metabolism.

> As serotonergic systems have been implicated in the control or modulation of sleep, food intake, sexual behavior, anxiety, and mood, disruption due to cell loss could have major consequences. The actual functional consequences of MDMA exposure remain to be determined.[16]

Compounds that are sold on the street as mescaline are often not mescaline at all but rather LSD, one of the synthetic mescaline derivatives, or phencyclidine. Users must be careful (caveat emptor), because higher doses of any of these substitute drugs can be dangerous and may be toxic.

Myristin and Elemicin

Myristin and *elemicin*, the pharmacologically active ingredients in nutmeg and mace, are responsible for the psychedelic action of these spices. Nutmeg and mace are obtained, respectively, from the dried seed and the seed coat of the East Indian nutmeg tree (*Myristica fragrans*). Nutmeg and mace are occasionally encountered as drugs of abuse, usually when no other psychedelic substances are available.

Ingestion of large amounts (between 1 and 2 teaspoons, usually brewed in tea) may, after a delay of 2 to 5 hours, induce euphoria and changes in sensory perception, including visual hallucinations, acute psychotic reactions, and feelings of depersonalization and unreality.

Considering the close structural resemblance of myristin and elemicin to mescaline (see Figure 12.2), these psychedelic actions are not unexpected. However, both drugs produce many unpleasant side effects, including vomiting, nausea, and tremors. After nutmeg or mace has been taken to produce its psychedelic action, the side effects usually dissuade users from trying these agents a second time.

Serotonin-like Psychedelic Drugs

The serotonin-like psychedelic drugs include lysergic acid diethylamide (LSD), psilocybin and psilocin (both from the mushroom *Psilocybe mexicana)*, dimethyltryptamine (DMT), and bufotenine (Figure 12.3). Because of this structural resemblance, and because

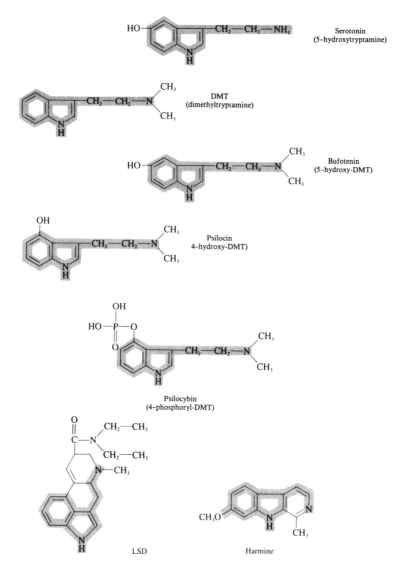

FIGURE 12.3   Structural formulas of serotonin (a chemical transmitter) and six serotoninlike psychedelic drugs. These six drugs are structurally related to serotonin (as indicated by the shading) and are thought to exert their psychedelic actions through alterations of serotonin synapses in the brain. Although LSD is structurally much more complex than serotonin, the basic similarity of the two molecules is apparent.

LSD antagonizes many of the peripheral actions of serotonin, an early hypothesis asserted that the psychedelic effects of LSD might be related to the antagonism of serotonin in the CNS. However, psychedelic effects persisted after these serotonin neurons were destroyed, suggesting that the effect must be exerted directly on the postsynaptic receptors for serotonin. As discussed earlier, LSD is likely a partial agonist of serotonin$_2$ receptors, triggering a series of responses that involve other neurotransmitter systems (hence, the overlap between the serotonin and the catecholamine psychedelics). Eventually these actions result in the *psychedelic syndrome* that is characteristic of all these drugs.

> One speculation about the manner by which hallucinogens manifest their impressive alterations of mood, perception, and thought is that the pontine raphe, a major center of 5-HT [serotonin] activity, serves as a filtering station for incoming sensory stimuli. It screens the flood of sensations and perceptions, eliminating those that are unimportant, irrelevant, or commonplace. A drug like LSD may disrupt the sorting process, allowing a surge of sensory data and an overload of brain circuits. Dehabituation, in which the familiar becomes novel, is noted under LSD. It may also be caused by lowering the sensory gates by inhibition of the raphe activity.[4]

Because LSD-like psychedelics may act as partial agonists of serotonin$_2$ receptors, drugs that block serotonin receptors may be useful in ameliorating or antagonizing the psychedelic effects of psychedelic drugs, especially when a "bad trip" is encountered. Such a reaction usually consists of paranoid ideation, depression, undesirable hallucinations, and/or a confusional state resembling a drug-induced dementia. Indeed, the antipsychotic drugs (Chapter 11) have been used successfully to treat patients who are experiencing an LSD-induced psychosis. However, because the neuroleptics may cause additional problems, they are not routinely used for this purpose. However, they are still used to treat otherwise uncontrollable persons who are suffering from psychedelic drug intoxication. In milder cases of intoxication, the patient is reassured and protected until the effects of the drug subside.

Lysergic Acid Diethylamide (LSD)

During the 1960s and early 1970s, lysergic acid diethylamide (LSD) became one of the most remarkable and controversial drugs known. LSD, in doses that are so small that they might even be considered infinitesimal, is capable of inducing remarkable psychological change in a person, enhancing self-awareness and altering internal reality, while causing relatively few alterations in the general physiology of the body.

Historical Background LSD was first synthesized in 1938 by Albert Hoffman, a Swiss chemist, as part of an organized research program to investigate possible therapeutic uses of compounds obtained from ergot. Ergot is a natural product derived from a fungus (*Claviceps purpurea*), which grows as a parasite on rye in grainfields of Europe and North America. The active products that are extracted from ergot are derivatives of lysergic acid. The pharmacological actions of these derivatives do not usually include hallucinations, but they do include constriction of blood vessels and increased contractions of the uterus. Therapeutically, ergot alkaloids are used to treat migraine headaches and to control postpartum hemorrhaging.

Early pharmacological studies of LSD in animals failed to reveal anything unusual, and the compound was almost forgotten. The psychedelic action was neither sought nor expected, because most derivatives of ergot are not psychoactive. Thus, LSD remained on the laboratory shelf unnoticed from 1938 until 1943, when Doctor Hoffman had an unusual experience. He later described that experience:

> In the afternoon of 16 April, 1943, . . . I was seized by a peculiar sensation of vertigo and restlessness. Objects, as well as the shape of my associates in the laboratory, appeared to undergo optical changes. I was unable to concentrate on my work. In a dreamlike state I left for home, where an irresistible urge to lie down overcame me. I drew the curtains and immediately fell into a peculiar state similar to drunkenness, characterized by an exaggerated imagination. With my eyes closed, fantastic pictures of extraordinary plasticity and intensive color seemed to surge toward me. After two hours this state gradually wore off.[17]

Hoffman correctly hypothesized that his experience resulted from the accidental ingestion of LSD. He decided to ingest some of the compound under controlled conditions and to describe the experience more completely. Using the dose of other drugs as a guide, he administered what seemed to be a minuscule oral dose (only 0.25 milligram). However, we now know that this dose is about 10 times the dose required to induce psychedelic effects in most persons. As a result of this miscalculation, his response was quite spectacular:

> After 40 minutes, I noted the following symptoms in my laboratory journal: slight giddiness, restlessness, difficulty in concentration, visual disturbances, laughing. . . . Later, I lost all count of time. I noticed with dismay that my environment was undergoing progressive changes. My visual field wavered and everything appeared

deformed as in a faulty mirror. Space and time became more and more disorganized and I was overcome by a fear that I was going out of my mind. The worst part of it being that I was clearly aware of my condition. My power of observation was unimpaired. . . . Occasionally, I felt as if I were out of my body. I thought I had died. My ego seemed suspended somewhere in space, from where I saw my dead body lying on the sofa. . . . It was particularly striking how acoustic perceptions, such as the noise of water gushing from a tap or the spoken word, were transformed into optical illusions. I then fell asleep and awakened the next morning somewhat tired but otherwise feeling perfectly well."[17]

For several years, LSD remained a laboratory and clinical curiosity. In 1949 the first North American study of LSD in humans was conducted, and during the 1950s large quantities of LSD were distributed to pharmacologists and physicians throughout the world for research purposes. A significant impetus to that research was the notion that the effects of LSD might constitute a model for psychosis, which would provide some insight into the biochemical and physiological processes of mental illness and its treatment. Also, some therapists tried LSD as an adjunct to psychotherapy to help patients verbalize their problems and gain some insight into the underlying causes.[18] However, this has not proven to be an effective treatment: "Such therapeutic use has waned, perhaps because psychiatrists—like the rest of us—found it too difficult to draw valid conclusions from the productions of chemically disordered brains."[19]

This early work with LSD on human volunteers introduced the LSD experience to college campuses and, from there, to a wider audience. The drug reached its peak in popularity during the late 1960s, after which its use decreased markedly. Considering the long history of other psychedelic drugs, it is unlikely that the recreational use of LSD will ever disappear completely.

Pharmacokinetics LSD is usually taken orally, and it is rapidly absorbed by that route. Usual doses range from about 25 micrograms to over 300 micrograms. Because such amounts are so small, LSD is often added to other substances, such as squares of paper, the backs of stamps, or sugar cubes, which can be handled more easily. LSD is absorbed within about 60 minutes, reaching peak blood levels in about 3 hours. It is distributed rapidly and efficiently throughout the body; it diffuses easily into the brain and readily crosses the placenta. The largest amounts of LSD in the body are found in the liver, where the drug is metabolized before it is excreted. The duration of action is about 6 to 8 hours.

Because of its extreme potency, only minuscule amounts can be detected in urine. Thus, conventional urine-screening tests are inadequate to detect LSD. When the use of LSD is suspected, urine is collected (up to 30 hours after ingestion) and an ultrasensitive radio-immunoassay performed to verify the presence of the drug.

Physiological Effects Although the LSD experience is character-ized by its psychological effects, subtle physiological changes also occur. Persons who take LSD may experience a slight increase in body temperature, dilatation of the pupils, slightly increased heart rate and blood pressure, increased levels of glucose (sugar) in the blood, and dizziness, drowsiness, nausea, and other effects that, although notice-able, seldom interfere with the psychedelic experience.

LSD is known to possess a low level of toxicity. Gable estimates for LSD an effective dose of 50 micrograms and a lethal dose of 14,000 micrograms.[20] These figures provide a therapeutic ratio of 280, making the drug a remarkably nonlethal compound. Such calculation does not include any fatal accidents or suicides that might occur when persons are intoxicated by LSD. The use of LSD during pregnancy is certainly unwise because of possible adverse effects on the fetus.[21]

Psychological Effects Although the physiological alterations usually produced by LSD are quite mild, the psychological effects are intense. The exact response that a person may have to using LSD is unpredictable and is influenced by a variety of factors, including the personality of the user, his or her expectations, previous experience with LSD and other psychoactive drugs, attitudes toward the use of LSD or any other illicit drug, motivations for using the drug, the set-ting in which the drug is administered, and the persons with whom the user interacts during the LSD experience.

Nevertheless, predictable responses to LSD include alterations in mood and emotion, in which laughter or sorrow may be evoked easily and even simultaneously. Both euphoria and dysphoria can be experi-enced, even by the same person during the same "trip." The principal psychological effects involve perceptual changes, especially visual hal-lucinations and perceptual distortions. True auditory hallucinations are rare.

The LSD-induced psychedelic experience can be divided into three phases:

1. The *somatic phase* occurs after absorption of the drug and consists of CNS stimulation and autonomic changes that are predom-inantly sympathomimetic in nature.

2. The *sensory* (or *perceptual*) *phase* is characterized by sensory distortions and pseudohallucinations, which are the effects desired by the drug user.

3. The *psychic phase* signals a maximum drug effect where changes in mood, disruption of thought processes, altered perception of time, depersonalization, true hallucinations, and psychotic episodes may occur. Experiencing the latter phase would be considered a "bad trip."[3]

Jaffe describes the second and third phases as follows:

> In the second or third hour, visual illusions, wavelike recurrences of perceptual changes (e.g., micropsia, macropsia), and affective symptoms may occur. Afterimages are prolonged, and the overlapping of present and preceding perceptions occurs. Some subjects recognize these confluences, whereas others elaborate them into hallucinations. In contrast to naturally occurring psychoses, auditory hallucinations are rare. Synesthesias, the overflow from one sensory modality to another, may occur. Colors are heard and sounds may be seen. Subjective time is also seriously altered, so that clock time seems to pass extremely slowly. The loss of boundaries and the fear of fragmentation create a need for a structuring or supporting environment and experienced companions. During the "trip," thoughts and memories can vividly emerge under self-guidance or unexpectedly, to the user's distress. Mood may be labile, shifting from depression to gaiety, from elation to fear. Tension and anxiety may mount and reach panic proportions. After about 4 to 5 hours, if a major panic episode does not occur, there may be a sense of detachment and the conviction that one is magically in control.[22]

Tolerance and Dependence Tolerance (a need to increase the dose to obtain the same effect) of both the psychological and physiological alterations that are induced by LSD readily and rapidly develops, and cross tolerance occurs between LSD and other catecholamine-like and serotonin-like psychedelics. This tolerance is lost within several days after the user stops taking the drug.

Physical dependence on LSD does not develop, even when the drug is used repeatedly for a prolonged period of time. In fact, most heavy users of the drug say that they ceased using LSD because they tired of it, had no further need for it, or had had enough. Even when the drug is discontinued because of concern about bad trips or about physical or mental harm, no withdrawal signs are exhibited. Laboratory animals do not self-administer LSD.

Adverse Reactions and Toxicity   The adverse reactions attributed to LSD generally fall into four categories: (1) the effects on the psychological state of the user, (2) the possibility of permanent damage to the brain, (3) the possible effects on the fetus when the drug is taken by a pregnant woman, and (4) the deleterious effects on society if use of the drug were widespread.

Concerning effects on the psychological state of the user, Dimijian wrote:

> Unpleasant experiences with LSD are relatively frequent and may involve an uncontrollable drift into confusion, dissociative reactions, acute panic reactions, a reliving of earlier traumatic experiences, or an acute psychotic hospitalization. Prolonged nonpsychotic reactions have included dissociative reactions, time and space distortion, body image changes, and a residue of fear or depression stemming from morbid or terrifying experiences under the drug. . . . With the failure of usual defense mechanisms, the onslaught of repressed material overwhelms the integrative capacity of the ego, and a psychotic reaction results. It appears that this [LSD-induced] disruption of long-established patterns of adapting may be a lasting or semipermanent effect of the drug.[23]

LSD reduces a person's normal ability to control emotional reactions, and drug-induced alterations in perception can become so intense that they overwhelm one's ability to cope. Because LSD can eliminate normal defense (or coping) mechanisms, it may precipitate psychotic episodes that would normally be suppressed.

There is also the possible problem of persistent flashbacks, which may occur weeks or even months after the last use of the drug. The mechanism that underlies flashbacks is unknown, but it may involve a long-lasting impairment of psychological defense mechanisms, which causes a periodic emergence of repressed feelings.

> Recurrences of drug effects without the drug—"flashbacks"—are a puzzling phenomenon; they occur in more than 15 percent of users. Commonly precipitated by use of marihuana, anxiety, fatigue, or movement into a dark environment, "flashbacks" may persist intermittently for several years after the last exposure to LSD. They are exacerbated by the use of phenothiazines. In some individuals the use of psychedelics can precipitate serious depressions, paranoid behavior, or prolonged psychotic episodes. Whether such episodes would have occurred without the drug is not clear. Prolonged psychotic episodes following repeated use of LSD tend to resemble naturally occurring schizophreniform psychotic states, and the prognosis appears to be similar. . . . It is possible that repeated use of LSD can induce subtle deficits in the capacity for abstract thinking.[22]

Rang and Dale elaborated on effects of LSD on mental health:

> There has been much concern over reports that LSD and other psychotomimetic drugs, as well as causing potentially dangerous "bad trips," can lead to more persistent mental disorders. There are recorded instances in which altered perception and hallucinations have lasted for up to 3 weeks following a single dose of LSD, and also reports of a persistent state resembling paranoid schizophrenia, which responds to antipsychotic drugs but may recur later. It is not at all clear whether this is due to a long-term effect of LSD, or whether LSD-taking is more likely in subjects destined to develop schizophrenia. The cautious view must be that LSD is causative. This, coupled with the fact that the occasional "bad trip" can result in severe injury through violent behavior, means that LSD and other psychotomimetics must be regarded as highly dangerous drugs.[24]

Whether long-term, frequent, high-dose use of LSD results in discernible damage to the brain has not been determined, but it is generally agreed that occasional use of LSD does not induce physical damage. Possible hazards to the fetus when a pregnant woman takes LSD are also unknown and seemingly unlikely. Although massive doses of LSD may cause chromosomal breakage (in laboratory models), usual doses do not appear to do so. In fact, data indicate that the incidence of fetal abnormalities in offspring of LSD users is the same as that in the normal population. Although there is some evidence of an increased incidence of structural abnormalities in infants born of parents who use LSD, those same parents tend to take a variety of other drugs as well, which makes it impossible to blame one specific compound.

Fears of long-term damage to society as a result of widespread use of LSD appear to be unsubstantiated. Even though some users experience psychological dependence, most persons eventually cease taking LSD and return to less potent drugs. Thus, despite the extreme potency and unusual psychedelic effects of LSD, the social use of other psychoactive drugs that have potent behavior-reinforcing properties (such as alcohol, nicotine, cocaine, amphetamine, and the opiates) should continue to cause more concern.[25]

LSD-like Tryptamine Derivatives

Dimethyltryptamine (DMT) is a naturally occurring psychedelic compound that is structurally related to serotonin. DMT can produce LSD-like effects in the user, and like LSD, it has been shown to bind to serotonin$_2$ receptors. Widely used throughout much of the world, DMT is an active ingredient of various types of South American snuff, such as cohoba (prepared from the beans of the *Piptadenia peregrina*) and epena (prepared from the bark of trees found in the upper Amazon River valley), as well as yopo (a similar product from the West Indies). DMT is partly responsible for the hallucinations and confusional syndrome that follow inhalation of these powders, but the presence of the drug bufotenine (5-hydroxy-DMT) also contributes to the effect. Unlike LSD, DMT is not absorbed when it is taken orally; it must be smoked or sniffed to be effective.

The psychedelic properties of DMT appear to result predominantly from alterations in visual perception or the occurrence of true hallucinations. Euphoria and behavioral excitability often accompany the sensory alterations. The duration of action of DMT is extremely short—usually only about 1 hour (hence its slang name, "businessman's LSD").

Psilocybin (4-phosphoryl-DMT) and *psilocin* (4-hydroxy-DMT) are two psychedelic agents that are found in at least 15 species of mushrooms that belong to the genera *Psilocybe, Panaeolus,* and *Conocybe.* These mushrooms grow throughout much of the world, including Central America and the northwestern portion of the United States.[26] *Psilocybe mexicana* (also referred to as *teonanacatl,* or "God's flesh") has a long and colorful history of use as a sacramental throughout Central America.

Psilocin and psilocybin are approximately 1/200 as potent as LSD, and their effects last about 6 to 10 hours. Unlike DMT, psilocin and psilocybin are absorbed effectively when taken orally; the mushrooms are eaten raw to induce psychedelic effects. There is great variation in the concentration of psilocybin and psilocin among the different species of mushrooms, as well as significant differences among mushrooms of the same species. For example, the usual oral dose of *Psilocybe semilanceata* ("liberty caps") may consist of 10 to 40 mushrooms, while the dose for *Psilocybe cyanescens* may be only 2 to 5 mushrooms. Thus, the species must be properly identified. Also, some extremely toxic species of mushrooms are not psychoactive, but they bear a superficial resemblance to the mushrooms that contain psilocybin and psilocin. Thus, to avoid unpleasant experiences, one must be familiar with all hallucinogenic and poisonous species of mushrooms. Since the effects of psilocybin so closely resemble those produced by LSD, the "psilocybin" sold on the street is almost always LSD, and ordinary mushrooms laced with LSD may be sold as "magic mushrooms."[27]

For a long time, psilocin and psilocybin were thought to be pharmacologically active. However, as Figure 12.3 shows, the only difference between the two compounds is that psilocybin contains a molecule of phosphoric acid. After the mushroom has been ingested, phosphoric acid is apparently removed from psilocybin, thus producing psilocin, the active psychedelic agent.

Although the psychedelic effects of *Psilocybe mexicana* have long been part of Indian folklore, *Psilocybe* intoxication was not described until 1955, when Gordon Wasson, a New York banker, traveled through Mexico. He mingled with native tribes and was allowed to participate in a *Psilocybe* ceremony, in which he consumed the magic mushroom. Wasson said:

> It permits you to travel backwards and forward in time, to enter other planes of existence, even to know God. . . . Your body lies in the darkness, heavy as lead, but your spirit seems to soar and leave the hut, and with the speed of thought to travel where it listeth, in time and space, accompanied by the shaman's singing . . . at least you know what the ineffable is, and what ecstasy means. Ecstasy! The mind harks back to the origin of that word. For the Greeks, *ekstasis* meant the flight of the soul from the body. Can you find a better word to describe this state?[28]

As might be predicted, the hallucinations and distortions of time and space that are caused by psilocybin resemble those produced by LSD. Weil narrates his personal experiences with the psilocybin mushroom.[29]

Ololiuqui (morning glory seeds) is yet another naturally occurring agent that is used by Central and South American Indians both as an intoxicant and as a hallucinogen. The drug is used ritually as a means of communicating with the supernatural, as are extracts of most plants that contain psychedelic drugs. The use of ololiuqui seeds in Central and South America was first described by the Spaniard Hernandez, who stated, "When the priests wanted to commune with their Gods . . . [they ate ololiuqui seeds and] a thousand visions and satanic hallucinations appeared to them."[30]

The seeds were analyzed in Europe by Albert Hoffman (the discoverer of LSD), who identified several ingredients. One ingredient was lysergic acid amide (not lysergic acid diethylamide, LSD). The lysergic acid amide that Hoffman identified is approximately 1/10 as active as LSD as a psychoactive agent. However, considering the extreme potency of LSD, lysergic acid amide is still quite potent.

Accompanying the psychedelic action of ololiuqui are the usual side effects of serotonin psychedelic drugs: nausea, vomiting, headache, increased blood pressure, dilated pupils, sleepiness, and so on. These side effects are usually quite intense and serve to limit the recreational use of ololiuqui. Ingestion of 100 or more seeds produces sleepiness, distorted perception, hallucinations, and confusion. Flashbacks have been reported, but they are infrequent.

Harmine is a psychedelic agent that is obtained from the seeds of *Peganum harmala*, a plant native to the Middle East. These seeds have been used as intoxicants for centuries. Intoxication by harmine is usually accompanied by nausea and vomiting, sedation, and finally sleep. The psychic excitement that users experience consists of visual distortions that are similar to those induced by LSD.

Psychedelic Anesthetic Drugs: Phencyclidine and Ketamine

Phencyclidine (PCP or "angel dust") and ketamine are referred to as *psychedelic anesthetic drugs* (Figure 12.4). These two drugs are structurally unrelated to the other psychedelic compounds and psychoactive drugs and likely do not act by modifying serotonin neurotransmission. Recently the receptors to which these two drugs bind and, as a consequence, produce their characteristic effects of amnesia, analgesia, and psychedelic dissociation were identified and termed "PCP receptors."[31]

Background

Phencyclidine was developed in 1956 as a potent analgesic-amnestic-anesthetic agent. It was briefly used as an anesthetic in humans before being abandoned because of a high incidence of bizarre and serious psychiatric reactions, including agitation, excitement, delirium, disorientation, and hallucinatory phenomena. The perception of body changes, disorganized thought, suspiciousness, confusion, and lack of cooperation that were exhibited resembled a schizophrenic state that consisted of both production (positive) and deficit (negative) symptoms.

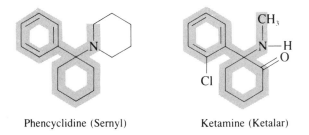

Phencyclidine (Sernyl)   Ketamine (Ketalar)

FIGURE 12.4 Structural formulas of the psychedelic anesthetic drugs phencyclidine and ketamine.

Phencyclidine is still used as a veterinary anesthetic, primarily for use in primates as an immobilizing agent. Ketamine, which is structurally related to phencyclidine (see Figure 12.4), induces a phencyclidinelike anesthetic state in low doses with only a moderate incidence of the bothersome psychiatric side effects. Ketamine is occasionally used in humans to provide anesthesia in patients who cannot tolerate the cardiovascular depressant effects of other anesthetics, such as individuals with hemorrhagic shock who have experienced severe physical injury.

Small amounts of phencyclidine became available in the "drug culture" in 1967, when it was referred to as the "peace pill" (PCP). Between 1971 and 1975, most PCP was available as a component of various illicit drug mixtures. In 1975, however, the use of illicit phencyclidine resurged, and it became one of the most abused drugs in the United States. By the early 1980s, the use of PCP had peaked, and it has now decreased markedly, although there are still periodic uprisings in use.

Phencyclidine has appeared on the illicit market in the form of powder, tablets, leaf mixtures, and 1-gram "rock" crystals and is commonly sold as "crystal," "angel dust," "hog," "PCP," "THC," "cannabinol," or "mescaline." When phencyclidine is sold as crystal or angel dust (terms also used for methamphetamine), the drug is usually in concentrations that vary between 50 and 100 percent. When it is purchased under other names or in concoctions, the amount of phencyclidine falls to between 10 and 30 percent, with the typical street dose being about 5 milligrams.[32] Phencyclidine can be taken orally, smoked, snorted, or injected intravenously.

Pharmacokinetics

PCP is well absorbed whether taken orally or smoked. When it is smoked, peak effects occur in about 15 minutes, when about 40 percent of the dose appears in the user's bloodstream. Oral absorption is slower; maximum blood levels are not reached until about 2 hours after the drug has been taken. In the stomach, phencyclidine exists in a water-soluble form that is poorly absorbed. However, when the drug passes into the intestine, which is less acidic, it becomes more lipid soluble and is readily absorbed through the intestinal lining into plasma. With such kinetics, after absorption and distribution throughout the body, much is secreted back into the stomach, carried to the intestine, and reabsorbed. This process of enterohepatic recirculation can markedly prolong its duration of action in the body, providing a prolonged and fluctuating course of clinical intoxication.[32]

Phencyclidine is metabolized in the liver, and its metabolites are excreted through the kidneys. The elimination half-life averages about 18 hours but varies widely, presumably because of the enterohepatic recirculation. Interestingly, this recirculation can be utilized to therapeutic advantage in treating phencyclidine overdosage. Since the drug repeatedly appears in the stomach in a water-soluble (ionized) form (see Chapter 2), activated charcoal can be given orally. This substance has been shown to bind phencyclidine and diminish its toxicity.[33]

A positive urine assay for PCP is assumed to indicate that PCP was used within the previous week. Blood and saliva tests for PCP can also be done. Because false-positive test results are common, a positive assay requires secondary confirmation.

Mechanism of Action

In 1979 experiments in rats demonstrated that phencyclidine binds to specific receptors in the brain. Within the next few years the binding sites were found to include the anterior forebrain (neocortex and olfactory structures), dentate gyrus, hippocampus, and the dorsal horns of the spinal cord. By 1990 it was concluded that these PCP receptors are located postsynaptically rather than presynaptically.[34] Phencyclidine binds to a specific binding site located within a channel whose molecular structure resembles that of the benzodiazepine-GABA complex (Chapter 4). Here the channel is an N-methyl-D-aspartic-acid- (NMDA-) type glutamate receptor channel, with glutamate being the major excitatory transmitter within the CNS. This NMDA-activated receptor is a specialized type of glutamate receptor.

> These receptors, which are ligand- [neurotransmitter-] gated cation channels, are involved in synaptic plasticity and in long-term enhancement of synaptic efficacy (i.e., long-term potentiation), thought to be the basis of processes involved in learning and memory.[35]

This NMDA/PCP-glutamate receptor has binding sites on the portion of the receptor complex exterior to the postsynaptic membrane (facing the synaptic cleft) for NMDA and for glutamate, both of which serve to open the channel and allow the influx of calcium ions (Figure 12.5).[36] These ions, in turn, activate intracellular processes in the postsynaptic cell.

Of importance here is a third binding site on this receptor complex, the binding site for phencyclidine (the PCP receptor), which is actually located within the transmembrane channel. By binding to this site, phencyclidine antagonizes the actions of NMDA and glutamate, preventing the channel from opening and thus preventing the influx of

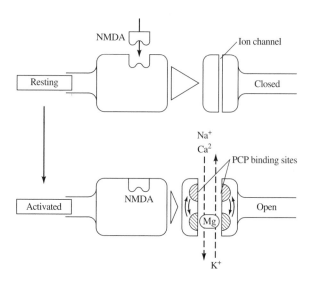

FIGURE 12.5 Model of NMDA receptor complex in resting state and after activation by attachment of NMDA. The intrachannel binding site for PCP (the stippled PCP receptors) is illustrated. Not illustrated are the intracellular processes caused by an influx of sodium (Na^+) and calcium (Ca^{+2}) ions. [Figure modified from Kemp, Foster, and Wong.[36]]

calcium and ultimately preventing activation of the neuron. Such action (i.e., as a noncompetitive antagonist of the NMDA-glutamate receptor) mediates the analgesic, psychotomimetic, and amnesic effects of phencyclidine.*

Psychological Effects

Phencyclidine and ketamine are referred to as *dissociative anesthetics,* because patients may feel dissociated from themselves and their environment. In humans, both drugs are unique among all the anesthetic drugs that have been studied. They induce an unresponsive state with intense analgesia and amnesia, although the patient's eyes remain open (blank stare), and he or she may even appear to be awake.

---

*Ikin and coworkers[35] isolated and analyzed the NMDA/PCP receptor complex. The receptor has a molecular weight of 203,000 and is composed of four membrane-spanning polypeptides (molecular weights of 67,000, 57,000, 46,000, and 33,000) which cluster together to form an ion channel that resembles the benzodiazepine-GABA receptor (Chapter 4). Here, however, the drug-binding site (the PCP receptor) is located within the lumen of the ion channel. Attachment of PCP to the receptor "plugs" the channel and inhibits ion (Ca^{+2}) influx when the transmitter (glutamate) attaches to its receptor on the outer surface.

When not used under controlled conditions, phencyclidine in low doses produces mild agitation, euphoria, disinhibition, or excitement in a person who appears to be grossly drunk and exhibits a blank stare. The subject may be rigid and unable to speak. In many cases, however, the patient is communicative, although he or she does not respond to pain.

> PCP acutely induces a psychotic state in which subjects become withdrawn, autistic, negativistic, and unable to maintain a cognitive set, and manifest concrete, impoverished, idiosyncratic, and bizarre responses to proverbs and projective testing. Some subjects show catatonic posturing. These schizophrenic-like alterations in brain functioning went beyond the symptom level. . . . Any person under the influence of even a small amount of PCP . . . will have profound alterations of higher emotional functions affecting judgment and cognition. . . . "[37]

Krystal and coworkers, in a recent study of ketamine, concluded that this drug (as well as phencyclidine) produces a broad range of symptoms, behaviors, and cognitive deficits that resemble aspects of endogenous psychoses, particularly schizophrenia and dissociative states.[38]

High doses of phencyclidine or ketamine induce a state of coma or stupor. However, abusers tend to "titrate" their dose to maximize the intoxicant effect while attempting to avoid unconsciousness. Blood pressure usually becomes elevated, but respiration does not become depressed. The patient may recover from this state within 2 to 4 hours, although a state of confusion may last for 8 to 72 hours. The disruption of sensory input by PCP causes unpredictable exaggerated, distorted, or violent reactions to environmental stimuli. Such reactions are augmented by PCP-induced analgesia and amnesia.

Massive oral overdoses, involving up to 1 gram of street-purchased phencyclidine, result in prolonged periods of stupor or coma. This state may last for several days and may be marked by intense seizure activity, increased blood pressure, and a depression of respiration that is potentially lethal. Following this stupor, a prolonged recovery phase, marked by confusion and delusions, may last as long as 2 weeks. In some persons, this state of confusion may be followed by a psychosis that lasts several weeks to a few months.

Side Effects and Toxicity

The course of recovery from any drug-induced schizophrenia-like psychotic state is variable for reasons that are poorly understood.

Flashbacks from phencyclidine may represent either recurrence of psychosis or mobilization of stored phencyclidine from adipose tissues (since the drug is very fat soluble and thus readily stored in body fat). Any flashbacks resulting from the latter mechanism should be expected to dissipate within a few weeks, however; after this time period the drug should be eliminated from the body.

The intoxicated state produced by phencyclidine use leads to such behavioral complications as severe anxiety, aggression, panic, paranoia, and rage. A user can also display violent reactions to sensory input, leading to such problems as falls, drowning, burns, driving accidents, and aggressive behavior.

Self-inflicted injuries and injuries sustained while physical restraints are applied are frequent, and the potent analgesic action certainly contributes to the lack of response to pain. Respiratory depression, generalized seizure activity, and pulmonary edema have all been reported. PCP has been implicated in a number of deaths by drowning, violent behavior, automobile accidents, and suicide.

Tolerance, Dependence, and Abuse

PCP is the only psychedelic drug self-administered by monkeys. In man, this pattern of compulsive abuse is also seen. By inference, therefore, phencyclidine seems to stimulate brain reward areas and therefore places the user at risk of compulsive abuse despite negative health consequences.

Tolerance develops in laboratory animals, and twofold dose increases have been observed. Physiological withdrawal is poorly studied in man; however, animals given unlimited access to phencyclidine for one month or longer demonstrate withdrawal signs. In summary, "research has established a compelling case that PCP is a strongly addicting drug."[37]

Therapy for PCP intoxication is aimed at reducing the systemic level of the drug, keeping the individual calm and sedated, and preventing any of several severe adverse medical effects. Such therapy involves (1) minimization of sensory inputs by placing the intoxicated individual in a quiet environment; (2) oral administration of activated charcoal, which can bind any PCP present in the stomach and intestine; (3) precautionary physical restraint to prevent self-injury; and (4) sedation with either a benzodiazepine (such as lorazepam) or a neuroleptic (such as haloperidol). Hyperthermia, hypertension, convulsion, renal failure, and other medical consequences should be treated as necessary by medical experts. PCP-induced psychotic states may be long-lasting (even for several weeks), especially in individuals with schizophrenia.

Study Questions

1. What is a psychedelic drug?
2. What differentiates a psychedelic drug from a behavioral stimulant, such as amphetamine or cocaine?
3. List four different types (classes) of psychedelic drugs.
4. Differentiate between mescaline and LSD.
5. How does LSD exert psychedelic actions?
6. What is the psychedelic syndrome?
7. What are some of the problems associated with the use of LSD?
8. How does phencyclidine differ from a nonselective CNS depressant? How does phencyclidine differ from LSD?
9. Phencyclidine is used as an animal tranquilizer or immobilizer. What properties of phencyclidine contribute to this use?

Notes

1. J. T. Ungerleider and R. N. Pechnick, "Hallucinogens," in J. H. Lowinson, P. Ruiz, R. B. Millman, and J. G. Langrod, eds., *Substance Abuse: A Comprehensive Textbook,* 2nd ed. (Baltimore: Williams & Wilkins, 1992), pp. 280–289.
2. J. H. Jaffe, "Drug Addiction and Drug Abuse," in A. G. Gilman, T. W. Rall, A. S. Nies, and P. Taylor, eds., *Goodman and Gilman's The Pharmacological Basis of Therapeutics,* 8th ed. (New York: Pergamon, 1990), p. 553.
3. H. W. Hitner, "Psychotomimetic Drugs," in J. R. DiPalma and G. J. DiGregorio, eds., *Basic Pharmacology in Medicine,* 3rd ed. (New York: McGraw-Hill, 1990), pp. 242–244.
4. S. Cohen, *The Chemical Brain: The Neurochemistry of Addictive Disorders* (Irvine, Ca.: Care Institute, 1988), pp. 66–67.
5. B. L. Jacobs, "How Hallucinogenic Drugs Work," *American Scientist* 75 (1987): 386–392.
6. Ibid., p. 387.
7. R. A. Glennon, M. Teitler, and J. D. McKenney, "Evidence for 5-HT$_2$ Involvement in the Mechanism of Action of Hallucinogens," *Life Sciences* 35 (1984): 2505–2511.
8. R. A. Glennon, "Do Classical Hallucinogens Act as 5-HT$_2$ Agonists or Antagonists?" *Neuropsychopharmacology* 3 (1990): 509–517.
9. R. A. Glennon, M. Teitler, and E. Sanders-Bush, "Hallucinogens and Serotonergic Mechanisms," *NIDA Research Monograph Series* 119 (1992): 131–135.
10. M. Teitler, S. Leonhardt, N. M. Appel, E. B. DeSouza, and R. A. Glennon, "Receptor Pharmacology of MDMA and Related Hallucinogens," *Annals of the New York Academy of Sciences* 600 (1990): 626–639.
11. S. G. Potkin and others, "Phenethylamine in Paranoid Chronic Schizophrenia," *Science* 206 (1979): 470.

12. A. Goldstein, *Addiction: From Biology to Drug Policy* (New York: W. H. Freeman and Company, 1994), p. 197.

13. M. E. Molliver, U. V. Berger, L. A. Mamounas, D. C. Molliver, E. O'Hearn, and M. A. Wilson, "Neurotoxicity of MDMA and Related Compounds: Anatomic Studies," *Annals of the New York Academy of Sciences* 600 (1990): 640–661.

14. E. B. DeSouza, G. Battaglia, and T. R. Insel, "Neurotoxic Effects of MDMA on Brain Serotonin Neurons: Evidence from Neurochemical and Radioligand Binding Studies," *Annals of the New York Academy of Sciences* 600 (1990): 682–697.

15. G. A. Ricaurte, K. T. Finnegan, I. Irwin, and J. W. Langston, "Aminergic Metabolites in Cerebrospinal Fluid of Humans Previously Exposed to MDMA: Preliminary Observations," *Annals of the New York Academy of Sciences* 600 (1990): 699–708.

16. Ungerleider and Pechnick, "Hallucinogens," p. 287.

17. *Interim Drug Report of the Commission of Inquiry into the Nonmedical Use of Drugs* (Ottawa: Information Canada, 1970), pp. 58–59.

18. R. Yensen, "LSD and Psychotherapy," *Journal of Psychoactive Drugs* 17 (1985): 267–277.

19. Goldstein, *Addiction*, p. 202.

20. R. S. Gable, "Toward a Comparative Overview of Dependence Potential and Acute Toxicity of Psychoactive Substances Used Nonmedically," *American Journal of Drug and Alcohol Abuse* 19 (1993): 263–281.

21. L. P. Finnegan and K. O. Fehr, "The Effects of Opiates, Sedative-Hypnotics, Amphetamines, Cannabis, and Other Psychoactive Drugs on the Fetus and Newborn," in O. J. Kalant, ed., *Research Advances in Alcohol and Drug Problems*, vol. 5 (New York: Plenum Press, 1980), pp. 653–723.

22. Jaffe, "Drug Addiction and Drug Abuse," p. 556.

23. G. G. Dimijian, "Contemporary Drug Abuse," in A. Goth, ed., *Medical Pharmacology*, 11th ed. (St. Louis: Mosby, 1984), p. 156.

24. H. P. Rang and M. M. Dale, *Pharmacology*, 2nd ed. (Edinburgh: Churchill Livingstone, 1991), pp. 743–744.

25. R. A. Wise, "The Role of Reward Pathways in the Development of Drug Dependence," *Pharmacology and Therapeutics* 35 (1987): 227–263.

26. J. Ott, *Hallucinogenic Plants of North America* (Berkeley: Wingbow Press, 1979).

27. Goldstein, *Addiction*, p. 195.

28. M. E. Crahan, "God's Flesh and Other Pre-Columbian Phantastica," *Bulletin of the Los Angeles County Medical Association* 99 (1969): 17.

29. A. Weil, *The Marriage of the Sun and the Moon* (Boston: Houghton Mifflin, 1980), pp. 73–79.

30. E. M. Brecher and Consumer Reports editors, *Licit and Illicit Drugs* (Mt. Vernon, N.Y.: Consumers Union, 1972), p. 345.

31. S. R. Zukin and R. S. Zukin, "Phencyclidine," in J. H. Lowinson, P. Ruiz, R. B. Millman, and J. G. Langrod, eds., *Substance Abuse: A Comprehensive Textbook*, 2nd ed. (Baltimore: Williams & Wilkins, 1992), pp. 290–302.

32. Ibid., p. 295.

33. Ibid., p. 297.
34. J. W. Bekenstein, J. P. Bennett, Jr., G. F. Wooten, and E. "Autoradiographic Evidence that NMDA Receptor-Coupled Channels Located Postsynaptically and Not Presynaptically in the Perforant Path-Dentate Granule Cell System of the Rat Hippocampal Formation," *Brain Research* 514 (1990): 334–342.
35. A. F. Ikin, Y. Kloog, and M. Sokolovsky, "N-Methyl-D-Aspartate/Phencyclidine Receptor Complex of Rat Forebrain: Purification and Biochemical Characterization," *Biochemistry* 29 (1990): 2290.
36. J. A. Kemp, A. C. Foster, and E. H. F. Wong, "Non-competitive Antagonists of Excitatory Amino Acid Receptors," *Trends in Neurological Sciences* 10 (1987): 294–298.
37. Zukin and Zukin, "Phencyclidine," p. 296.
38. J. H. Krystal, L. P. Karper, J. P. Seibyl, G. K. Freeman, R. Delaney, J. D. Bremmer, G. R. Heninger, M. B. Bowers, and D. S. Charney, "Subanesthetic Effects of the Noncompetitive NMDA Antagonist, Ketamine, in Humans: Psychotomimetic, Perceptual, Cognitive, and Neuroendocrine Responses," *Archives of General Psychiatry* 51 (1994): 199–214.

CHAPTER 13

MARIJUANA: A UNIQUE SEDATIVE-EUPHORIANT-PSYCHEDELIC DRUG

The ancient preparation called marijuana has sedative, euphoriant, and (in large doses) hallucinogenic properties. The hemp plant *Cannabis sativa* from which marijuana comes grows throughout the world and flourishes in most temperate and tropical regions. It is one of humanity's oldest cultivated nonfood plants. The major psychoactive ingredient of the marijuana plant is delta-9-tetrahydrocannabinol (THC). THC and other natural and synthetic cannabinoids produce the characteristic motor, cognitive, psychedelic, and analgesic effects that are described in this chapter. THC is most concentrated in the resin obtained from the flowers of the female plant.

Names for *Cannabis* products include *marijuana, hashish, charas, bhang, ganja,* and *sinsemilla.* Hashish and charas, which consist of the dried resinous exudate of the female flowers, are the most potent preparations with a THC content averaging between 7 and 14 percent. Ganja and sinsemilla refer to the dried material found in the tops of the female plants, where the THC content averages about 4 to 5 percent (rarely over 7 percent). Bhang and marijuana are low-grade preparations taken from the dried remainder of the plant, and their THC content can be as low as 1 percent. Thus, marijuana products that are commercially available vary in THC concentration from about 1 percent to about 4 to 7 percent. The usual range of potency for marijuana seems to be 2 to 5 percent.

Until recently marijuana was classified according to its behavioral effects. Thus, marijuana and its active ingredients (principally THC) were classified as mild sedative-hypnotic agents (at least at low to moderate doses), with clinical effects being similar to those of alcohol

330

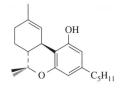

FIGURE 13.1   Structure of delta-9-tetrahydrocannabinol (THC).

and the antianxiety agents. Unlike the sedative-hypnotic compounds, however, higher doses of THC may also produce euphoria, hallucinations, and heightened sensations—effects that are similar to a mild LSD experience. Further, very high doses of THC do not produce anesthesia, coma, or death (also unlike the sedatives). Little cross tolerance occurs between THC and LSD or between THC and the sedative-hypnotic compounds. Thus, while THC seems to bear superficial resemblance to both the sedatives and the psychedelics, it is remarkably different from both sets of drugs.

In chemical structure, THC does not resemble either the sedatives or the psychedelics (Figure 13.1), nor does it resemble any known or suspected neurotransmitter. If any structural comparison is made, it is usually to steroid molecules; this fact is a point of interest since THC has significant effects on sex-hormone-mediated body functions. It was once thought that THC might act like a general anesthetic, affecting neuronal membranes to increase membrane fluidity (an action that has not been correlated with psychedelic action). This has now been dismissed as a mechanism of action. However, the 1990s have yielded

> new and truly exciting developments...in several areas of cannabis and cannabinoid research. These include substantial strides in our understanding of pharmacological, biochemical, and behavioral mechanisms of action for the cannabinoid compounds and of the smoked material.[1]

This research is of such importance that we discuss THC's mechanism of action after we review the history of marijuana.

History

In a recent review on the history of marijuana use, Grinspoon and Bakalar noted that the use of *Cannabis sativa* dates from about 2700 B.C.[2] Marijuana in ancient times was used primarily as a mild intoxicant and was a subject of controversy even in those days. It is somewhat milder than alcohol and much less useful for religious and psychedelic experiences than the naturally occurring psychedelic drugs (since cannabis produces much less sensory distortion). Over the years, products from *Cannabis sativa* have been claimed to have a wide variety of medical uses, although few persist in native cultures. Today, however, our society is reexamining potential therapeutic uses of THC and its derivatives.

Cannabis sativa is rather new to Western culture. During the American colonial period, in the 1700s, the plant was grown widely in Virginia, presumably for its fiber, which was used for rope. Even George Washington grew hemp for fiber and, possibly, for its medicinal and other properties.

Hemp cultivation flourished in the United States for many years but then declined when more profitable crops, such as cotton, were introduced and the importation of cheap hemp from the Far East began. During World War II, cultivation of hemp was expanded when imports became severely limited. However, hemp need not be cultivated, because *Cannabis sativa* grows wild and does not need to be tended.

Marijuana—at least until the beginning of the twentieth century—was not widely used for either medical or recreational purposes. Its psychoactive properties had been discovered but had not attracted much attention. The use of marijuana was restricted primarily to the "less desirable" elements in society. During the early 1920s, the news media portrayed marijuana as being evil and part of "underground" activities. In 1926 a New Orleans newspaper exposed the "menace of marijuana," claiming that an association existed between marijuana and crime; laws were subsequently passed in Louisiana to outlaw its use. During the next five years other states began to pass laws against the use of marijuana.

Probably the greatest impetus to the outlawing of marijuana was provided during the early 1930s. The federal commissioner of narcotics had an intense interest in encouraging the states and the Bureau of Narcotics to enforce vigorously the laws against using marijuana. During the next few years, marijuana began to be looked on as a narcotic—an agent responsible for crimes of violence and a great danger to public safety. These attitudes were popularized throughout the 1930s by numerous news articles, which convinced the public that marijuana was indeed evil. By 1940 the country was convinced that marijuana was a "killer drug" and a potent narcotic that (1) induced people to commit crimes of violence, (2) led to heroin addiction, and (3) was a great social menace.

The emotional campaign against marijuana continued through the 1950s. At that time, the use of marijuana was still restricted primarily to the lower classes of society. However, during the late 1950s and early 1960s, marijuana and other psychoactive drugs became extremely popular among middle- and upper-class youths. Throughout the 1960s, the use of marijuana by American youths steadily increased. However, the rate of experimentation with marijuana did not explode with the same rapidity as experimentation with LSD, and the use of marijuana did not really become widespread until the late 1960s and early 1970s, when the use of LSD and other potent psychedelic drugs had begun to decline.

By 1972 at least 2 million Americans used marijuana daily; marijuana use exceeded the use of alcohol among many young adults. In 1977 a national survey on drug use showed that persons between 18 and 25 years old used marijuana the most, with a precipitous drop in use among persons older than 35 years of age. An estimated 43 million Americans had tried marijuana by the spring of 1977.

Surveys taken from 1975 through 1986 revealed that the percentage of high school seniors who smoked marijuana had declined steadily since the peak period of use, between 1977 and 1979 (Table 13.1). Also, daily use of marijuana by high school seniors declined from a peak of 11 percent in 1978 to less than 4 percent.[3] Disquieting, however, were the observations that the number of students who smoked cigarettes had not declined, use of alcohol had continued unabated, and use of cocaine had increased steadily. Marijuana was (and still is) rarely used by persons over the age of 50. In 1990 an estimated 6 to 10 million Americans smoked marijuana at least once every week.

TABLE 13.1 Percentage of high school seniors using drugs within the past 30 days.

	1975	1976	1977	1978	1979	1980	1981	1982	1983	1984	1985	1986
Marijuana, hashish	27.1	32.2	35.4	37.1	36.5	33.7	31.6	28.5	27.0	25.2	25.7	23.4
Cocaine	1.9	2.0	2.9	3.9	5.7	5.2	5.8	5.0	4.9	5.8	6.7	6.2
Alcohol	68.2	68.3	71.2	72.1	71.8	72.0	70.7	69.7	69.4	67.2	65.9	65.3

Source: University of Michigan Institute for Social Research. Conducted for the National Institute on Drug Abuse, 1987.
Note: Survey was based on a confidential questionnaire administered nationwide.

Finally, a survey in late 1993 revealed that the apparent decline in marijuana use had ceased, and a small resurgence was occurring. Alcohol and cigarette use also continued unabated. Among high school seniors, 26 percent had used marijuana in the previous year (up from 22 percent in 1992) and 19 percent smoked cigarettes daily. Among eighth-grade students, 8 percent had used marijuana within the past year and 14 percent smoked cigarettes daily. These figures do not include significant numbers of school dropouts, who traditionally exhibit a much higher incidence of drug use.

Thus, drug use may be making a comeback among the newest generation of students. Further, the combined effects of alcohol and marijuana are a cause of continuing concern;[4] this topic will be elaborated upon later.

Mechanism of Action

Evidence gathered through the mid-1980s led to the hypothesis that THC and other cannabinoids act via a pharmacologically distinct set of receptors. Where or what these receptors were, however, was unknown. Howlett and coworkers demonstrated in 1986 that THC inhibited the intracellular enzyme adenylate cyclase and that such inhibition required the presence of a guanine-nucleotide-binding protein complex.[5] THC does not directly inhibit the enzyme;[6,7] rather, it acts on a specific, unidentified receptor in such a way that the enzyme is ultimately inhibited.

Matsuda and coworkers further studied this cannabinoid receptor.[8] They were able to isolate and clone from rat cerebral cortex a protein-complex receptor that both inhibited adenylate cyclase and bound cannabinoids. They then determined that the amino acid sequence of the protein is a chain of 473 amino acids with seven hydrophobic domains. Based on this finding, Howlett and coworkers in 1991 proposed that the membrane receptor to which cannabinoids bind comprise seven membrane-spanning regions that extend through the cell membrane (Figure 13.2); each region (or cylinder) is composed of one hydrophobic domain.[9] When THC binds to the outer portion of the receptor, the cyclic nucleotide second-messenger system is activated to inhibit adenylate cyclase. THC effects are not exerted through actions on GABA receptors[10] or through alterations in dopamine release.[11]

Thus, the cannabinoid receptor has been isolated and cloned, its transmembrane structure proposed, and its cellular transduction

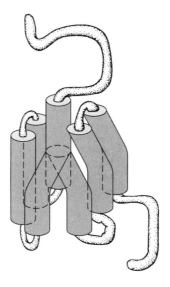

FIGURE 13.2   Predicted tertiary structure of the cannabinoid receptor. The primary structure of the cannabinoid receptor deduced from the cDNA nucleotide sequence comprises seven relatively hydrophobic domains (depicted as cylinders) that extend through the plasma membraine. The N-terminal extracellular (above) and C-terminal intracellular (below) extensions and intervening loops are depicted as stippled regions. [From Howlett, Champion-Dorow, McMahon, and Westlake.[9]]

mechanisms delineated (i.e., inhibition of adenylate cyclase). Two important points remained to be demonstrated:

1. identification of a naturally occurring "ligand," or agonist neurotransmitter, which binds to the cannabinoid receptor and thus might function as a "natural THC"

2. localization of THC receptors in the brain, with correlation of such localization with marijuana's behavioral and cognitive effects

In the search for a naturally occurring ligand, Devane and coworkers in 1992 isolated from porcine brain an arachidonic acid derivative, named anandamide (Figure 13.3), which specifically binds to the cannabinoid receptor and produces cannabinoidlike pharmacological effects.[12] Fride and Mechoulam,[13] Felder and coworkers,[14] and Bornheim and coworkers[15] in 1993 extended the work on anandamide, demonstrating that this substance produces behavioral, hypothermic, and analgesic effects that parallel those caused by psychotropic

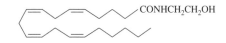

FIGURE 13.3 Structure of anandamide, a proposed, naturally occurring (endogenous) agonist (ligand) of the cannabinoid receptor.[12]

cannabinoids. Indeed, anandamide appears to exhibit the essential criteria required to be classified as a cannabinoid/anandamide receptor agonist.[14] Certainly, much more will be forthcoming about this newly identified natural ligand for the cannabinoid receptor, which is now called the anandamide receptor.[16]

In the late 1980s, it was hypothesized that the hippocampus, cerebral cortex, cerebellum, and basal ganglia ("striatum") were the loci of action of THC and other cannabinoid drugs because these structures are involved in cognition and memory, mood, and higher intellectual functions, as well as motor functions.[6] Herkenham and coworkers delineated the unique pattern of localization of cannabinoid/anandamide receptors in the brain (Figures 13.4 and 13.5).[17–19] First, large numbers of receptors are found in the basal ganglia and cerebellum, which are involved in many forms of movement control that are affected by smoking marijuana. Second, the cerebral cortex, especially the frontal cortex, is rich in cannabinoid receptors. Binding of THC here likely mediates at least some of the psychoactive effects of the drug, including the drug-induced "high," the characteristic distortions of the sense of time (discussed later), alterations in the ability to concentrate, and production of a dreamlike state.[18] Cannabinoid/anandamide receptors are also dense in the hippocampus; this fact may account for THC-induced disruption of memory, memory storage, and coding of sensory input. Because brain stem structures do not bind cannabinoids, THC does not affect basal body functions, including respiration. Indeed, the lack of cannabinoid/anandamide receptors in the brain stem explains the relative nonlethality of THC, which is a remarkably nonfatal drug.

In 1994 Lynn and Herkenham studied the peripheral effects of cannabinoids, reporting that, outside the brain, cannabinoid receptors are found only in specific components of the immune system (confined to beta-lymphocyte-enriched areas such as the spleen).[20] Nonspecific binding of cannabinoids was found in several areas, including the heart, lungs, endocrine system, and reproductive organs. Thus, both the specific receptor binding in the immune system and the widespread nonspecific binding account for the side effects of marijuana, which are discussed below.

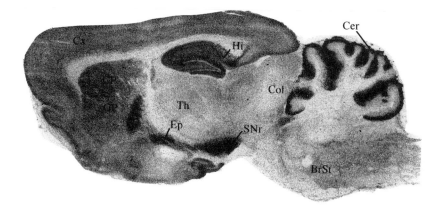

FIGURE 13.4 Autoradiographic binding of a potent cannabinoid to cannabinoid receptors in the rat brain. Br St, brain stem; Cer, cerebellum; Col, colliculi; CP, caudate-putamen; Cx, cerebral cortex; Ep, entopeduncular nucleus; GP, globus pallidus; Hi, hippocampus; SNr, substantia nigra; Th, thalamus.

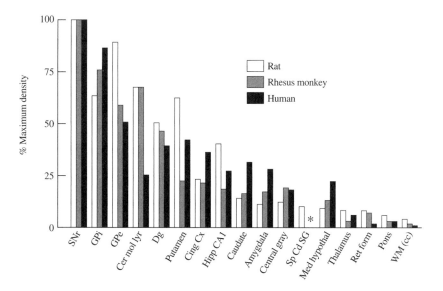

FIGURE 13.5 Relative densities of cannabinoid receptors across brain structures in rat, rhesus monkey, and human. Cer Mol Lyr, cerebellum, molecular layer; Cing Cx, cingulate cortex; DG, dentate gyrus; GPe, external globus pallidus; GPi, internal globus pallidus; Hipp CA1, hippocampal field CA1; Med Hypothal, medial hypo-thalamus; Ret Form, reticular formation; Sp Cd SG, substantia gelatinosa of spinal cord (*only rat measured); WM (cc), white matter of corpus callosum.

Pharmacokinetics

Most marijuana available in the United States has a THC content that rarely exceeds 7 percent and usually averages about 3 to 4 percent.[21] In the United States, THC is usually administered in the form of a hand-rolled marijuana cigarette (the average marijuana cigarette contains between 0.4 and 1 gram of plant material). Thus, if a marijuana cigarette contains 1 gram of plant material with a THC content of about 5 percent, the cigarette contains approximately 50 milligrams of THC. Because THC is usually administered by smoking marijuana, the quantity of drug absorbed into the bloodstream varies considerably with the previous smoking experience of the user, the amount of time that the smoke is held in the lungs, and the number of persons smoking the same cigarette.

Usually persons who have previously smoked marijuana can hold the smoke in their lungs longer than can novices, which allows more THC to be absorbed into the bloodstream before the smoke is exhaled. Similarly, persons who habitually smoke tobacco cigarettes can usually hold marijuana smoke in their lungs longer than can nonsmokers. Further, the fewer persons who share a marijuana cigarette, and the closer the cigarette is smoked to the "butt," the more THC is available to each smoker.

In general, about one-fourth to one-half of the THC present in a marijuana cigarette is actually available in the smoke. Thus, if a cigarette contains 50 milligrams of THC, about 12 to 25 milligrams are available in the smoke. It is extremely unlikely, however, that even a single person smoking one cigarette would absorb 100 percent of the THC in that cigarette. In practice, the amount of THC absorbed into the bloodstream as a result of the social smoking of one marijuana cigarette is probably in the range of 0.4 to 10 milligrams.[22] Perez-Reyes and coworkers estimate a "bioavailability" (amount of THC in the cigarette actually present in plasma) of about 14 percent, ranging from a low of 1.4 percent to a maximum of 34.5 percent.[21]

As discussed in Chapter 2, the absorption of inhaled drugs is rapid and complete. The onset of behavioral effects of THC in smoked marijuana occurs within minutes after smoking begins and corresponds with the rapid attainment of peak concentrations in plasma (Figure 13.6). Unless more is smoked, the effects seldom last longer than 3 to 4 hours (Figure 13.7).

THC is also absorbed when it is administered orally, but the absorption is slow and incomplete. The onset of action usually takes 3 to 60 minutes, with peak effects occurring 2 to 3 hours after ingestion. Its effects persist for 3 to 5 hours or even longer. THC is approximately 3 times more effective when it is smoked than when it is taken orally.

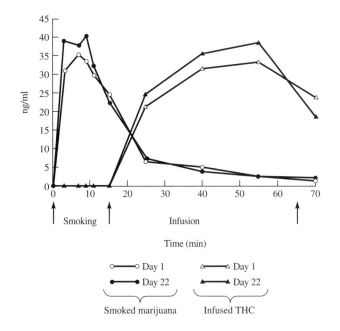

FIGURE 13.6 Mean plasma concentrations of total THC for smoked marijuana and infused THC on days 1 and 22. One marijuana cigarette was smoked from 0 to 15 minutes and was followed by intravenous infusion from 15 to 65 minutes, as indicated by the arrows. Results from day 22 were obtained after daily smoking of marijuana and suggest that tolerance failed to develop. [From Perez-Reyes, White, McDonald, Hicks, Jeffcoat, and Cook.[21]]

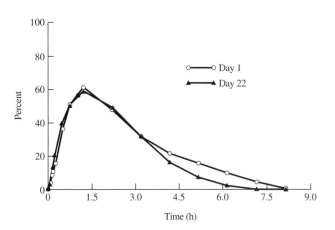

FIGURE 13.7 Mean ratings of "high" from the combination of smoked marijuana and infused THC on days 1 and 22.[21] As in Figure 13.6, the lack of development of tolerance is apparent.

Because marijuana products are crude preparations that are not soluble in water, they should not be administered by injection. Indeed, injection of any product of *Cannabis sativa* or any other plant is extremely dangerous. Finally, it should be noted that when a product is sold illicitly as "THC," it virtually never contains THC but rather a number of other psychedelic agents.

Once THC is absorbed, it is distributed to the various organs of the body, especially those that have significant concentrations of fatty material. Thus, THC readily penetrates the brain; the blood–brain barrier does not appear to hinder its passage. Similarly, THC readily crosses the placental barrier and reaches the fetus. It is almost completely metabolized to an active product (11-hydroxy-delta-9-THC) that is converted to an inactive metabolite; this metabolite is then excreted.[22]

After the initial period of intoxication, THC levels fall rapidly for about 1 hour to a low level (because of the high solubility of THC in body fat) that persists for days. The metabolism of THC is quite slow; an elimination half-life of about 30 hours is generally accepted, although some researchers report a half-life of about 4 days.[23] Thus, THC persists in the body for several days or even weeks. Such a delay tends to prolong and intensify the activity of subsequently smoked marijuana, which may at least partially explain why regular users achieve a "high" more quickly, more easily, and with a smaller amount of the drug than do intermittent users (a phenomenon that was formerly and incorrectly called "reverse tolerance").

Because only minute quantities of THC are found in the urine of persons who use the drug, tests for THC focus primarily on isolating its metabolites. Such detection tests are complex and involve specialized chemical techniques, such as immunoassay, chromatography, or spectrometry. Although acute or occasional use is detected for about 1 to 3 days, chronic smokers (even if they smoke only two to three times weekly) have persistently positive urine tests for THC metabolites. A heavy smoker who stops smoking may show positive urine tests for about one month after cessation. Thus, a positive urinalysis can indicate either recent use or use that occurred several weeks earlier. Multiple sampling may be necessary to differentiate the results. Thus, a single positive urine test does not mean that a person was under the influence of marijuana at the time the urine specimen was collected.

Pharmacological Effects

In animals, THC and other cannabinoids

> produce a unique syndrome of behavioral effects in a wide variety of animal species. At low doses, they produce a mixture of depressant

and stimulatory effects, and at higher doses, predominantly CNS depression. . . . A state of hyperreflexia or hyperstimulation is observed during the depressive portion of the syndrome. Higher doses . . . produce a more classical type of depression in rodents, including catalepsy. . . . Cannabinoids produce a combination of hypoactivity, hypothermia, antinociception, and catalepsy in mice. Other animal [effects] are dog static ataxia, monkey overt behavior, and drug discrimination.[24]

Thus, in animals, THC is sedative and analgesic, decreases spontaneous motor activity, decreases body temperature, calms aggressive behavior, potentiates the effects of barbiturates and other sedatives, blocks convulsions, and depresses reflexes. In primates, THC decreases aggression, decreases the ability to perform complex behavioral tasks, seems to induce hallucinations, and appears to cause temporal distortions. THC causes monkeys to increase the frequency of their social interactions. High doses can depress ovarian function, lower the concentration of female sex hormones, decrease ovulation, and possibly decrease sperm production. These effects likely result from the nonspecific binding of cannabinoid discussed above.

In humans THC primarily affects the functioning of the cardiovascular system and the CNS. An increase in pulse rate is the most commonly observed physiological effect of THC, although blood pressure is little affected. Blood vessels of the cornea can dilate, which results in the bloodshot eyes that can be observed in persons who have just smoked marijuana. THC users frequently report increased appetite, dry mouth, occasional dizziness, and slight nausea. Respiratory depression is not observed.

> Although the increased heart rate could be a problem for people with cardiovascular disease, dangerous physical reactions to marijuana are almost unknown. No human being is known to have died of an overdosage. By extrapolation from animal experiments, the ratio of lethal to effective (intoxicating) dose is estimated to be on the order of thousands to one.[25]

The behavioral effects of THC in humans vary with dose, route of administration, setting, the experience and expectation of the user, and individual vulnerability to the CNS alterations. In general, all the senses may be enhanced, and the perception of time is usually altered. Users report an increased sense of well-being, mild euphoria, relaxation, and relief from anxiety. The "high," or euphoria, is frequently followed by a period of drowsiness or sedation. "The subjective effects include dissociation of ideas. Illusions and hallucinations occur infrequently."[26]

At higher doses of THC (several cigarettes or moderate doses of hashish taken orally), the user experiences an intensification of emotional responses and alterations in sensation that resemble mild sensory distortions and even mild hallucinations. Few persons who smoke marijuana socially are seeking these effects. Only a small percentage of persons who smoke marijuana use it to induce a pronounced state of sensory distortion.

At higher doses, acute depressive reactions, acute panic reactions, or mild paranoia have been observed.[24] These reactions are likely due to the alterations in perception produced by THC; some panic responses may follow the feeling of a loss of mental control. Only at psychotoxic doses of THC does one see delusions, paranoia, hallucinations, confusion and disorientation, depersonalization, altered sensory perception, and loss of insight. Such reactions are unusual and generally short lasting. Common predisposing factors include preexisting personality disturbances. Jaffe discusses the effects of such large doses:

> Higher doses of THC can induce frank hallucinations, delusions, and paranoid feelings. Thinking becomes confused and disorganized; depersonalization and altered time sense are accentuated. Anxiety reaching panic proportions may replace euphoria, often as a result of the feeling that the drug-induced state will never end. With high enough doses, the clinical picture is that of a toxic psychosis with hallucinations, depersonalization, and loss of insight. . . . Most users are able to regulate their intake in order to avoid the excessive dosage that produces these unpleasant effects. . . . Use of marihuana may also cause an acute exacerbation of symptomatology in stabilized schizophrenics, and it is an independent risk factor for the development of schizophrenia.[27]

The effects of marijuana on cognition, learning, and attention have been the focus of significant study. Acute use impairs the ability to perform complex functions requiring attention and mental coordination (e.g., driving), although simple reflex activities are less affected. Solowij and coworkers studied chronic users and concluded that such users

> have difficulty in setting up an accurate focus of attention and in filtering out irrelevant information. The data suggest a dysfunction in the allocation of attentional resources and stimulus evaluation strategies. These results imply that long-term cannabis use may impair the ability to efficiently process information.[28]

The authors of the study were unable to assess to what extent this deficit might be due to chronic buildup of THC and whether functioning would return to normal upon prolonged discontinuation of use. An obvious question is to what extent the smoking of marijuana might affect or potentiate the attentional deficits seen in attention deficit disorders of childhood and adolescence.

Block and coworkers in 1992 studied the acute effects of marijuana smoking on cognition, reporting significant impairment in learning, associative processes, and psychomotor performance.[29] Notably, marijuana "altered associative processes, encouraging more uncommon associations."[29] A freer, less logically controlled flow of thought followed smoking. Abstraction and vocabulary were less affected. Other reported cognitive deficits following marijuana use include impaired memory and deficits in concept formation, learning, attention, and signal detection.[26]

Early studies of the effects of cannabis on memory ascribed drug-induced deficits to alterations in cholinergic activity. The memory deficits likely result from direct actions on the cannabinoid/anandamide receptors, with any cholinergic deficits occurring as a secondary event.

Finally, to understand the behavioral effects and attractiveness of a psychoactive drug, one must evaluate the interaction of that drug with the brain reward systems. Gardner and Lowinson recently reviewed marijuana's interactions with these systems, particularly loci in the dopamine-mediated, medial forebrain bundle projection. They state that

> acute enhancement of brain reward mechanisms appears to be the single essential commonality of abuse prone drugs, and the hypothesis that recreational and abused drugs act on these brain mechanisms to produce the subjective reward that constitutes the "high" or "rush" or "hit" sought by drug users is, at present, the most compelling hypothesis available on the neurobiology of recreational drug use and abuse.[30]

Furthermore, they emphasize that brain reward is, in fact, critically dependent on the functional integrity of dopamine neurotransmission within the mesotelencephalic dopamine systems.[31]

Also involved are synaptic interconnections of opioid and many other neurotransmitters. Indeed, Gardner and Lowinson argue that THC acts on this system as do other abused drugs, inducing the release of dopamine in reward loci including the basal ganglia, the nucleus accumbens, and the prefrontal cortex.[30] However, their data were obtained in a single strain of rodents; the three other strains of rodents that they studied failed to demonstrate THC-induced dopamine release. Thus, as summarized by Abood and Martin, because "these effects have been reported in one strain of rat, their extrapolation to human abuse is tentative at best."[32]

Finally, as emphasized in earlier chapters, before a drug can be implicated in neuropsychological dysfunction, the individual must be examined in a nonintoxicated state; in the case of THC, this state may require a drugfree period of weeks or months. Only then can one assess the individual for psychopathology that is unrelated to drug use (i.e., comorbidity). The question of cause and effect (whether the use of marijuana or another drug causes or unmasks psychopathology) will likely continue unanswered for the foreseeable future.

Therapeutic Uses

Currently there are one approved and several possible therapeutic uses for THC and its various derivatives. *Dronabinol* (Marinol, which is THC formulated in sesame oil) and *nabilone* (Cesamet, a synthetic cannabinoid) are available for use in the treatment of nausea and vomiting associated with chemotherapy in cancer patients.

Recently dronabinol has been shown to stimulate the appetite and promote weight gain in both symptomatic HIV (AIDS) and cancer patients.[33] These effects, together with the anti-emetic effect, can enhance the overall quality of life in these terminally ill patients.[33]

THC also exhibits mild analgesic properties, is anti-epileptic, decreases intraocular pressure in patients with glaucoma, and can relieve bronchospasm in asthmatics. Other drugs, however, are available for treating these conditions. Therefore, it is unlikely that the FDA will approve marijuana or THC for these purposes in the foreseeable future.

Side Effects and Toxicity

Changes in behavior that result from intoxication constitute a major side effect. Marijuana impairs a person's ability to drive an automobile safely much as alcohol does. It differs significantly, however, in that with marijuana one may not feel intoxicated even when one is. Thus one may feel capable of driving yet still be impaired.

> The impairment persists for 4–8 hours, well beyond the time that the user perceives the subjective effects of the drug. The impairment is apparent to trained observers: 94% of subjects failed a roadside sobriety test 90 minutes after smoking marijuana; 60% still failed after 150 minutes."[27]

Soderstrom and coworkers studied patients, 67 percent of whom were injured in motor vehicle accidents and 33 percent of whom suffered from nonvehicular trauma.[4] Marijuana was detected in 35 percent of subjects, and alcohol was present in 33 percent. Sex (male) and age (younger than 30 years) correlated with an increased incidence of marijuana use. A combination of both marijuana and alcohol were present in 16.5 percent of subjects, marijuana alone was present in 18 percent, alcohol alone was present in 16 percent, and neither drug was present in 49 percent.

The effects of marijuana and alcohol on a person's ability to drive and perform other complex tasks are additive. Because nearly 50 percent of regular marijuana users drink alcoholic beverages when using marijuana, persons who drive should be concerned about the further deterioration in driving ability that occurs when marijuana is used along with alcohol.

As discussed, marijuana exerts significant effects on learning, memory, and cognitive functioning. Obviously, chronic marijuana use (enough to maintain some level of drug in plasma and/or dissolved in body fat) would interfere with intellectual accomplishment. Also of concern would be drug use in individuals with preexisting cognitive or attentional deficits.

Over the years, much concern has been expressed about a marijuana-induced "amotivational syndrome" as well as marijuana-induced brain damage. However, there is no supporting evidence for either of these conditions occurring in humans.[2,22] Westlake and coworkers examined cannabinoid receptors in the basal ganglia, cerebral cortex, hippocampus, and cerebellum of rats and monkeys chronically exposed to THC and marijuana.[34] They could find no evidence of irreversible alteration of these receptors as a result of chronic exposure.

Some concern has been expressed that cannabis use might precipitate or exacerbate psychotic episodes. Recently Linszen and coworkers examined the effects of marijuana use on young schizophrenic patients.[35] Marijuana use was associated with significantly more and earlier psychotic relapses or exacerbations of symptoms, and a causal relationship seemed likely. Although the number of subjects was small, the results support the concept that "heavy cannabis misuse is at least a stressor for psychotic relapse, and possibly a premorbid precipitant." At the very least, treatment strategies for schizophrenic patients should include discouragement of cannabis use.

Relatively few serious physical health consequences seem to be associated with the use of marijuana.

As for toxicity associated with chronic marijuana use, there has been some evidence of alterations in the reproductive system, immune system, and lungs. However, convincing evidence has yet to emerge from well-controlled studies that marijuana is solely responsible for any alterations that have been observed in these organ systems.[24]

Nevertheless, we may still be in a prodromal state, where toxicity to major body organs has not yet become apparent.

Since the major route of administration of THC is by smoking marijuana cigarettes, analysis of the effects of smoking seems pertinent. Also, given the documented effects of THC on the reproductive and immune systems, we review the effects of marijuana on these organs.

Pulmonary Effects

The gaseous and particulate components of both marijuana and tobacco smoke provide some insights into the potential for marijuana to cause pulmonary damage (Table 13.2).[36] Note that with the exception of the presence of THC in marijuana and nicotine in tobacco, both inhalants are remarkably similar. In determining the significance of the toxins in marijuana smoking, we must remember that the amount of tobacco used by the average cigarette smoker is 10 to 20 times the amount of marijuana used by the average marijuana smoker. On the other hand, when a person smokes marijuana, he or she inhales more deeply and holds the smoke in the lungs longer.

Reports of altered lung function due to smoking marijuana show evidence of bronchial irritation and inflammation, airway narrowing with increased reactivity to irritants (as in asthma), reduced macrophage and ciliary activity (leading to a reduced ability to clear the lungs of inhaled particulate matter), and signs of early stages of emphysema.[37] These pulmonary changes should not be surprising, because they result from the persistent and repetitive inhalation of the gases and particulate products contained in marijuana smoke (see Table 13.2).

Aside from its irritant effects, the obvious question is whether marijuana smoke causes lung cancer. No direct evidence shows that chronic marijuana smoking causes lung cancer; but cancers of the upper respiratory tract and tongue have been noted in persons who smoke marijuana.[38] Also, it is possible that marijuana smokers are in a prodromal phase of *Cannabis*-induced lung cancer. Cellular changes that are consistent with early cancerous stages have been reported in biopsies of the bronchial tubes in heavy marijuana smokers and in a variety of animal models.[39]

TABLE 13.2 Gases and particulates in marijuana and tobacco smoke.

	Marijuana cigarette	Tobacco cigarette
GAS PHASE ANALYSIS		
Carbon monoxide (vol %)	3.99	4.58
(mg)	17.6	20.2
Carbon dioxide (vol %)	8.27	9.38
(mg)	57.3	65.0
Ammonia (µg)	228	178
HCN (µg)	532	498
Isoprene (µg)	83	310
Acetaldehyde (µg)	1200	980
Acetone (µg)	443	578
Acrolein (µg)	92	85
Acetonitrile (µg)	132	123
Benzene (µg)	76	67
Toluene (µg)	112	108
Dimethylnitrosamine (ng)	75	84
Methylethylnitrosamine (ng)	27	30
PARTICULATE MATTER ANALYSIS		
Phenol (µg)	76.8	138.5
o-cresol (µg)	76.8	24
m-, p-cresol (µg)	54.4	65
2,4- and 2,5-dimethylphenol (µg)	6.8	14.4
Cannabidiol (µg)	190	——
Delta-9-tetracannabinol	820	——
Nicotine	——	2850
Naphthalene (ng)	3000	1200
1-methylnaphthalene (ng)	6100	3650
2-methylnaphthalene (ng)	3600	1400
Benzo(a)anthracene (ng)	75	43
Benzo(a)pyrene (ng)	31	22.1

Source: D. Hoffman, K. D. Brunemann, G. B. Gori, and E. L. Wynder.[36]

Effects on the Immune System

Evidence has implicated long-term marijuana use with a degree of immunosuppression, which might render the smoker susceptible to infections, diseases, or even cancer.[40] Although data in this area are controversial and implications have not been proven, marijuana smoking, in some circumstances, can partially suppress immunity. The clinical significance of this occurrence is not known, but it should be noted also that other depressant drugs, such as alcohol, barbiturates, benzodiazepines, and anticonvulsants, share this immunosuppressive action.

Because both the spleen and the lymphocytes (white blood cells) are important organs in the body's immune response, they have been investigated to determine how they are affected by cannabinoids.

Kaminski and coworkers identified protein-binding cannabinoid receptors in the membranes of spleen cells.[41] When activated by THC, these receptors inhibit the intracellular adenylate cyclase second-messenger system and thereby reduce the ability of these spleen cells to function adequately in the immune response. Diaz, Specter, and Coffey reported similar effects on lymphocytes.[42] Finally, as discussed earlier, in 1994 Lynn and Herkenham reported that

> besides the nervous system, cannabinoid receptors were localized to certain tissues of the immune system in the rat. Whereas this finding has implications for human immunomodulation, it should be noted that rodents are more susceptible than humans to immunomodulation by cannabinoids, perhaps reflecting the substantially higher levels of receptor [presumably for the transmitter anandamide] in their immune cells. In humans, immune suppression is subtle and in many cases insignificant. There is little evidence for cannabinoid immunosuppression as a causative agent in disease.[43]

Undoubtedly studies of the effects of cannabinoids and cannabinoid receptors on the human immune will be forthcoming.

Effects on Reproduction

Evidence of THC-induced suppression of sexual function and reproduction is being gathered. The chronic use of marijuana by males can reduce levels of the hormone testosterone and inhibit sperm formation.[22] Reductions in male fertility and sexual potency, however, have not been reported. In females, the levels of the hormones FSH (follicle-stimulating hormone) and LH (luteinizing hormone) are reduced by the use of marijuana. Menstrual cycles can be affected and anovulatory cycles have been reported. All these actions seem to be reversible when drug use is discontinued.[44]

THC affects reproduction both through the brain (at the level of the pituitary gland and hypothalamus [discussed in Chapter 14]) and through non-receptor-mediated, nonspecific effects on the testis and ovary.[20]

Finally, like all psychoactive drugs, marijuana freely crosses the placenta, and so its use should be avoided during pregnancy. Fetal damage due to marijuana smoking is difficult to assess because pregnant women who use marijuana generally use other drugs (especially alcohol, caffeine, and nicotine) as well.

Tolerance and Dependence

Tolerance to *Cannabis* is well substantiated and is thought to result from an adaptation of the brain to the continuous presence of the drug (so-called pharmacodynamic or receptor tolerance). The development of tolerance can reach 100-fold in animals, although this degree of receptor tolerance has not been demonstrated even in the heaviest users of marijuana.[22]

It is generally thought that physical dependence on THC does not develop: "It is well established that chronic heavy use of cannabis does not result in a withdrawal syndrome with severe symptomatology. However, the occurrence of some form of psychological dependence or craving is more probable than physical dependence."[45]

Cessation of drug intake can be accompanied by irritability, restlessness, nervousness, decreased appetite, weight loss, insomnia, rebound increase in REM sleep, tremor, chills, and increased body temperature. Overall the syndrome is relatively mild, beginning within a few hours after cessation of drug administration and lasting about 4 to 5 days.[22] Thus, the development of tolerance and physical dependence is a theoretical possibility, but its practical significance (if any) is probably slight.

Psychological dependence on a psychoactive drug can usually be predicted by whether an animal will self-administer the drug when allowed free access. Also, the ability of a drug to stimulate central reward pathways can explain the compulsive abuse of and psychological dependence upon the drug. Earlier in this chapter, we discussed Gardner and Lowinson's thesis that marijuana is a potent activator of central reward systems.[30] However, animals tend not to self-administer THC-containing products, and THC does not substitute for drugs with strong reinforcing properties. According to Abood and Martin, "This observation suggests limited potential for development of physical dependence, as well as limited psychological dependence due to the weak reinforcing properties of delta-9-THC."[32]

As with other psychoactive drugs, marijuana dependence is determined by three critical elements:

1. preoccupation with the acquisition of the drug
2. compulsive use of the drug
3. relapse to, or recurrent use of, the drug

To date, these have not been major problems with marijuana alone; the criteria are far more commonly met in polydrug dependence. Therefore, few treatment programs are oriented solely toward marijuana abuse. Treatments such as psychotherapy can be appropriate for frequent users of marijuana, but this is not therapy for marijuana abuse. Instead, it is for an underlying psychopathology, one symptom of which is the abuse of cannabis. Grinspoon and Bakalar wrote, "Being attached to cannabis is not so much a function of any inherent psychopharmacologic property of the drug as it is emotionally driven by the underlying psychopathology. Success in curtailing cannabis use requires dealing with that pathology."[46] Miller, Gold, and Pottash describe a 12-step program for treating persons who exhibit marijuana dependence.[47]

Marijuana and Public Safety

The first reports that causally linked the use of marijuana to aggression, violence, and crime appeared during the 1930s. It was felt (with little factual basis) that marijuana led to antisocial acts, to crimes of violence and aggression, and even to the use of opiates. Respected governmental commissions over the past 100 years (the first being the "Indian Hemp Commission Report of 1894") have all concluded that marijuana is not the demon that it is often perceived to be. Nevertheless, the laws against marijuana are often excessively harsh, with a marked discrepancy between the true danger to society and perceived danger.[44]

Only the unsophisticated today believe that marijuana leads to violence and crime.[2] Indeed, marijuana is much less likely than alcohol to precipitate aggressive behavior.

> Instead of inciting criminal behavior, cannabis may tend to suppress it. The intoxication induces a mild lethargy that is not conducive to any physical activity, let alone the commission of crimes. The release of inhibitions results in fantasy and verbal rather than behavioral expression. During the high, marijuana users may say and think things they would not ordinarily say and think, but they generally do not do things that are foreign to their nature. If they are not already criminals, they will not commit crimes under the influence of the drug.[48]

If there is any relation between drug use and crime, psycho-active drugs that produce aggressive behavior (such as alcohol, co-caine, and the amphetamines) are probably more responsible.

How should society respond to marijuana? There is now enough information on the pharmacological and toxicological effects of marijuana to begin formulating a new legal policy. Many states, in fact, have already done this by removing felony penalties for simple pos-session of small amounts. As the National Commission on Marijuana and Drug Abuse reported as early as 1972, "The State is obliged to justify restraints on individual behavior."[49]

To date, the reports of all governmental commissions that have investigated marijuana have not opposed legally restricting cannabis, nor do they suggest that cannabis is a safe drug for general use.[44] However, they do question the severity of punishment when the per-ceived danger to society is far greater than the actual dangers to either society or the individual.

What, then, should society do about the harshness of existing legal penalties? The most conservative course of action might be that pro-posed by the National Commission on Marijuana and Drug Abuse, which recommended in 1972 the following changes in Federal law:

> Possession of marijuana for personal use would no longer be an offense, but marijuana possessed in public would remain contra-band subject to summary seizure and forfeiture. Casual distribution of small amounts of marijuana for no remuneration, or insignificant remuneration not involving profit, would no longer be an offense.[50]

The commission further recommended that a plea of marijuana intoxi-cation not be a defense for any criminal act committed when a person was under its influence and that proof of such intoxication not consti-tute a negation of specific intent.

These changes would essentially decriminalize the possession of small amounts of marijuana in all states—persons apprehended who possess small quantities would no longer be subject to a punishment that many regard as more severe than the offense. Nevertheless, the product would not be legalized, and the government would continue to discourage its use.

The call for the legalization of marijuana was restated in a discus-sion of the Dutch experience with controlled legalization of marijuana: "A legal market for marijuana . . . could help steer young people away from hard drugs by breaking the connection between marijuana smok-ers and drug pushers."[51]

Although marijuana is not a "killer weed," it is not an innocuous substance that is devoid of toxicity. The legal statutes should protect users, nonusers who might be affected by intoxicated users, and juveniles who might not be able to make rational decisions concerning the risks and benefits of the drug. It is up to society to determine what kind of protection should be offered. Society appears to be accepting and tolerating (although not yet approving) the social use of marijuana as a recreational drug, but legal guidelines for recreational use are still far from decided.

Study Questions

1. Describe the potencies (concentrations) of THC in various preparations of marijuana.
2. How are the effects of THC similar to those of the nonselective depressants? How are the effects of THC dissimilar to those of the nonselective depressants?
3. How are the effects of THC similar to those of the psychedelic drugs? How are the effects of THC dissimilar to those of the psychedelic drugs?
4. How does the half-life of THC in the body reflect a person's ability to become intoxicated more easily and with a smaller amount of the drug after repeated use of marijuana?
5. Discuss some of the concerns and side effects that are associated with varying degrees of marijuana use by young adults.
6. Discuss the involvement of marijuana use in traumatic incidents and crimes of violence.
7. Discuss the concerns about long-term side effects that may be associated with the chronic use of marijuana.
8. Discuss the concept of a "cannabinoid receptor."
9. How might a treatment program be organized for persons who are dependent on marijuana?
10. What do you think society's response would be to the continued illicit use of marijuana? Should marijuana be legalized? If so, how should it be regulated or restricted?

Notes

1. R. E. Musty, P. Consroe, A. Makriyannis, "Introduction," *Pharmacology, Biochemistry & Behavior* 40 (1991): 457–459.
2. L. Grinspoon and J. B. Bakalar, "Marijuana," in J. H. Lowinson, P. Ruiz, R. B. Millman, and J. G. Langrod, eds., *Substance Abuse: A Comprehensive Textbook*, 2nd ed., (Baltimore: Williams & Wilkins, 1992), pp. 236–246.
3. T. R. Okrie, "Three Positive Shifts Away from Marijuana Use, 1979–1988," *Journal of School Health* 59 (1989): 34–36.

4. C. A. Soderstrom, A. L. Trifillis, B. S. Shanker, and W. E. Clark, "Marijuana and Alcohol Use among 1023 Trauma Patients: A Prospective Study," *Archives of Surgery* 123 (1988): 733–737.

5. A. C. Howlett, J. M. Qualy, and L. L. Khachatrian, "Involvement of G_i in the Inhibition of Adenylate Cyclase by Cannabimimetic Drugs," *Molecular Pharmacology* 29 (1986): 307–313.

6. M. Bidaut-Russell, W. A. Devane, and A. C. Howlett, "Cannabinoid Receptors and Modulation of Cyclic AMP Accumulation in the Rat Brain," *Journal of Neurochemistry* 55 (1990): 21–26.

7. C. A. Audette, S. H. Burstein, S. A. Doyle, and S. A. Hunter, "G-Protein Mediation of Cannabinoid-Induced Phospholipase Activation," *Pharmacology, Biochemistry & Behavior* 40 (1991): 559–563.

8. L. A. Matsuda, S. J. Lolait, M. J. Brownstein, A. C. Young, and T. I. Bonner, "Structure of a Cannabinoid Receptor and Functional Expression of the Cloned cDNA," *Nature* 346 (1990): 561–564.

9. A. C. Howlett, T. M. Champion-Dorow, L. L. McMahon, and T. M. Westlake, "The Cannabinoid Receptor: Biochemical and Cellular Properties in Neuroblastoma Cells," *Pharmacology, Biochemistry & Behavior* 40 (1991): 565–569.

10. R. G. Pertwee, S. E. Browne, T. M. Ross, and C. D. Stretton, "An Investigation of the Involvement of GABA in Certain Pharmacological Effects of Delta-9-Tetrahydrocannabinol," *Pharmacology, Biochemistry & Behavior* 40 (1991): 581–586.

11. E. Castaneda, D. E. Moss, S. D. Oddie, and I. Q. Whishaw, "THC Does Not Affect Striatal Dopamine Release: Microdialysis in Freely Moving Rats," *Pharmacology, Biochemistry & Behavior* 40 (1991): 587–592.

12. W. A. Devane, L. Hanus, A. Breuer, R. G. Pertwee, L. A. Stevenson, G. Griffin, D. Gibson, A. Mandelbaum, A. Etinger, and R. Mechoulam, "Isolation and Structure of a Brain Constituent That Binds to the Cannabinoid Receptor," *Science* 258 (1992): 1946–1949.

13. E. Fride and R. Mechoulam, "Pharmacological Activity of the Cannabinoid Receptor Agonist, Anandamide, a Brain Constituent," *European Journal of Pharmacology* 231 (1993): 313–314.

14. C. C. Felder, E. M. Briley, J. Axelrod, J. T. Simpson, K. Mackie, and W. A. Devane, "Anandamide, an Endogenous Cannabimimetic Eicosanoid, Binds to the Cloned Human Cannabinoid Receptor and Stimulates Receptor-Mediated Signal Transduction," *Proceedings of the National Academy of Sciences of the United States of America* 90 (1993): 7656–7660.

15. L. M. Bornheim, K. Y. Kim, B. Chen, and M. A. Correia, "The Effects of Cannabidiol on Mouse Hepatic Microsomal Cytochrome P450-Dependent Anandamide Metabolism," *Biochemical & Biophysical Research Communications* 197 (1993): 740–746.

16. W. A. Devane, "New Dawn of Cannabinoid Pharmacology," *Trends in Pharmacological Sciences* 15 (1994): 40–41.

17. M. Herkenham, A. B. Lynn, M. D. Little, M. R. Johnson, L. S. Melvin, B. R. deCosta, and K. C. Rice, "Cannabinoid Receptor Localization in Brain,"

Proceedings of the National Academy of Sciences, USA 87 (1990): 1932–1936.

18. M. Herkenham, A. B. Lynn, M. R. Johnson, L. S. Melvin, B. R. deCosta, and K. C. Rice, "Characterization and Localization of Cannabinoid Receptors in Rat Brain: A Quantitative *in Vitro* Autoradiographic Study," *Journal of Neuroscience* 11 (1991): 563–583.

19. M. Herkenham, "Cannabinoid Receptor Localization in Brain: Relationship to Motor and Reward Systems," *Annals of the New York Academy of Sciences* 654 (1992): 19–32.

20. A. B. Lynn and M. Herkenham, "Localization of Cannabinoid Receptors and Nonsaturable High-Density Cannabinoid Binding Sites in Peripheral Tissues of the Rat: Implications for Receptor-Mediated Immune Modulation by Cannabinoids," *Journal of Pharmacology and Experimental Therapeutics* 268 (1994): 1612–1623.

21. M. Perez-Reyes, W. R. White, S. A. McDonald, R. E. Hicks, A. R. Jeffcoat, and C. E. Cook, "The Pharmacological Effects of Daily Marijuana Smoking in Humans," *Pharmacology, Biochemistry & Behavior* 40 (1991): 691–694.

22. J. W. Jaffe, "Drug Addiction and Drug Abuse," in A. G. Gilman, T. W. Rall, A. S. Nies, and P. Taylor, eds., *Goodman and Gilman's The Pharmacological Basis of Therapeutics*, 8th ed. (New York: Pergamon, 1990), pp. 549–553.

23. E. Johansson, M. M. Hardin, S. Agurell, and L. E. Dollister, "Terminal Elimination Plasma Half-life of Delta-1-Tetrahydrocannabinol in Heavy Users of Marijuana," *European Journal of Clinical Pharmacology* 37 (1989): 273–277.

24. M. E. Abood and B. R. Martin, "Neurobiology of Marijuana Abuse," *Trends in Pharmaceutical Sciences* 13 (1992): 202.

25. Grinspoon and Bakalar, "Marijuana," p. 241.

26. Abood and Martin, "Neurobiology of Marijuana Abuse," p. 201.

27. J. W. Jaffe, "Drug Addiction and Drug Abuse," in A. G. Gilman, T. W. Rall, A. S. Nies, and P. Taylor, eds., *Goodman and Gilman's The Pharmacological Basis of Therapeutics*, 8th ed. (New York: Pergamon, 1990), p. 551.

28. N. Solowij, P. T. Michie, and A. M. Fox, "Effects of Long-Term Cannabis Use on Selective Attention: An Event-Related Potential Study," *Pharmacology, Biochemistry & Behavior* 40 (1991): 683.

29. R. I. Block, R. Farinpour, and K. Braverman, "Acute Effects of Marijuana on Cognition: Relationships to Chronic Effects and Smoking Techniques," *Pharmacology, Biochemistry & Behavior* 40 (1992): 907–917.

30. E. L. Gardner and J. H. Lowinson, "Marijuana's Interaction with Brain Reward Systems: Update 1991," *Pharmacology, Biochemistry & Behavior* 40 (1991): 571.

31. Ibid., p. 572.

32. Abood and Martin, "Neurobiology of Marijuana Abuse," p. 203.

33. T. F. Plasse, R. W. Gorter, S. H. Krasnow, M. Lane, K. V. Shepard, and R. G. Wadleigh, "Recent Clinical Experience with Dronabinol," *Pharmacology, Biochemistry & Behavior* 40 (1991): 695–700.

34. T. M. Westlake, A. C. Howlett, S. F. Ali, M. G. Paule, A. C. Scallet, and W. Slikker, Jr., "Chronic Exposure to Delta 9-Tetrahydrocannabinol Fails to

Irreversibly Alter Brain Cannabinoid Receptors," *Brain Research* 544 (1991): 145–149.

35. D. H. Linszen, P. M. Dingemans, and M. E. Lenior, "Cannabis Abuse and the Course of Recent-Onset Schizophrenic Disorders," *Archives of General Psychiatry* 51 (1994): 273.

36. D. I. Hoffman, K. D. Brunemann, G. B. Gori, and E. L. Wynder, "On the Carcinogenicity of Marijuana Smoke," *Recent Advances in Phytochemistry* 9 (1975): 63–81.

37. H. Gong, Jr., S. Fligiel, D. P. Tashkin, and R. G. Barbers, "Tracheobronchial Changes in Habitual, Heavy Smokers of Marijuana with and without Tobacco," *American Review of Respiratory Disease* 136 (1987): 142–149.

38. G. A. Caplan and B. A. Brigham, "Marijuana Smoking and Carcinoma of the Tongue: Is There an Association?" *Cancer* 66 (1990): 1005–1006.

39. U.S. Department of Health and Human Services, *The Health Consequences of Smoking: The Changing Cigarette. A Report of the Surgeon General* (Washington, D.C.: U.S. Government Printing Office, 1981), pp. 81–85.

40. L. E. Hollister, "Marijuana and Immunity," *Journal of Psychoactive Drugs* 20 (1988): 3–8.

41. N. E. Kaminski, M. E. Abood, F. K. Kessler, B. R. Martin, and A. R. Schatz, "Identification of a Functionally Relevant Cannabinoid Receptor on Mouse Spleen Cells That Is Involved in Cannabinoid-Mediated Immune Modulation," *Molecular Pharmacology* 42 (1992): 736–742.

42. S. Diaz, S. Specter, and R. G. Coffey, "Suppression of Lymphocyte Adenosine 3':5'-Cyclic Monophosphate (cAMP) by Delta-9-Tetrahydro-cannabinol," *International Journal of Immunopharmacology* 15 (1993): 523–532.

43. Lynn and Herkenham, "Localization of Cannabinoid Receptors," p. 1621.

44. A. Goldstein, *Addiction: From Biology to Drug Policy* (New York: W. H. Freeman and Company, 1994), pp. 174–176.

45. Abood and Martin, "Neurobiology of Marijuana Abuse," p. 204.

46. Grinspoon and Bakalar, "Marijuana," p. 243.

47. N. S. Miller, M. S. Gold, and A. C. Pottash, "A 12-Step Treatment Approach for Marijuana (*Cannabis*) Dependence," *Journal of Substance Abuse Treatment* 6 (1989): 241–250.

48. Grinspoon and Bakalar, "Marijuana," p. 239.

49. National Commission on Marihuana and Drug Abuse, *Marihuana: A Signal of Misunderstanding* (New York: Signet, 1972), p. 159.

50. Ibid., p. 85.

51. A. Kupfer, "What to Do about Drugs," *Fortune,* June 20, 1988, pp. 39–41.

CHAPTER 14

FERTILITY-REGULATING DRUGS AND ANABOLIC-ANDROGENIC STEROIDS

Neurons interact with one another through the release of chemical neurotransmitters. In its simplest form, a neurotransmitter is secreted from the presynaptic terminal of one neuron; it diffuses across a narrow synaptic cleft and then acts on the postsynaptic membrane of the next neuron. These chemical transmitters are also appropriately called *neurohormones* because, by definition, a hormone is a substance that is released by one type of cell and then exerts its effect on a different organ or structure. However, the neurotransmitters travel only a very short distance from their sites of release to their sites of action (across the synaptic cleft). The normal hormones of the body (compounds such as estrogen, insulin, thyroid hormone, growth hormone, and testosterone) are released by secretory cells into the bloodstream and then are transported to target organs that are a great distance away.

Besides a physiological similarity between hormones and neurotransmitters, the brain regulates the synthesis and release of both. As we will see, the hypothalamus releases a "releasing factor" hormone that travels only a short distance to the pituitary gland, where it induces the release of a second hormone. This hormone is released from the cells of the pituitary gland into the bloodstream and travels to distant sites in the body where it acts on various body organs to affect the functioning of target organs. Figure 14.1 illustrates this process. When the plasma level of a body hormone, such as estrogen or testosterone (two of the sex hormones), falls, cells in the hypothalamus

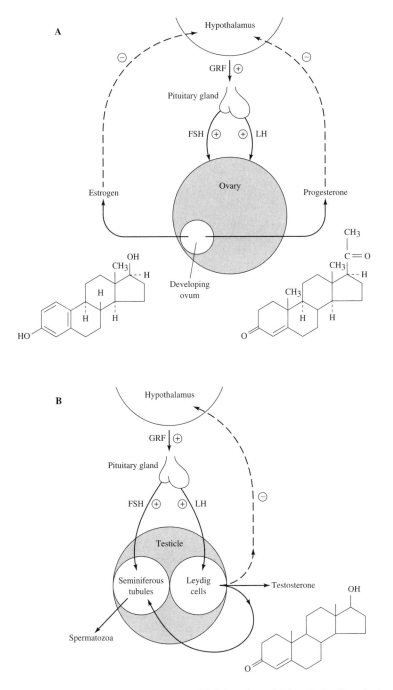

FIGURE 14.1   Hormonal regulation of **(A)** female and **(B)** male fertility. The brain (hypothalamus and pituitary gland) is involved in the control of male and female fertility. However, fertility in the male is not subject to periodic cycling as it is in the female. The structures of naturally occurring estrogen (estradiol), progesterone, and testosterone are also shown. GRF, gonadotropin-releasing factor; FSH, follicle-stimulating hormone; LH, luteinizing hormone. *Solid arrows,* stimulation; *dashed arrows,* inhibition.

(which have "receptors" for the hormone) are activated. As a result, the hypothalamus releases a second hormone that causes stimulation of body organs to produce and release the hormone. This process is called a hormone feedback loop, which is the mechanism that regulates the levels of many hormones in the body.

Two examples of such a hormone feedback loop are pertinent to the topics of drug education and drug misuse, and these will be discussed in this chapter. The first is the regulation of female fertility by estrogen and progesterone, two reproductive hormones that can be suppressed or increased by drugs. Contraceptive drugs suppress the release of fertility-inducing hormones from the hypothalamus and pituitary gland and therefore suppress fertility and decrease the possibility of pregnancy; drugs that increase fertility perform in the opposite way. The second example involves the anabolic-androgenic steroids, testosterone and its derivatives. These compounds (1) block the normal CNS regulation of testosterone, male fertility, and the process of spermatogenesis and (2) exert peripheral hormonal actions to enhance physical appearance, athletic performance, muscle building, fighting ability, and aggressive competition. In recent years, the abuse of the anabolic-androgenic steroids by both men and women has become a topic of much concern.

PHARMACOLOGICAL REGULATION OF FERTILITY

Figure 14.2 illustrates the principal organs of the human female reproductive system. These organs include the ovaries, the fallopian tubes, the uterus, and the vagina. In the process of reproduction, ova (eggs) develop in the ovaries. Once developed, a single ovum is released and taken up (captured) by extensions of the fallopian tubes, called fimbriae, which gather the ovum into the fallopian tube. The ovum is then transported down the tube into the uterus. If the ovum becomes fertilized by a sperm (usually as the ovum passes down the fallopian tube), it implants itself on the inner wall of the uterus, where it develops into a fetus and placenta.

The Monthly Ovarian Cycle

After puberty and the development of ovarian function, a woman normally secretes various sex hormones in a rhythmic monthly pattern; as

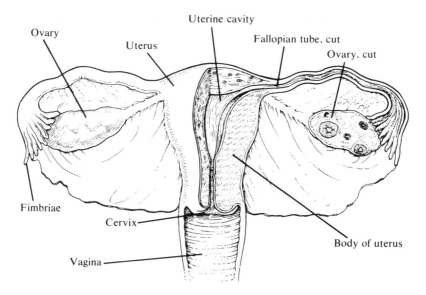

Uterine cavity

Ovary

Uterus

Fallopian tube, cut

Ovary, cut

Fimbriae

Cervix

Body of uterus

Vagina

FIGURE 14.2 Principal organs of the female reproductive system.

levels of these hormones change, corresponding changes occur in the activity of the female sexual organs. The duration of this cycle averages 28 days, but it may vary from 20 days to as long as 45 days.

In order to accomplish the two most important aims of this cycle—the development and release of a single ovum and the proliferation of a uterine endometrium that is prepared for the implantation of a fertilized ovum—a coordinated sequence of hormonal events must occur. This sequence of events is illustrated in Figure 14.3. At the beginning of the cycle, the levels of both estrogen and progesterone in the bloodstream are low, the endometrium that was built up during the preceding cycle begins to slough, and the woman menstruates for several days. Because the levels of estrogen and progesterone are low, the cells in the hypothalamus begin to release the gonadotropin-releasing factor (GRF) hormone. GRF is a 10-amino-acid peptide (a small protein), which, on release, is transported in the bloodstream from the hypothalamus to the pituitary gland, where it induces release of the follicle-stimulating hormone (FSH) and the luteinizing hormone (LH).[1] In response to FSH in the bloodstream, one or a few ovarian follicles (each one containing an ovum) begin to enlarge. Then, after 5 or 6 days, one of these ovarian follicles begins to develop more rapidly than the others, and the ovum begins to mature.

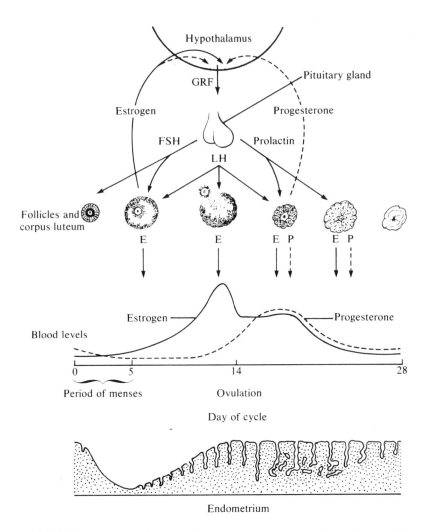

FIGURE 14.3 Sequence of events in brain, ovaries, and uterus during the monthly ovarian cycle in females. GRF, gonadotropin-releasing factor; FSH, follicle-stimulating hormone; LH, luteinizing hormone; E, estrogen; P, progesterone. *Solid arrows,* stimulation; *dashed arrows,* inhibition.

The maturing ovum then begins to release small quantities of estrogen into the circulating blood. The estrogen inhibits further secretion of GRF from the hypothalamus, therefore inhibiting further release of FSH from the pituitary gland. As a result of this inhibition, the other follicles that had also started to develop regress. The secretion of estrogen by the one maturing ovum and the follicle in which it is contained reaches a peak just before midcycle (day 14). Near the end of this preovulatory phase, LH release peaks and prepares the ovarian follicle for ovulation by stimulating it to grow rapidly. The follicle swells until it eventually ruptures, and the developed ovum is released. This occurrence is referred to as the time of ovulation. Because LH is necessary for the final preovulatory development of the follicle and subsequent ovulation, the follicle will not rupture and ovulation will be inhibited if LH is not present (even with large quantities of FSH).

After ovulation, the ovum is gathered by the fimbriae into one of the fallopian tubes, where a sperm may fertilize it. Whether fertilized or not, the ovum then enters the uterus. The follicle from which the ovum was released changes to become a structure (called the corpus luteum) that secretes both estrogen and progesterone. These hormones released from the corpus luteum maintain the uterus in a state conducive to receiving a fertilized ovum. This state is established by the maintenance of a highly vascular endometrial lining (or endometrium) on the uterine wall. In addition, the estrogen and progesterone that are released from the corpus luteum act on the hypothalamus to inhibit the release of GRF. During the next 10 days, the corpus luteum regresses and, within about 12 days, ceases to function. At this point it no longer releases estrogen and progesterone, menstruation begins, and a new cycle follows if the ovum was not fertilized. If the ovum was fertilized and implanted, the endometrium begins to secrete large quantities of hormones that act to maintain pregnancy and prevent menstrual sloughing.

Oral Contraceptives

Oral contraceptives are the most effective pharmacological technique for preventing pregnancy. They typically contain an orally absorbable estrogen derivative and/or progesterone derivative (called a *progestin*).* Available preparations can be classified according to their steroid content (Table 14.1; Figure 14.4):

1. fixed combinations that contain constant amounts of an estrogen (usually ethinyl estradiol) and progestin (for example, norethindrone)

---

*Naturally occurring estrogen and progesterone cannot be utilized, since neither of them is absorbed following oral administration. Thus, synthetically produced derivatives that are effectively absorbed from the gastrointestinal tract are used. Two estrogen derivatives and five progestins are currently marketed (Table 14.1).

TABLE 14.1 Oral contraceptives available in the United States.

		Steroid composition			
Trade name	Manufacturer	Progestin	mg	Estrogen	µg
Brevicon	Syntex	Norethindrone	0.5	Ethinyl estradiol	35
Demulen 1/35	Searle	Ethynodiol	1.0	Ethinyl estradiol	35
Demulen 1/50	Searle	Ethynodiol	1.0	Ethinyl estradiol	50
Desogen	Organon	Desogestrel	0.15	Ethinyl estradiol	30
Levlen	Berlex	Levonorgestrel	0.15	Ethinyl estradiol	30
Lo/Ovral	Wyeth	Norgestrel	0.3	Ethinyl estradiol	30
Loestrin-1/20	Parke-Davis	Norethindrone	1.0	Ethinyl estradiol	20
Loestrin-1.5/30	Parke-Davis	Norethindrone	1.5	Ethinyl estradiol	30
Micronor	Ortho	Norethindrone	0.35	——	——
Modicon	Ortho	Norethindrone	0.50	Ethinyl estradiol	35
Nor-Q.D.	Syntex	Norethindrone	0.35	——	——
Nordette	Wyeth	Levonorgestrel	0.15	Ethinyl estradiol	30
Norethin 1/35	Searle	Norethindrone	1.0	Ethinyl estradiol	35
Norethin 1/50	Searle	Norethindrone	1.0	Ethinyl estradiol	50
Norinyl 1 & 35	Syntex	Norethindrone	1.0	Ethinyl estradiol	35
Norinyl 1 & 50	Syntex	Norethindrone	1.0	Mestranol	50
Norlestrin-1/50	Parke-Davis	Norethindrone	1.0	Ethinyl estradiol	50
Norlestrin-2.5/50	Parke-Davis	Norethindrone	2.5	Ethinyl estradiol	50
Ortho-Novum 1/35	Ortho	Norethindrone	1.0	Ethinyl estradiol	35
Ortho-Novum 1/50	Ortho	Norethindrone	1.0	Mestranol	50
Ortho-Novum 1/80	Ortho	Norethindrone	1.0	Mestranol	80
Ortho-Novum 10/11	Ortho	Norethindrone	0.5, 1.0	Ethinyl estradiol	35
Ortho-Novum 2	Ortho	Norethindrone	2.0	Mestranol	100
Ortho-Novum 7/7/7	Ortho	Norethindrone	0.5, 0.75, 1	Ethinyl estradiol	35
Ovcon-35	Mead Johnson	Norethindrone	0.4	Ethinyl estradiol	35
Ovcon-50	Mead Johnson	Norethindrone	1.0	Ethinyl estradiol	50
Ovral	Wyeth	Norgestrel	0.5	Ethinyl estradiol	50
Ovrette	Wyeth	Norgestrel	0.075	——	——
Tri-Levlen	Berlex	Levonorgestrel	0.5, 0.075, 0.125	Ethinyl estradiol	30 40, 30
Tri-Norinyl	Syntex	Norethindrone	0.5, 1, 1.5	Ethinyl estradiol	35
Triphasil	Wyeth	Levonorgestrel	0.5, 0.075, 0.125	Ethinyl estradiol	30

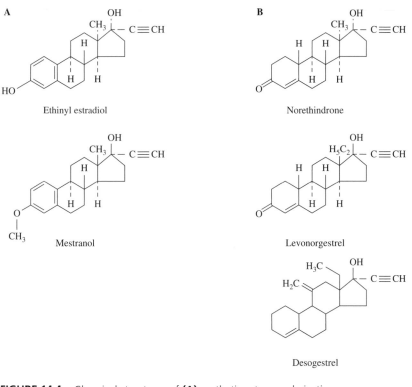

FIGURE 14.4 Chemical structures of **(A)** synthetic estrogen derivatives and **(B)** synthetic progestins. Note the similarity in the structures.

2. multiphasic combinations that contain constant amounts of estrogen and variable amounts of progestin (the dose of progestin changes from week to week)

3. "minipills" that contain constant amounts of progestin only[2]

During the early 1960s, the availability of orally absorbed estrogen and progestin fueled the technology to develop pharmacological control of ovulation as a means of preventing pregnancy. The problem was to find an appropriate combination of estrogen and progestin that would effectively suppress ovulation but limit the number and intensity of side effects. Excessive amounts of estrogen and progestin produce abnormal menstrual bleeding, whereas insufficient amounts do not completely inhibit the release of GRF, which could result in an unwanted pregnancy. Today, four decades after the introduction of these agents, close to optimal balances have been achieved. Contemporary oral contraceptives are extremely safe and very effective at blocking conception. Indeed, we are probably at or near the lowest dose levels that can be achieved without sacrificing efficacy.

Combination Products

All but three of the oral contraceptive products that are currently available contain a combination of estrogen and progestin in low, regular, or variable doses. The low-dose combination pills contain 30 to 35 micrograms of ethinyl estradiol and afford a reasonable compromise between the toxicities that are produced by too much estrogen and the bothersome breakthrough bleeding that results from too little. Because the regular-dose products contain 50 micrograms of ethinyl estradiol, their use is diminishing rapidly in favor of the low-dose products, which appear to be equally effective in preventing pregnancy while causing only mild increases in breakthrough bleeding. A small number of products contain more than 50 micrograms of estrogen (usually mestranol), and these products are used even less frequently (most are among the earliest products marketed).

The variable-dose products are either *biphasic* or *triphasic,* depending on the number of variations in dosage during a given month's cycle. These products are designed to reduce the total hormone content that is administered to the body throughout the menstrual cycle while still providing contraception that is as effective as that obtained from products that contain higher doses.

The combination oral contraceptives are taken for 21 days of the menstrual cycle (usually days 5 to 24, counting the first day of menstruation as day 1). This is followed by one week without medication, toward the end of which withdrawal bleeding (menstruation) occurs.

By combining estrogen and progestin, combination pills block release of both FSH and LH (by means of negative feedback effects on both the pituitary gland and the hypothalamus); ovarian follicles do not develop, and no ovulation occurs. The estrogen primarily inhibits the release of FSH. The progestin suppresses the release of LH and acts directly on the uterus to produce an endometrium that will not accept the implantation of a fertilized ovum. The progestin thickens the normal mucus discharge of the cervix so that sperm cannot gain access to the uterus and fallopian tubes, where fertilization occurs. In addition to suppressing the release of FSH, the estrogen also stabilizes the uterine lining (the endometrium) so that irregular shedding and unwanted breakthrough bleeding does not occur. The estrogen also potentiates the action of the progestin.[3] All these actions minimize the likelihood of conception and implantation as long as the pills are taken faithfully.

Progestational Contraceptives

During the early 1980s, there was concern that long-term use of the estrogen contained in the combination estrogen–progestin contraceptives might be harmful. These fears prompted the use of continuous progestational therapy without concomitant administration of estrogen.

A progestational agent given alone produces an endometrium that is not receptive to an ovum and a thick cervical mucus that is impervious to sperm transport, although an ovarian follicle still might mature. Thus, even if fertilization does occur, the progestin tends to prevent implantation of the fertilized ovum in the endometrium.

However, the administration of progestin alone (three such products are currently available; they are taken early and continuously) is not quite as reliable as the administration of a combination product; statistics indicate an approximately threefold increase in the incidence of unwanted pregnancies. Nevertheless, for women who experience significant side effects when using combination products, the administration of progestin-only products affords better contraceptive protection than do foams, creams, jellies, or rhythm, and it is certainly far better than no contraception at all. Table 14.2 lists the pregnancy rates for various forms of contraception.

TABLE 14.2 Pregnancies per 100 woman-years.

Contraception method	Pregnancies
Oral contraceptive pills, combination	1
Oral contraceptive pills, progestin only	2–3
Intrauterine device (IUD)	1–6
Diaphragm with spermicidal cream or gel	2–20
Condom	3–36
Spermicidal aerosol foams	2–29
Spermicidal gels and creams	4–36
Periodic abstinence ("rhythm")	
All types	1–47
Calendar method	14–47
Temperature method	1–20
Mucus method	1–25
No contraception	60–80

Undesirable Effects

The frequent, mild side effects that are induced by combination-type oral contraceptives resemble those that are experienced during early pregnancy and are generally attributed to the estrogen content. These effects include nausea, occasional vomiting, headache, dizziness, and breast discomfort. Because these side effects are usually related to the dose, products that have less estrogen generally have milder side effects. However, the incidence of breakthrough bleeding increases with decreasing doses of estrogen.

Other side effects are generally not too bothersome; they include weight gain and psychological changes that may result in depression in some women. These side effects are most frequently seen when progestin-only pills are taken. Vaginal infections appear to be more common and more resistant to treatment in women who take oral contraceptives than in women who do not.

When oral contraceptives are no longer taken, normal cyclic periods are usually resumed, but they are often not reestablished immediately. It may take several months or even longer, presumably because the hypothalamus, pituitary gland, and ovaries have been suppressed for prolonged period of time. Approximately 95 percent of women whose menstrual periods were normal before taking oral contraceptives resume normal periods within a few months after they stop taking the drug. In women who discontinue oral contraceptives to become pregnant, 50 percent conceive within three months; more important, after two years, only 7 to 15 percent fail to conceive. Thus, infertility does not seem to occur often, if at all, in women who discontinue the use of oral contraceptives.

Serious Side Effects

The possibility that oral contraceptives cause serious side effects has been a source of concern. These side effects include (1) cardiovascular risks (arteriosclerosis, venous blood clots and emboli [thromboembolism], heart attacks, stroke, high blood pressure, and lipoprotein and cholesterol imbalance), (2) cancer risks (especially uterine, cervical, liver, and breast), (3) diabetes mellitus (sugar diabetes), and (4) adverse effects on a fetus if the drugs are taken during pregnancy.

No group of pharmacological agents has been studied more than the oral contraceptives.[4] All efforts have been directed at maximizing the benefits of drug use while minimizing potential risks, especially those involving the cardiovascular system. Decreasing the amount of estrogen from 100–150 micrograms per tablet (levels in the pills of the 1960s) to 30–35 micrograms per tablet (levels of today) has drastically

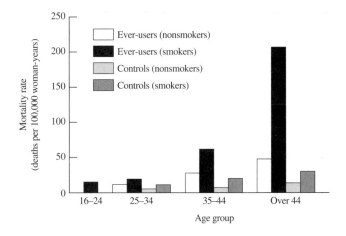

FIGURE 14.5 Circulatory disease mortality rates by age, smoking status, and oral contraceptive use.

reduced the cardiovascular risks. In healthy women who are not predisposed to these conditions, the risks of blood clots, stroke, heart attack, hypertension, and atherosclerosis are minimal.[5–10] All reports state that women who use oral contraceptives can reduce their risk of cardiovascular disease by reducing or eliminating cigarette smoking.[11] Indeed, smoking increases all the potential risks in women who take oral contraceptives (Figure 14.5).

Data now demonstrate that concern over the risks of cancer is unwarranted. Concern arose during the 1960s, when high-dose oral contraceptives were shown to be associated with a slightly increased risk of cervical cancer. Today this risk is no longer considered significant. Almost all investigators now believe that use of low-dose oral contraceptives does not increase the risk of breast or cervical cancer.[12,13] Indeed, the use of oral contraceptive products actually reduces a woman's risk of uterine and ovarian cancer by 40 to 50 percent.[13,14]

Other risks once thought to be associated with the use of oral contraceptives include the altered metabolism of glucose, altered utilization of insulin, and the possible development of diabetes mellitus (sugar diabetes).[15] These issues are no longer major causes for concern. Speroff, Glass, and Kase summarize:

> Insulin and glucose changes with the low dose monophasic and multiphasic pills are so minimal that it is now believed that they are of no clinical significance. . . . It can be stated definitively that birth control use does not produce an increase in diabetes mellitus. The hyperglycemia associated with oral contraception is not deleterious and is

completely reversible. Even women who have risk factors for diabetes in their history do not seem to be affected.[3]

Reproductive problems after oral contraception has been ended have been a concern, but they have not been substantiated. After cessation of oral contraceptive use, there is no increase in the occurrence of spontaneous abortions, pregnancy complications, or congenital malformations.[16]

Conclusions and Contraindications

Stolley, Strom, and Sartwell offer reasonable guidelines for the use of oral contraceptives:[11]

1. Women over 35 years of age should avoid the use of these products.
2. Women who smoke cigarettes should avoid the use of these products and users should not smoke.
3. The product that is effective at the lowest dose of estrogen that does not cause unacceptable breakthrough bleeding should be chosen.
4. Women with high blood pressure or a tendency toward migraine headaches should be carefully educated and monitored.

Oral contraceptives are contraindicated in women with any of the following conditions:

1. venous thrombophlebitis, thromboembolic disorders, cerebral vascular disease, or coronary artery disease
2. impaired liver function or jaundice
3. known or suspected cancer of the breast or uterus
4. abnormal genital bleeding
5. known or suspected pregnancy
6. congenitally elevated blood cholesterol or lipid levels
7. an addiction to cigarettes (for women over the age of 35 years)

Additional information about oral contraceptives may be obtained from a physician or pharmacist. The insert that is packaged with oral contraceptives is written in layman's terms and expands on the information given here.

Alternatives to Oral Contraceptives

A few effective pharmacological alternatives to birth control pills do exist for women who want to avoid pregnancy but do not want to take a daily oral contraceptive tablet. These proven techniques and devices include the following:

1. a long-acting, injected progestin (Depo-Provera)

2. implanted plastic tubes containing a long-acting, progestin-releasing contraceptive (Norplant)

3. diaphragms, condoms, intrauterine devices, and contraceptive creams (vaginal spermicides)

Diaphragms, condoms, and intrauterine devices (IUDs) are only approximately 90 to 95 percent effective. Even less effective are vaginal spermicides and the nonpharmacological strategies of the rhythm method, coitus interruptus, and douching. The most effective nonpharmacological technique for the temporary prevention of unwanted pregnancy is abstention. For permanent prevention, sterilization of men (vasectomy) and women (tubal ligation) are 100 percent effective but should not be considered reversible.

Depo-Provera

Certain long-acting injectable products can be used as contraceptive agents. The most important is medroxyprogesterone acetate, marketed under the trade name Depo-Provera. Depo-Provera is a progestin approved for use in the United States in 1992 after being used for many years by millions of women worldwide as an effective contraceptive. A single dose of 150 milligrams is injected intramuscularly every 3 to 6 months. The advantages of this form of contraception include freedom from taking daily tablets, freedom from the side effects of estrogen, and the maintenance of normal FSH activity. Depo-Provera inhibits ovulation by blocking the midcycle surge of LH. It induces thickening of the cervical mucus and inhibits the development of the lush uterine endometrium that is necessary for the fertilized ovum to survive. Follicular development is not suppressed, because the normal estrogen cycle is maintained. The contraceptive protection that Depo-Provera provides is approximately equal to that afforded by the combination-type oral contraceptives. Disadvantages and side effects associated with Depo-Provera include breakthrough bleeding ("spotting"), weight gain, depression, headaches, and abdominal bloating.

As Figure 14.6 illustrates, up to eight months may be required for Depo-Provera to be totally eliminated from the body after injections are discontinued. Thus, regular menstrual periods take several months to return, and fertility during that period is unpredictable.

Norplant

Also approved in 1992 was a novel hormonal contraceptive device that delivers pregnancy-preventing progestin (levonorgestrel) for a maxi-

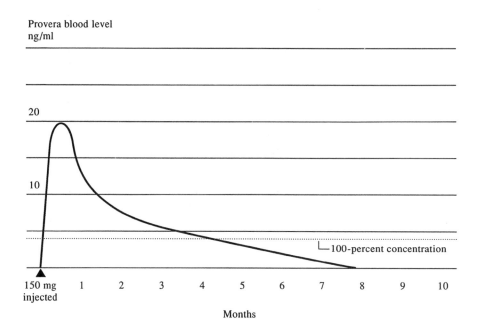

FIGURE 14.6 Blood levels of Depo-Provera following intramuscular injection. [From Speroff, Glass, and Kase,[3] p. 489.]

mum of five years following its surgical implantation under the skin of a woman's upper arm. The device consists of six flexible silicone rubber tubes, each of which is filled with progestin and is about the size of a matchstick. The tubes are inserted in a fanlike manner through a small skin incision. This implant has the advantage of being removable. Sufficient drug is released over a five-year period to protect against pregnancy. The gross cumulative pregnancy rate at five years is 2.6 pregnancies per 100 woman-years.[17]

Side effects are usually minimal and resemble those observed in women who take progestin-only oral contraceptives (that is, irregular periods and breakthrough bleeding). Because this is the most disturbing side effect for many users, counseling prior to insertion is of paramount importance.[17]

Postcoital Contraceptives

After unprotected intercourse, certain pharmacological measures may be used to prevent an unwanted pregnancy. Older postcoital techniques included high doses of estrogen in preparations that were often referred to as "morning after" pills. In one such regimen, large doses (e.g., 25 milligrams of diethylstilbestrol) were administered twice daily for five days. This pharmacological regimen apparently reduced the time required for a fertilized ovum to pass down the fallopian tube into the uterus, thus impairing the viability of the fertilized ovum in the uterus. In newer regimens, high doses of either ethinyl estradiol (the oral contraceptive Ovral) or conjugated estrogens (Premarin) are prescribed to accomplish much the same purpose.

Although postcoital regimens may be effective for contraception, routine use of them may be dangerous. In emergencies where there is a great desire to avoid pregnancy, such as for women who have been subjected to rape or incest, they can be very useful. Severe nausea, vomiting, and breast tenderness are frequently noted following treatment.

Mifepristone (RU-486), a Pharmacological Abortifacient

As discussed, progesterone is required to maintain the uterine lining (endometrium) in a state suitable for supporting a fertilized ovum. Pharmacological blockade of progesterone receptors in the uterus will provoke endometrial necrosis and shedding (menstruation). Thus, if a woman is in the early stages of pregnancy, the growing fetus will be aborted if she takes a progesterone antagonist. Today older techniques of postcoital contraception (in reality, early pharmacological abortion, or "contragestion"[18]) have been supplanted by the newer agent mifepristone. Mifepristone (RU-486) is the first clinically available progesterone antagonist, currently being used in Europe (especially in France) and in the Far East.[19] In studies reported in the late 1980s, the administration of mifepristone was accompanied by a later dose of prostaglandin, which induced uterine contractions to insure successful abortion.

In a recent study of 800 women and female adolescents, Glasier and coworkers compared the effectiveness of mifepristone as an abortifacient (without the prostaglandin) with the sequential administration of high doses of ethinyl estradiol and norgestrel.[20] Administered within 72 hours after unprotected intercourse, none of the 402 females who received mifepristone became pregnant, while 4 of the 398 females who received ethinyl estradiol and norgestrel did. The authors concluded that "the drug has the potential to avert unwanted and unplanned pregnancy. More widely available contraceptive services that included mifepristone as a postcoital agent would help reduce the demand for therapeutic abortion."[21]

Mifepristone has been the source of a moral controversy since the initial reports demonstrated its efficacy as an abortifacient. Consequently, the drug is not available in the United States. How this debate is resolved will determine whether this and similar compounds will become available for clinical use in this country. In an editorial accompanying the Glasier report, Grimes and Cook argue that mifepristone is actually not an abortifacient:

> Pregnancy begins when implantation [in the uterus of a fertilized ovum] is complete. Implantation begins five to six days after fertilization and is complete eight days later. When a woman's oocyte [egg] is fertilized *in vitro,* she cannot claim to be pregnant until the conceptus is implanted successfully [by artificial means] in her uterus. The same holds for fertilization *in vivo.* Since the postcoital contraceptive action of mifepristone occurs before implantation, it is not an abortifacient when used this way.[22]

A letter to the editor in the same journal (followed by a rebuttal by Grimes and Cook) challenged the statement:

> Many people feel that a fertilized ovum constitutes a new human life and that preventing its implantation constitutes abortion. This is the central issue about mifepristone. . . . Redefining the meaning of contraception to include the prevention of implantation does not change the fact that preventing implantation is what many people find problematic with the drug.[23]

I will leave conclusions to the reader. When after fertilization of the ovum is a woman pregnant? Is the nonimplanted ovum a living being? Is early pharmacological abortion (contragestion) the same as later surgical abortion of an implanted, fertilized ovum? The studies cited here do not answer these questions, but they do raise them.

Agents That Increase Fertility

Women who are having difficulty becoming pregnant may be candidates for drugs that can increase fertility. Infertility, as a medical diagnosis, may be caused by many factors, physical and psychological, in either the man or the woman. Certain types of infertility in women can be pharmacologically manipulated.

One such pharmacological approach is an extension of the scheme illustrated in Figure 14.3. When estrogen acts on the hypothalamus, the release of GRF is inhibited, the release of FSH and LH by the pituitary gland is decreased, and follicular development is inhibited. If the action of estrogen on the hypothalamus were blocked, GRF would be released; this action would, in turn, stimulate the release of FSH and LH from the pituitary gland. Subsequently, one or more ovarian follicles would develop, and eventually at least one ovum would be released. For a drug to block the inhibitory action of estrogen on the hypothalamus, it would have to attach to normal estrogen receptors (thus blocking the normal access of estrogen to the receptor) without causing any changes in cellular behavior (in pharmacological terms, it would have affinity for the receptors but be devoid of intrinsic activity).

Clomiphene

Clomiphene (Clomid), a compound that is frequently referred to as a "fertility pill," is a drug that binds to estrogen receptors without intrinsic activity. Clomiphene has enabled many women who were previously unable to conceive to become pregnant. Clomiphene has also been responsible for causing multiple births; sometimes four or five ova are released and fertilized in women who take the drug. However, the possibility of bearing more than one child is usually not considered a problem for couples who have not been able to conceive by other methods. Because clomiphene acts on the hypothalamus, the pituitary gland and ovaries must be functional if the drug is to improve a woman's chances of conception. Thus, the drug is ineffective if infertility is caused by a deficit in the man or when the woman's infertility is caused by pituitary or ovarian dysfunction.

Ordinarily the administration of clomiphene is started on day 5 of the menstrual period (day 1 being the first day of menses); it is then taken daily for 5 days. The drug is then stopped until the next menstrual cycle if the woman does not become pregnant. The procedure is then repeated, often with slowly increasing doses. Approximately 35 percent of formerly infertile women become pregnant when they take clomiphene. Side effects of clomiphene include ovarian cysts (14 percent), multiple pregnancies (8 percent), and birth defects (2.4 percent). The incidence of birth defects in nontreated women who conceive without the aid of clomiphene is approximately 1 percent.

Alternatives to Clomiphene

If a woman does not become pregnant after several trials on clomiphene, Pergonal (human postmenopausal hormone), Follutein (chorionic gonadotropin), or bromocriptine can be tried.

Pergonal is a commercial product that contains FSH and LH, which are extracted from the urine of postmenopausal women.

Follutein, a hormone produced by the human placenta, is extracted from the urine of pregnant women. It exerts actions that are virtually identical to those of pituitary LH. Thus, sequential injections of Pergonal and then Follutein can, in anovulatory women, simulate the normal FSH and LH release found in fertile women. Pergonal is injected daily for 9 to 12 days, and then, after a day of rest, the woman is given a single injection of Follutein. Approximately 75 percent of women who are treated by this method ovulate, and approximately 25 percent of them become pregnant.

Bromocriptine is an agonist (stimulant) of dopamine receptors that inhibit the pituitary secretion of prolactin, restoring gonadotropin function and ovarian responsiveness. It seems to increase a woman's responsiveness to clomiphene.[3]

ANABOLIC-ANDROGENIC STEROIDS

The anabolic-androgenic steroids (A-ASs) are a group of drugs that include the male sex hormone *testosterone* and several synthetically produced structural derivatives of testosterone. The term anabolic-androgenic steroids arises because these substances have both body-building (anabolic) and masculinizing (androgenic) effects.[24] In the past few decades, the A-ASs have become very controversial because they have been used illicitly by both men and women to promote athletic performance and to improve physical appearance. Indeed, public concern rose to the point where Congress passed the Anabolic Steroids Act of 1990 to control the distribution and sale of the drugs. This act added these drugs to Schedule III of the Controlled Substances Act of 1990, classifying them as drugs with abuse potential that may lead to dependence.

Figure 14.7 illustrates the chemical structures of testosterone and several available derivatives. These differ from each other primarily in their resistance to metabolic degradation by liver enzymes. After oral administration, testosterone is effectively absorbed from the intestine. However, following absorption, it is rapidly transported in blood to the liver, where it is immediately metabolized; as a result, little testosterone reaches the systemic circulation.[25] Administered by injection, some of this "first-pass metabolism" is blunted, and it is the metabolic product, androstanolone, that is most active as an anabolic substance.[25]

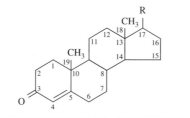

Compound	R
Testosterone	—OH
Testosterone propionate	—O—COCH₂CH₃
Testosterone enanthate	—O—CO(CH₂)₅CH₃
Testosterone cypionate	—O—COCH₂CH₂— (cyclopentyl)
Nandrolone decanoate	—O—CO(CH₂)₈CH₃ (no methyl group at position 19)
Nandrolone phenpropionate	—O—CO(CH₂)₂— (phenyl) (no methyl group at position 19)

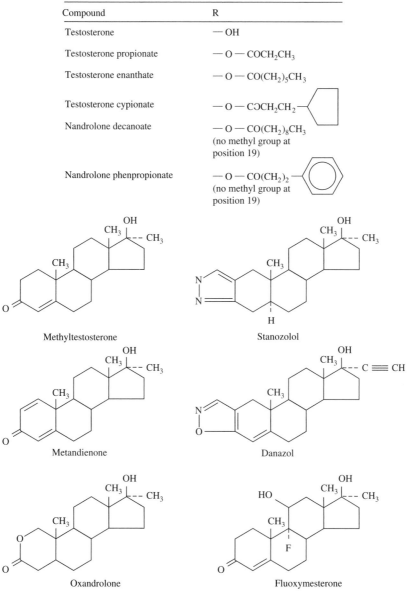

Methyltestosterone

Stanozolol

Metandienone

Danazol

Oxandrolone

Fluoxymesterone

FIGURE 14.7 Structures of some common parenteral (left) and oral (right) anabolic-androgenic steroids. [Reproduced with permission from Lucas.[25]]

TABLE 14.3   Anabolic-androgenic steroids.

Name	Route	Brand name
U.S. APPROVED		
Testosterone cypionate	im	Depo-Testosterone, Virilon
Nandrolone phenpropionate	im	Durabolin
Nandrolone decanoate	im	Deca-Duraboli
Danazol	po	Danocrine
Fluoxymesterone	po	Halotestin
Methyltestosterone	po	Android, Metandren, Testred, Virilon
Oxymetholone	po	Anadrol-50
Slanozolol	po	Winstrol
OUTSIDE U.S.		
Testosterone enanthate	im	Delatestryl
Testosterone propionate	im	Testex, Oreton propionate
Methenolone enanthate	im	Primobolan Depot
Ethylestrenol	po	Maxibolan
Mesterolone	po	
Methandrostenolone	po	Dianabol
Methenolone	po	Primobolan
Norethandrolone	po	
Oxandrolone	po	Anavar
Oxymesterone	po	Oranabol
VETERINARY		
Bolasterone	im	Finiject 30
Boldenone undecylenate	im	Equipoise
Stanozolol	im	Winstrol
Mibolerone	po	

Reproduced with permission from K. B. Kashkin.[26]
Note: i.m., intramuscular; p.o., oral.

Structural modification of the testosterone molecule can reduce metabolic degradation and thus improve the effectiveness of both oral and intramuscular administration.

Importantly, not all these drugs are illicit substances. Eight synthetic A-AS substances (Table 14.3) are approved in the United States for therapeutic uses, which include testosterone replacement in hypogonadal males, the treatment of certain blood anemias and severe muscle loss following trauma, and, in females, the treatment of endometriosis and fibrocystic disease of the breast.[26]

Mechanism of Action

The mechanism of testosterone and other A-AS drugs is quite well understood. The natural hormone is synthesized principally in a specialized type of cell (the Leydig cell) of the testes. This occurs under the influence of gonadotropin-releasing hormone (GRH) released from the hypothalamus, which stimulates the synthesis and release of luteinizing hormone (LH) from the pituitary gland; the latter acts on the Leydig cells to stimulate testosterone production (see Figure 14.1).

Once in the bloodstream, testosterone (or an exogenous A-AS) passes through the cell walls of its target tissues and attaches to steroid receptors in the cytoplasm of the cell (Figure 14.8). This hormone–receptor complex is translocated into the nucleus of the cell and attached to the nuclear material (the DNA). A process of genetic transcription follows, and new messenger RNA is produced. Translation of this RNA results in the production of specific new proteins that leave the cell and mediate the biological functions of the hormone. Thus, the effects of A-AS on target cells are mediated by intracellular receptors and the synthesis of new proteins. The increased levels of circulating testosterone (or other A-AS drugs) exert a negative feedback effect on the hypothalamus, inhibiting further stimulation of testosterone

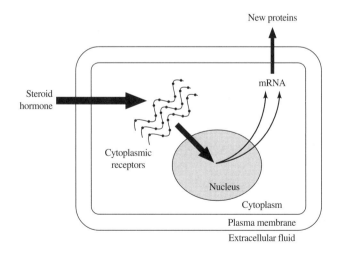

FIGURE 14.8 Mechanism of action of steroid hormones on cells. The hormone passes through the cell wall of its target tissue and binds to steroid receptors in the cytoplasm. The hormone–receptor complex moves into the nucleus and binds to sites on the chromatin, which is transcribed to give specific messenger RNA (mRNA). The mRNA is translated into specific new proteins that mediate the function of the hormone. [Reproduced with permission from Lucas.[25]]

release (the same as occurred with estrogen and the progestin in the oral contraceptives).

What, then, are the consequences of the above described process?

> Anabolic steroids, under proper circumstances, may increase both the size and strength of the athlete and may thereby improve performance in athletic activities that require size and strength. Anabolic steroids have no positive effects on aerobic performance of the athlete.[27]

Effects on Athletic Performance

A-ASs induce size and strength gains through anticatabolic, anabolic, and motivational effects on the athlete. Table 14.4 summarizes the constellation of effects and side effects. The anticatabolic effect means that the A-ASs block the action of natural cortisone, which normally functions to increase energy stores during periods of stress and training. Cortisone makes available such energy stores by breaking down proteins into their constituent amino acids. Carried to excess, muscle wasting can occur. This action is blocked by the A-ASs. Indeed, the anticatabolic action may be the major mechanism by which these drugs ultimately increase body mass.[27]

The anabolic effects follow from the above described mechanism to induce the synthesis of new protein in muscle cells. Effects also follow from A-AS–induced release of endogenous growth hormone, which has anabolic effects as well.[27] It is important to note, however, that the doses commonly used by athletes are 10 to 200 times the therapeutic dosage for testosterone deficiency. Often this involves the "stacking" or "pyramiding" of multiple drugs, even combining oral and injectable substances through cycles of several weeks' duration.[26]

According to Bauer, "There is near, but incomplete, scientific consensus that AASs do increase muscle strength and lean body mass when combined with intensive training and a proper diet."[28] Kashkin summarizes as follows:

> It is known that androgens can increase the rate of RNA transcription above that found with exercise alone and that androgens can induce the formation of new myofilaments (the contractile filaments in muscle) and cause enlarging myofibrils (muscle cells) to divide.[29]

The motivational effects are profound, and at least a part of this effect is certainly a placebo effect. In addition, athletes taking A-AS drugs often develop very aggressive personalities, a condition nicknamed "'roid rage." Such an effect can also be reproduced in animals

TABLE 14.4 Effects of anabolic-androgenic steroids.

Positive effects
    Transient increase in muscular size and strength
    Treatment of catabolic states
        Trauma
        Surgery
Adverse effects
    Cardiovascular
        Increase in cardiac risk factors
            Hypertension
            Altered lipoprotein fractions
            Increase in LDL/HDL ratio
        Reported strokes/myocardial infarctions
    Hepatic effects associated with oral compounds
        Elevated liver enzymes
        Peliosis hepatis (greater than 6 months' use)
        Liver tumors
            Benign
            Malignant (greater than 24 months' use)
    Reproductive system effects
        In males
            Decreased testosterone production
                Abnormal spermatogenesis
                Transient infertility
                Testicular atrophy
        In females
            Altered menstruation
    Endocrine effects
        Decreased thyroid function
    Immunologic effects
        Decreased immunoglobulins IgM/IgA/IgC
    Musculoskeletal effects
        Premature closure of bony growth centers
        Tendon degeneration
            Increased risk of tendon tears
    Cosmetic
        In males
            Gynecomastia
            Testicular atrophy
            Acne
            Acceleration of male pattern baldness
        In females
            Clittoral enlargement
            Acne
            Increased facial/body hair
            Coarsening of the skin
            Male pattern baldness
            Deepened voice
    Psychologic
        Risk of habituation
        Severe mood swings
        Aggressive tendencies
        Psychotic episodes
        Depression
        Reports of suicide
    Legislation
        Classified as Schedule III controlled substance

Reproduced with permission from H. A. Haupt.[27]

fed large doses of these drugs. Lucas notes, "For some sports, such as football, these steroids may serve the dual purpose of increasing strength and performance as well as enhancing combativeness."[30]

In the female athlete, A-AS drugs exert the same anabolic and anti-catabolic effects found in male athletes. However, these drugs also induce in females masculinizing and other effects, which include increases in facial and body hair, lowered voice, enlarged clitoris, coarser skin, and menstrual cycle cessation or irregularity. Cessation of steroid use results in a variable and often incomplete return of the altered functions.

These drugs are also widely used (and abused) by young male (usually noncompetitive) athletes who take them to develop the muscular physique considered fashionable. Haupt estimates that about 6 percent of male high school seniors under age 18 have used or currently use A-ASs.[27] This figure represents between 250,000 and 500,000 young adult males. Unlike competitive athletes who may choose to terminate drug use when competition ends, such youth may continue to take A-ASs in order to maintain the cosmetic effect. As we will see, dire consequences can result.

Endocrine Effects

Males taking A-ASs experience a hypogonadal state, which is characterized by atrophy of the testicles, impaired production of sperm, and infertility. These effects are generally thought to be reversible upon cessation of drug use. However, such reversibility is not guaranteed.[26] Other endocrine effects in the male include early male pattern baldness, reduced libido, acne, and the development of gynecomastia (femalelike breast growth). The latter effect, the result of some of the A-ASs being metabolized to the female hormone estradiol, may not be reversible with drug discontinuation.

Cardiovascular Effects

Adverse effects on the cardiovascular system have been of concern, with two published reports of fatal myocardial infarctions (heart attacks) occurring in users of A-ASs. Atherosclerosis-induced coronary artery disease was implicated in these deaths. Thus, analysis of the potential correlation between A-ASs and atherosclerosis is important. Here, the effect of these steroids on blood cholesterol as a predisposing factor to atherosclerotic coronary artery disease must be considered. Cholesterol is of two types: "bad" cholesterol (low-density lipoprotein cholesterol, or LDL) and "good" cholesterol (high-density lipoprotein cholesterol, or HDL). Decreasing HDL and increasing LDL is strongly correlated with an increased risk of coronary artery disease.

All A-ASs induce a reduction in serum HDL cholesterol and an elevation in LDL cholesterol. This suggests that individuals taking these drugs are at greater risk of suffering coronary artery disease. This condition can be expressed as myocardial infarctions, thrombo-embolic disease (blood clots and emboli), strokes, and hypertension. The actual risk of cardiovascular disease is unknown at this time, largely due to the young age of users, their relatively lean or muscular physiques, and the intermittent pattern of drug use. We may have to wait until these users are adults to determine whether they have been harmed by using A-ASs during their earlier years.

Effects on the Liver

The use of oral A-AS preparations has been associated with a risk of liver disorders, especially jaundice and tumors.[25] Increases in the blood levels of liver enzymes, indicative of possible liver dysfunction, are quite common among users of A-ASs.[26] Hepatitis is also not uncommon. In addition, several dozen cases of liver carcinomas of unusual type have been reported. The incidence of developing these potentially fatal carcinomas is estimated to be 1 to 3 percent within two to eight years of exposure to the orally administered agents.

Psychological Effects

As noted above, an increase in aggression, competitiveness, and com-bativeness is characteristic in athletes using large doses of A-ASs. It is now well established that areas of the brain that influence mood and judgment contain steroid receptors and that sharp fluctuations in the levels of steroid hormones have profound psychological effects.[26] Steroid receptors are widely distributed in the CNS, especially in the hypothalamus and the limbic regions. In the hypothalamus, they autoregulate their own reproductive actions (through the negative feedback system discussed earlier). Hypothalamic actions also mod-ulate other vegetative systems of the body, a matter of importance during steroid withdrawal. The limbic receptors appear to account for the effects of steroids on mood.

Thus, A-ASs administered in regular large doses are indeed mood-altering chemicals. They differ markedly from other mood-altering drugs, however, in their delayed onset of effect. This delay occurs because their mechanism of synthesizing new proteins takes days or weeks. Because their effects are not immediate, they may not be perceived as being a consequence of drug ingestion. Questions have been raised about immediate effects on opioid, GABA, and other receptors, but these effects are little understood.[26] Haupt summarizes:

> There are significant adverse psychological effects associated with the use of anabolic steroids although the effects are not easily measured by current psychological inventories. Athletes taking anabolic steroids suffer some degree of personality change that may range from simple mood swings to a psychosis requiring hospitalization for treatment. A Jekyll-and-Hyde personality is common, where even the slightest provocation can cause an exaggerated, violent, and often uncontrolled response. The users of anabolic steroids often suffer disturbed personality relationships that may include separations from family and friends and even divorce. Arrest records are not uncommon. Fortunately these psychological effects are reversible when the steroids are discontinued, but the social scars may be permanent.[31]

Kashkin reviews these psychological effects at length, adding that about half of a small population of interviewed weightlifters experienced depression and an even higher percentage experienced paranoid thoughts and some psychotic features.[26]

Abuse, Dependence, and Treatment

By definition, the ingestion or injection of A-AS drugs for athletic or cosmetic purposes constitutes drug abuse, since the drugs are used in doses far exceeding those needed for medical indications; such use persists despite recognized, unavoidable side effects and negative consequences for the physical and psychological health of the user.

The mechanisms responsible for dependence are largely unknown and may be psychological or physiological. Indeed, the muscle-building (anabolic and anticatabolic) effects of A-ASs may be sufficient psychological reinforcement to maintain self-administration, especially for those who link their appearance with their self-worth.

Physical dependence is characterized by withdrawal symptoms when the drug is removed. Withdrawal from large doses of A-ASs can be accompanied by psychological depression, fatigue, restlessness, insomnia, loss of appetite, and decreased libido. Other withdrawal symptoms that have been reported include drug craving, headache, dissatisfaction with body image, and (rarely) suicidal ideation. Despite these observations, no defined psychiatric withdrawal syndrome has been described; withdrawal psychosis or bipolar illness has not been reported, although depression is commonplace.

As with all other psychoactive drugs, treatment of A-AS dependence first requires removal of the drug. Thus, abstinence is the first treatment goal. During the early stage of abstinence, attention should be directed to any of the signs of withdrawal. Supportive therapy, including reassurance, education, and counseling, is the mainstay of withdrawal treatment.[24] Antidepressants may be indicated when withdrawal is complicated by major depression. A physician trained in endocrinology can best prescribe other therapies for hormonal alterations.

Following acute withdrawal, further therapy should focus on maintaining abstinence and addressing factors that may lead to relapse. Such therapy may be directed at (1) assisting abusers to free themselves of the association between physical appearance and self-esteem and (2) assisting development of a balance of physical and non-physical pursuits, which can foster feelings of competence.[24]

The abuse of A-ASs by athletes, bodybuilders, and body-conscious individuals poses a special challenge to society in general. While those drugs have psychoactive effects, they are not euphoric or mood altering immediately following administration (as are other illicit drugs). Perhaps the desire of individuals to take A-ASs has been fostered largely by our societal fixations on winning and on physical appearance. Thus, successful intervention must go beyond education, counseling, law enforcement, and drug testing. Ultimately a social environment that currently encourages the use of the anabolic-androgenic steroids may have to be changed.

Study Questions

1. Differentiate between a neurotransmitter and a neurohormone. Give examples of each.
2. Where does fertilization occur?
3. Classify the various types of oral contraceptives. How do the newer contraceptives differ from those that were available in the 1960s?
4. What circumstance prevents further reductions in the amount of estrogen that is contained in oral contraceptives?
5. How do the steroid hormones in oral contraceptives work to block fertility?
6. Over the past 30 years, there has been much discussion about long-term harmful effects of oral contraceptives. Discuss the areas of concern and the current views of such potential toxicity.
7. Differentiate among precoital contraception, postcoital contraception, and pharmacological abortifacients. Give examples of each.

8. What drugs are available to increase fertility in women?
9. What are androgenic-anabolic steroids? How do they affect body functions?
10. Describe the similarities and differences between dependence on anabolic steroids and the more traditional drugs of abuse.

Notes

1. L. Speroff, R. H. Glass, and N. G. Kase, *Clinical Gynecologic Endocrinology and Infertility*, 4th ed. (Baltimore: Williams & Wilkins, 1989), pp. 51–61.
2. D. B. Bartosik, "Female Sex Hormones, Oral Contraceptives, and Fertility Agents," in J. R. DiPalma and G. J. DiGregorio, eds., *Basic Pharmacology in Medicine*, 3rd ed. (New York: McGraw-Hill, 1990), p. 521.
3. Speroff, Glass, and Kase, *Clinical Gynecologic Endocrinology and Infertility*, pp. 461–481.
4. B. Hedon, "The Evolution of Oral Contraceptives. Maximizing Efficacy, Minimizing Risks," *Acta Obstetricia et Gynecologica Scandinavica* 152, suppl. (1990): 7–12.
5. D. R. Mishell, Jr., "The Pharmacologic and Metabolic Effects of Oral Contraceptives," *International Journal of Fertility* 34, suppl. (1989): 21–26.
6. P. G. Stubblefield, "Cardiovascular Effects of Oral Contraceptives: A Review," *International Journal of Fertility* 34, suppl. (1989): 40–49.
7. M. Thorogood and M. P. Vessey, "An Epidemiologic Survey of Cardiovascular Disease in Women Taking Oral Contraceptives," *American Journal of Obstetrics and Gynecology* 163 (1990): 274–281.
8. G. Samsioe and L. A. Mattsson, "Some Aspects of the Relationship between Oral Contraceptives, Lipid Abnormalities, and Cardiovascular Disease," *American Journal of Obstetrics and Gynecology* 163 (1990): 354–358.
9. E. P. Frohlich, "Vascular Complications in Women Using the Low Steroid Content Combined Oral Contraceptive Pills: Case Reports and Review of the Literature," *Obstetrical and Gynecological Survey* 45 (1990): 578–584.
10. R. J. Derman, "Oral Contraceptives and Cardiovascular Risk. Taking a Safe Course of Action," *Postgraduate Medicine* 88 (1990): 119–122.
11. P. D. Stolley, B. L. Strom, and P. E. Sartwell, "Oral Contraceptives and Vascular Disease," *Epidemiologic Reviews* 11 (1989): 241–243.
12. H. Olsson, "Oral Contraceptives and Breast Cancer. A Review," *Acta Oncologica* 28 (1989): 849–863.
13. K. Gast and T. Snyder, "Combination Oral Contraceptives and Cancer Risk," *Kansas Medicine* 91 (1990): 201–208.
14. D. R. Mishell, Jr., "Correcting Misconceptions about Oral Contraceptives," *American Journal of Obstetrics and Gynecology* 161 (1989): 1385–1389.
15. I. E. Godsland, D. Crook, and V. Wynn, "Low-Dose Oral Contraceptives and Carbohydrate Metabolism," *American Journal of Obstetrics and Gynecology* 163 (1990): 348–353.

16. L. Speroff, "The Effects of Oral Contraceptives on Reproduction," *International Journal of Fertility* 34, suppl. (1989): 34–39.

17. H. B. Croxatto, "NORPLANT: Levonorgestrel-Releasing Contraceptive Implant," *Annals of Medicine* 25 (1993): 155–160.

18. E. E. Baulieu, "Contragestion by the Progesterone Antagonist RU 486: A Novel Approach to Human Fertility Control," *Contraception* 36, suppl. (1987): 1–5.

19. I. M. Spitz, D. Shoupe, R. Sitruk-Ware, and D. R. Mishell, Jr., "Response to the Antiprogestogen RU 486 (Mifepristone) during Early Pregnancy and the Menstrual Cycle in Women," *Journal of Reproduction and Fertility* 37, suppl. (1989): 253–260.

20. A. Glasier, K. J. Thong, M. Dewar, M. Mackie, and D. T. Baird, "Mifepristone (RU 486) Compared with High-Dose Estrogen and Progestin for Emergency Postcoital Contraception," *New England Journal of Medicine* 327 (1992): 1041–1044.

21. Ibid., p. 1044.

22. D. A. Grimes and R. J. Cook, "Mifepristone (RU 486)—An Abortifacient to Prevent Abortion?" *New England Journal of Medicine* 327 (1992): 1088–1089.

23. R. P. Hamel and M. T. Lysaught, letter to the editor in *New England Journal of Medicine* 328 (1993): 354–355.

24. K. J. Bower, "Anabolic Steroids," *Psychiatric Clinics of North America* 16 (1993): 97–103.

25. S. E. Lucas, "Current Perspectives on Anabolic-Androgenic Steroid Abuse," *Trends in Pharmacological Sciences* 14 (1993): 61–68.

26. K. B. Kashkin, "Anabolic Steroids," in J. H. Lowinson, P. Ruiz, R. B. Millman, and J. G. Langrod, eds., *Substance Abuse: A Comprehensive Textbook*, 2nd ed. (Baltimore: Williams & Wilkins, 1992), pp. 380–395.

27. H. A. Haupt, "Anabolic Steroids and Growth Hormone," *American Journal of Sports Medicine* 21 (1993): 468–474.

28. Bower, "Anabolic Steroids," pp. 98–99.

29. Kashkin, "Anabolic Steroids," p. 386.

30. Lucas, "Current Perspectives," p. 63.

31. Haupt, "Anabolic Steroids and Growth Hormone," p. 470.

CHAPTER 15

DRUGS AND SOCIETY: PRIORITIES AND ALTERNATIVES

As far back as recorded history, every society has used drugs that produce effects on mood, thought, and feeling. Moreover, there were always a few individuals who digressed from custom with respect to the time, the amount, and the situation in which these drugs were to be used. Thus, both the nonmedical use of drugs and the problem of drug abuse are as old as civilization itself.[1]

Indeed, Genesis 9:20–23 describes Noah as becoming drunk with wine and being found in a drunken stupor in his tent.[2] Alcohol is not the only drug that has been used through the ages; every culture has used any naturally occurring substance available whose use alleviated anxiety, produced relaxation, provided relief from boredom, alleviated pain, increased strength or work tolerance, or provided temporary distortion of reality. In most cultures, only one or at most very few naturally occurring substances were available. Also, use of mind-altering chemicals was closely, even religiously, monitored, and only a relative minority of individuals "abused"drugs.

From the previous 14 chapters, several points that differentiate our current pattern of psychoactive drug use from the traditional one are readily apparent.

1. We have available in one culture all of the psychoactive drugs ever used throughout the world.

2. In most cases, the pharmacologically active ingredient in each natural product has been isolated, identified, and made available to those who desire the drug.

3. Synthetic derivatives can be manufactured that, in many cases, magnify the psychoactive potency of the natural substance by 100-fold or more.

4. Users have devised new methods of drug delivery, starting with the invention of the hypodermic syringe in the 1860s and ending with the development of "crack" cocaine and "ICE" methamphetamine in the 1980s and 1990s. These developments have markedly increased the delivered dose and decreased the time to onset of drug action.

Despite these problems regarding psychoactive drugs, all is not dismal. On the positive side have been remarkable advances:

1. Fifty years of research have provided marvelous drugs that can help control mental illnesses, including schizophrenia, major depression, bipolar disorder, major anxiety states and phobias, chronic pain, epilepsy, and insomnia.

2. Many of the same drugs are also useful in supplementing the psychotherapy of obsessive–compulsive disorder, panic disorder, bulimia, anorexia, and a variety of personality disorders. The use of drugs as adjuvants to psychotherapy is discussed at length in several reviews in a recent issue of the *Psychiatric Clinics of North America.*[3] The concomitant use of psychotherapy and psychopharmacology is discussed in Chapter 16.

As in past decades, caffeine, nicotine, and ethyl alcohol are the major addictive drugs used by the vast majority of people today. As Figure 15.1 shows, caffeine use is nearly universal, with 180 million of the 203 million Americans over the age of 11 using the drug weekly. Thankfully, little harm seems to follow from such use (Chapter 7).

Nicotine and alcohol are the next most widely used and abused addictive drugs; both agents cause enormous harm as measured by death and disability (Chapters 5 and 7). Goldstein reported that the probability of an American living today having a drug abuse or dependence disorder was 36 percent for nicotine and 14 percent for alcohol.[4] This compares with 4 percent for marijuana (it is a much less used and less harmful drug than either nicotine or alcohol; Chapter 13).

Finally, including all the other drugs shown in Figure 15.1, about 6 to 7 million people had "used any other illicit drug in the past week" of the study. These drugs include behavioral stimulants (cocaine and amphetamines), heroin and other opioids, and hallucinogens, tranquilizers, and volatile agents. Johnson and Muffler offer similar statistics,

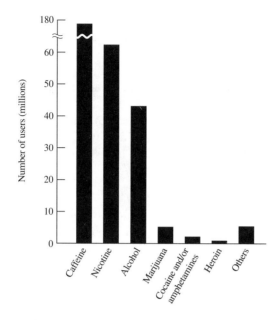

FIGURE 15.1 Use of addictive drugs in the United States in 1991. Numbers include people who used each drug at least weekly (heroin use at least once in past year). "Others" includes inhalants and hallucinogens. [Data from *National Household Survey on Drug Abuse*, U.S. Department of Health and Human Services, Public Health Service, Alcohol, Drug Abuse, and Mental Health Administration, DHHS Publication No. (ADM) 92-1887, Washington, D.C., 1992. [Source: Goldstein,[4] fig. 1.1, p. 6.]

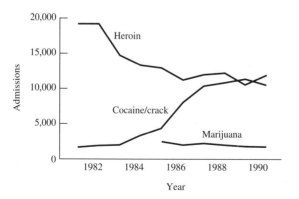

FIGURE 15.2 Primary drugs of abuse at admission to drug treatment programs in New York City, 1980–1990. [Source: Johnson and Muffler,[5] fig. 10.4, p. 12.]

providing illustrations and figures to describe lifetime use, past-year use, and past-30-days use.[5] Johnson and Muffler strongly emphasize the "crack era" of today; their figures reveal a leveling off or decrease in the use of other substances but remarkable increases in the use of cocaine (Figure 15.2).

About 2 percent of our population will have a drug abuse or dependency disorder with one of these other drugs during their lifetime.[6] Although this figure represents a large number of people, most of this discussion will focus on alcohol, caffeine, and nicotine—the agents that are the most widely used and that exact such an enormous toll on our society.

First, however, we must begin by discussing why people are attracted to certain psychoactive drugs and why they continue to use these drugs despite known hazards to their own health and life.

PSYCHOACTIVE DRUGS AS BEHAVIORAL REINFORCERS

In earlier chapters, we introduced the concept that drugs are widely abused because they activate brain mechanisms involved in reward and positive reinforcement. The systems and structures involved include (1) dopamine, serotonin, opioid, GABA, and cannabis neurons and/or receptors and (2) the median forebrain bundle, ventral tegmental area of the brain, hippocampus, frontal cortex, and nucleus accumbens. Here we attempt to use these facts to describe a neuroanatomical system that underlies the behavior-reinforcing actions of all these drugs. Since conditioning and learning processes are of central importance in drug addiction, we then explain drug-seeking behavior as an amalgam of positive reinforcement, discriminative effects, aversive effects, and stimuli associated with drug use.

Lessons from the Laboratory

Laboratory animals self-administer many psychoactive drugs in varying degrees. Indeed, the degree to which an animal self-administers a particular drug closely parallels the degree of abuse exhibited by human users of the drug.[7] In addition, if a drug is to maintain drug-seeking behavior, it must serve as a positive reinforcer.[8]

For example, cocaine is self-administered to excess by every species of animal that has been tested, including rats, squirrels, monkeys, rhesus monkeys, pigtail macaques, baboons, dogs, and humans.[9] Certainly, the same behavior in a variety of species is evidence of the impressive behavior-reinforcing property of cocaine.

> Animals will press a lever more than 4,000 times to get a single injection of cocaine, and when given free access, they generally self-administer high daily doses that may produce severe toxic effects and induce self-mutilating behavior. . . . Generally the animals die of toxic effects and inanition [starvation] after a period of several weeks of continuous use.[10]

The self-administration of strongly reinforcing drugs by several species dispels the notion that the drug abuser (compared to a casual user or a nonuser) has some kind of inherent pathological condition (for example, a preexisting psychopathology) that creates a propensity for abusing drugs. Thus, we must examine briefly the reinforcing properties of the major psychoactive drugs.

Cocaine and the amphetamines are the most powerful reinforcing drugs.[11] This reinforcing property of the potent behavioral stimulants is probably the most important factor in their compulsive abuse by humans, and it plays a major role in the drug's appeal to users.

Morphine, heroin, and other opioids are readily self-administered by animals but in a way that differs from the self-administration of cocaine and the amphetamines: "Animals self-administering morphine gradually raise the daily dose over a period of weeks, then self-administer the drug at a steady rate that avoids gross toxicity and withdrawal symptoms."[10] The initial increase in dose probably reflects the development of drug tolerance. The subsequent stabilization in dosage probably reflects a reduction in the pleasurable effect of the drug over time, with drug use being continued primarily to avoid withdrawal symptoms.

Nicotine is not initially self-administered by animals. Over time the rate of self-administration increases, but it decreases rapidly when saline is substituted for the drug.[12] Miller and Gold state that "nicotine also has been found . . . to be a positive reinforcer, although not to the same extent as cocaine."[13]

Caffeine is generally thought to be a relatively weak behavioral reinforcer. Some positive reinforcing effects are seen at low doses, but aversive effects are seen at higher doses. Both animals and humans demonstrate a preference for caffeine, but this preference decreases as the work required to obtain caffeine increases.[14,15]

Ethanol (ethyl alcohol) was shown in the early 1970s to be an effective behavioral reinforcer, although animals usually do not self-administer the drug without prior exposure to it. Formerly this reinforcing property was thought to be the result of its antianxiety or "disinhibiting" action, since the drug is neither euphoriant nor analgesic, nor is it a behavioral stimulant or a psychedelic. Recently, however, Miller and Gold reviewed an interesting hypothesis that the two-step metabolism of ethanol (by aldehyde dehydrogenase) induces a shift in the metabolism of the neurotransmitter dopamine to form a tetrahydroisoquinoline called *tetrahydropaperoline* (THP).[13] THP, in turn, is postulated to stimulate opioid receptors, which (as we will see) affects dopamine neurons. Other behavior-reinforcing actions of ethanol may be exerted through interactions with GABA neurons, which (as we will also see) also affect dopamine and the nucleus accumbens.[7]

Chlorpromazine and other neuroleptic drugs are never self-administered; in fact, animals learn to avoid behaviors that result in the receipt of an injection of a neuroleptic drug. Administration of a neuroleptic drug will often terminate or block the behavior-reinforcing properties of drugs such as cocaine. Similarly, the clinical antidepressants are not self-administered by animals; consequently, as stated in Chapter 8, they are not considered as drugs of abuse.

The cannabinoids (marijuana) and the psychedelics (such as PCP and LSD) are now considered to be behavioral reinforcers although these effects have been more difficult to demonstrate, especially with marijuana.[2,8]

Mechanism of Reinforcement Action

In recent years, it has become apparent that there are specific circuits in the brain dedicated to the neural mediation of reward and pleasure. The activation or enhancement of this reward mechanism seems to be the single feature shared by all abusable substances; drugs subject to compulsive abuse "act on these brain mechanisms to produce the subjective reward that constitutes the reinforcing 'high' or 'rush' or 'hit' sought by substance abusers."[16] Specifically, all abusable substances, through varied mechanisms and neurotransmitters, ultimately stimulate a mesotelencephalic–nucleus accumbens dopaminergic system that runs through the medial forebrain bundle. Drugs that have negative-reward effects (such as the phenothiazines) inhibit activity in or increase the thresholds of this same system.

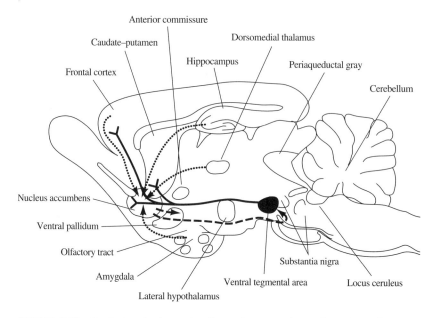

FIGURE 15.3 Sagittal rat brain section illustrating a cocaine and amphetamine neural reward circuit that includes a limbic–extrapyramidal motor interface. Dotted arrows indicate limbic afferents to the nucleus accumbens and dashed arrows represent efferents from the nucleus accumbens thought to be involved in psycho-motor stimulant reward. Solid arrows indicate projections of the mesocorticolimbic dopamine system thought to be a critical substrate for psychomotor stimulant reward. This system originates in the A10 cell group of the ventral tegmental area and projects to the olfactory tubercle of the nucleus accumbens and the ventral striatal domains of the caudate–putamen. [Adapted from G. F. Koob,[7] fig. 1, p. 178.]

Exactly what is this brain reward system, and how do drugs of such varying classes and neurotransmitter actions influence it? First, there are two major dopaminergic (dopamine-releasing) neuronal sys-tems in the midbrain (Figure 15.3). A primary, or first-stage, system comprises descending (or caudally projecting) fibers of dopaminergic neurons whose cell bodies are located in the nucleus accumbens and several limbic structures. These first-stage fibers run within the medial forebrain bundle and synapse onto second-stage dopaminergic neu-rons whose cell bodies are located in the ventral tegmental area (VTA) of the midbrain. The second-stage fibers are the axons of these VTA cells, and they ascend (travel rostrally) also in the medial forebrain bundle and project into neurons of the forebrain, largely in the nucleus accumbens, frontal cortex, amygdala, and septal area.

In essence, this two-neuron system comprises a dopaminergic loop between the forebrain and the VTA of the midbrain.[7,17] Exactly how this loop functions in reward mechanisms is not known, but Koob postulates that

> the mesocorticolimbic dopamine system appears to act as a modulator or a filtering and gating mechanism for signals from the limbic regions, signals mediating basic biological drives and motivational variables. These signals are thought ultimately to be translated into motor acts via the output of the extrapyramidal motor system.[18]

Cocaine and the amphetamines are now thought to act on both the first- and the second-stage neuronal terminals (located in the VTA and the nucleus accumbens). Here, the drugs essentially mimic the effects of direct electrical stimulation of these areas. The other drugs of abuse act only on the second-stage neurons, probably through endogenous opioid circuitry:

> Cell bodies, axons, and synaptic terminals of enkephalinergic and endorphinergic neurons are found in profusion throughout the extent of the reward-relevant mesotelencephalic dopamine circuitry.... Endogenous opioid peptide neurons synapse directly onto mesotelencephalic dopamine axon terminals, forming precisely the type of axo-axonic synapses one would expect of a system designed to modulate the flow of reward-relevant neural signals through the dopamine circuitry.[19]

As Figure 15.3 illustrates,

> the drug-sensitive dopamine "second stage" component of the reward circuitry is under the modulatory control of a wide variety of other neural systems, including the enkephalinergic mechanisms alluded to above, but also including GABAergic, seritonergic, noradrenergic, and neuropeptide neurotransmitter and neuromodulatory mechanisms.[20]

Koob states that it is quite apparent that

> dopamine forms a critical link for all reward, including opiates and sedative/hypnotics. While open to multiple neurotransmitter inputs and outputs, this view still holds a centrist position for dopamine in all reward. An emphasis on multiple independent neurochemical elements, ... places the focus on the nucleus accumbems and its circuitry as an important, perhaps critical, substrate for drug reward.[18]

It is important to recognize that enhancement of brain reward mechanisms explains only a portion of the motivation for compulsive

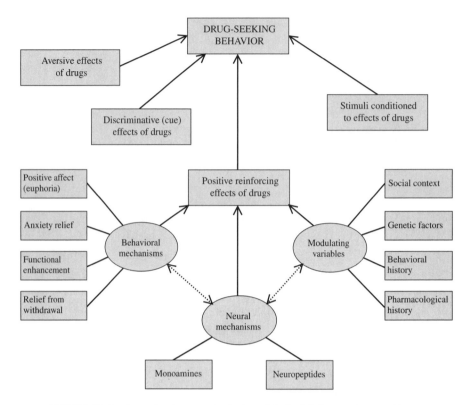

FIGURE 15.4 A psychopharmacological model of addiction as drug-seeking behavior controlled by four main processes: positive reinforcing and discriminative effects of drugs and of stimuli associated with them (which facilitate drug seeking), and aversive effects of drugs (which weaken the behavior). These four processes are common to drugs of many classes. A more detailed framework for analyzing positive reinforcing effects is shown (similar analyses could be made for discriminative and aversive effects); at this level it is envisaged that the relative importance of the different factors shown in the diagram will vary considerably between classes of drugs. [From Stolerman,[8] fig. 1, p. 171.]

abuse of drugs. Stolerman reviews the complementary mechanisms that underlie drug-seeking behavior.[8] As shown in Figure 15.4, a drug's ability to serve as a positive reinforcer is the minimum requirement for a drug to maintain drug-seeking behavior. Such positive reinforcement is maintained by three influences:

1. the neural mechanisms previously discussed

2. behavioral mechanisms, including drug-induced euphoria, relief from anxiety, functional enhancement, and relief from withdrawal

3. multiple modulating variables, including the social context in which the drug is used, genetic factors, attitudes, expectations, and the history of previous reinforcement and reward

Besides the positive reinforcing effects of drugs, discriminative (cue) effects of drugs contribute to drug-seeking behavior (Figure 15.4). Here, drug-seeking behavior is associated with its perceived effects. This factor contributes to drug relapse and withdrawal, possibly as an anxiogenic stimulus. These effects "have the potential to cue the appearance of drug-seeking behavior."[7]

Aversive effects of drugs tend to reduce drug-seeking behavior by means of negative reward and punishment mechanisms. These mechanisms "may set an upper limit to the amount of drugs that may be sought."[21]

Finally, environmental stimuli can become associated with drug-seeking behavior through classical conditioning responses. These stimuli strengthen behavior to a level greater than that obtained by the drug effect alone. For example, in cigarette dependency, the sight of other smokers and the taste and smell of cigarette smoke are powerful reinforcers, over and above the physiological effects of nicotine.

DRUG USE AND ABUSE

Our choice of methods is limited for reducing the level of drug abuse in our society. Over the years, we have passed laws designed to limit the availability of drugs and to punish drug users deemed dangerous to themselves or to society. When these laws are strictly enforced, they can reduce drug use by persons who fear reprisal. However, experience has shown that aggressive legislation does not control a person's desire for mind-altering drugs. Moreover, the legislation fails to address the legal drugs that cause the greatest amount of harm to individuals and society—alcohol and nicotine.

Widespread legalization of behavior-reinforcing drugs probably would not be effective, and it certainly is politically unlikely. Jonas states

> simple legalization of the currently illegal drugs, if properly implemented, could solve much of the drug-traffic-related crime problem. However, it would do nothing to solve the substance abuse problem, especially that major part of it caused by tobacco and alcohol.[22]

Our government, which has traditionally used a legalistic and moralistic approach to drug abuse, is adamantly against the relaxation of penalties for any currently illegal drug. For example, as stated in the 1989 White House report *National Drug Control Strategy:*

> In short, legalizing drugs would be an unqualified national disaster. In fact, any significant relaxation of drug enforcement—for whatever reason, however well-intentioned—would promise more use, more crime, and more trouble for desperately needed treatment and education efforts.[23]

Our current "war" against drugs focuses on only the illegal drugs and defines the drug abuse problem in terms of violations of the law rather than individual and public health. Such an approach is maintained despite a federal antidrug budget of almost $12 billion with about 50 percent dedicated to law enforcement.

Other traditional techniques for reducing drug abuse include education and developing negative attitudes toward drugs in both users and potential users. Such efforts have brought limited results without focusing on the real drug problem.

> Current national policy has a number of defects. Perhaps the most serious one is that it directs the bulk of its attention to the lesser of the harms. In 1989, there were about 500,000 deaths (in the United States) associated with the use of alcohol and tobacco. The 1990 NIDA Household Survey reported that the number of regular cocaine users has risen by 15%, from 292,000 to 335,000. Thus there were one-third fewer regular cocaine users in 1990 than there are alcohol and tobacco deaths each year. Yet the Office of National Drug Control Policy focuses exclusively on the former.[24]

With this in mind, it is time to take a public health approach to the problem of drug abuse. As advocated by Jonas, the primary goal of this approach is to

> reduce the use and abuse of all the recreational mood-altering drugs to provide for their safe, pleasurable use, consistent with centuries' old human experience, while minimizing to the greatest degree possible their harmful effects in individuals, the family, and society as a whole.[25]

To achieve this goal, we must acknowledge the following facts:

1. Many psychoactive drugs (and virtually all drugs of abuse) are potent behavioral reinforcers, and that fact alone will always lead to misuse.

2. There will always be a segment of society that will abuse behavior-reinforcing drugs.

3. Given a market, there will always be an available supply of drugs and people to distribute them.

4. A drugfree society should not be a goal of government policymakers.

5. Two legal drugs, alcohol and nicotine, are far more dangerous than many illegal drugs.

6. It is necessary to teach people how to coexist with potentially harmful drugs without being harmed by them.

One of the most heartening developments today is the widening effort to teach moral values in our nation's schools. The direness of the drug epidemic has provided immense impetus. Further, more Americans now realize that the best way to prevent drug addiction is to inculcate a sense of personal worth and personal integrity. No other item is more important in our students' curricula.[26]

Clearly, both the family and the community are vital in the effort to prevent drug abuse. Parents must set examples, show concern, exert influence, clarify values, provide open communication, and teach individual responsibility. Parents should certainly abstain from cigarettes, drink alcohol in moderation, and avoid driving after drinking. Parents can be positive educators if they act as good role models, provide accurate information, and show alternatives to the drug experience. Similarly, peer programs and peer influence can be effective in building a person's sense of self-worth and thus in reducing the attractiveness of drugs.

Shedler and Block expanded on this concept of values and upbringing as a factor in drug abuse.[27] They reported that adolescents who are frequent abusers of drugs had significant behavioral maladjustments before they began to use drugs. Drug use is therefore a symptom, not a cause, of personal and social maladjustment. These authors emphasized that drug use and abuse can be understood only in the context of an individual's personality structure and developmental history. Drug abuse is only part of a broad psychological syndrome that is not adequately explained in terms of peer influences. Social policy should not try to eliminate drug experimentation by adolescents. Indeed, adolescents with a history of drug experimentation but who are not frequent users of drugs can be quite stable and well adjusted. Instead, social policies should try to foster sensitive and empathic parenting, self-esteem, interpersonal relationships, and meaningful goals in life.

Drug Education

The classic approach to teaching people about the actions of psychoactive drugs is to describe (1) how the body absorbs, distributes, metabolizes, and excretes the drugs; (2) how the brain is organized and operates; (3) how neuronal function is related to behavior; and (4) how these functions are altered when drugs are ingested. Such a scheme avoids many of the complications that are inherent in an emotion-laden approach to drug education. The facts that are provided leave no room for mystery.

Of course, such an approach necessarily provides explicit directions for taking drugs. This result has been amply demonstrated in comprehensive drug education programs that increased the extent of drug use rather than decreased it. However, the goal of drug education is not only to decrease drug use but to provide accurate information. With such information, people can examine and modify their own risk-taking behavior and thus make the informed decisions necessary to lead a healthy life in the community at large.

No program of drug education can guarantee the elimination of —or even a drastic reduction in—the use of psychoactive drugs. However, such a program can teach society all the beneficial and harmful effects of a given drug (whether licit and illicit). As a result, society should be able to view drugs in proper perspective. However, education alone will not dissuade youth from experimenting with drugs, nor will it prevent some individuals from becoming drug dependent. A recent White Paper from the U.S. Office of National Drug Abuse Policy stated the following:

> Although [drug prevention] programs may not prevent someone from ever using drugs, they may well contribute toward a person ultimately leading a drug-free life. Furthermore, if a program can delay the onset of first use of a drug, while not the primary goal of prevention, it will decrease the likelihood of the user becoming addicted and a burden on society.[28]

To alter the behavior of youth requires both education and examples set by teachers, peers, parents, and, indeed, the whole community. As stated by Goldstein, three steps are necessary:

- Basic information has to be imparted—truthful information—to generate motivation for behavior change. Only honest, straightforward, and full information about the health risks of the addictive drugs will meet this requirement.
- The means for behavior change have to be provided. Here many techniques have proven effective, especially teaching children how

to resist peer pressure. It is important to promote a redefinition of drug-using peers as not "cool."

• Methods for reinforcing the new behaviors have to be employed. This means, in short, that children need recognition, praise, and other rewards for not using drugs. Emphasis on how drugs detract from a healthy body and an attractive appearance, for example, appeals to adolescents' interest in athletics as well as to their developing sexuality and their striving for intimate peer relationships.[29]

In essence, this approach is directed toward building one's self-esteem in a drugfree environment. While praiseworthy, this approach works best for those least likely to abuse drugs.[27] Youth from stable, non-drug-using, supportive families in communities not scarred by violence and drug trafficking are more likely to respond positively. The situation is vastly different for other populations:

> Adolescents whose lives have already been scarred by dysfunctional family situations, poverty, or exposure to violence may be unable to see how using or selling drugs could make matters any worse; and they may view drugs as a way to alleviate their pain and despair or as a quick route to material gain. These adolescents need drug prevention programs that are both more intensive and appropriate to their lives and experiences.[30]

Ultimately, prevention of drug abuse requires that adults be willing to set a consistent example by avoiding psychoactive drug use and enforcing the laws that restrict access of minors to psychoactive and dependency-producing drugs. Such action is particularly important regarding cigarettes and alcohol; the casualness with which we use these drugs and allow their promotion demonstrates both our personal ignorance and our hypocrisy about the use of addicting drugs.

In addition to prevention, we must address the problem of the treatment of drug-dependent individuals. First, individuals must be moved from addiction to a drugfree state, and second, they must be prevented from relapse. Primm quotes from a recent study[31] by the Institute of Medicine: "The study's conclusion that 'addiction is a chronic relapsing disorder that requires continuous aftercare and follow-up' may be the first time that a major scientific body has, after in-depth research and deliberation, accepted this concept."[32]

Practical and Immediate Efforts

Perhaps the most important element of the Public Health Approach is that there will be a single national policy for controlling the abuse of all the recreational mood-altering drugs. This policy will apply to each and every recreational mood-altering drug, whether it is currently legal or currently illegal. This policy will end the current "OK"/"not-OK" drug dichotomy.[33]

Such a policy must incorporate the following components:

1. a scientifically based system for classifying recreational, mood-altering drugs

2. a broad definition of "responsible use" that takes into account age, drug, time, place, and other risk factors

3. a rational price/tax structure for whatever drugs are legal

4. guidelines for pro-drug advertising

Deterring the use of cigarettes and alcohol, which extract a multi-billion-dollar toll in lives, health, and productivity, should be the top priority in a drug abuse campaign. These substances should be the major focus of educational, regulatory, and enforcement efforts.

In addition, we must be prepared to meet the challenge of the sudden and episodic emergence of fashionable, potent, and dangerous drugs, such as crack cocaine, methamphetamine, ICE methamphetamine, anabolic-androgenic steroids, and "designer" derivatives of psychedelics and narcotics.

Cigarettes

There is no "safe use" of cigarettes, and there is no such thing as responsible use of cigarettes.[22]

Cigarettes are the only product which, when used as directed, increase the risk of death and disease.[34]

The extent of people's addiction to cigarettes is clear. The many serious consequences that smoking has on the lungs and the cardiovascular system are described in Chapter 7.

The worst consequences of smoking by women are the effects on reproduction and children. Maternal smoking affects growth, intellectual and emotional development, and behavior of the newborn. A recent report notes a significant level of nicotine not only in the hair of infants whose mothers smoked but also in the hair of infants whose mothers reported having been exposed to environmental tobacco smoke while pregnant.[35] To give an unborn child the best chance of being normal both at birth and during later development, a mother-to-be must avoid cigarette smoking and exposure to environmental smoke.

Cigarette smoking by younger women began reaching crisis proportions in the 1980s;[36] the incidence of cigarette smoking among women today approaches that among men.[37] The increase in cigarette smoking by women has largely been attributed to cigarette advertisements:

> Over the past half century and with remarkable consistency, tobacco advertising has linked smoking with women's emancipation and achievement of equality with men. Themes like "You've come a long way, baby" and the introduction of a new cigarette "For women who know the meaning of free" testify to the continuing marketing appeal of stressing independence and equal right to enjoyment.[37]

Marketing to women includes special packaging and the introduction of "designer" cigarettes, promising sophistication, attractiveness, a slender body, and sex appeal.

> The health consequences of smoking are well documented, as is the addictiveness of the behavior that prevents many smokers from being able to successfully quit before these health consequences manifest. ... We have demonstrated that tobacco advertising has a temporal and specific relationship to smoking uptake in girls younger than the legal age to purchase cigarettes. Our findings add to the evidence that tobacco advertising plays an important role in encouraging young people to begin this lifelong addiction before they are old enough to fully appreciate its long-term risks.[37]

Such promotional efforts are directed not only at young, impressionable females but also at their male counterparts:

> By sponsoring auto races, tennis tournaments, and other sporting events, tobacco companies maintain a high profile among young impressionable fans. Such sponsorship helps to associate tobacco with success, glamour, social popularity, and lots of fun, rather than with deadly drug addiction.[38]

Blum notes that sponsorship of motor racing has become one of the major promotional activities used by the tobacco industry.[39] During a one-and-a-half-hour televised auto race, the Marlboro logotype was shown 5933 times for a total exposure of 46 minutes. Indeed, the surgeon general's 23rd report on smoking and health, *Preventing Tobacco Use among Young People*, published in 1994, addresses the problem of smoking by youth.[40]

Cigarette smoking is clearly the most widespread example of drug dependence, the most preventable cause of disease and disability, and the most unnecessary of modern epidemics in the world today. Forty-six million Americans still smoke, and cigarettes cause more illness and death than any other drug. The major problem is that most of the severe consequences of smoking have a delayed onset—often 20 years or more, at which time much of the damage is irreversible. Smoking and dependence develop early in life, usually during adolescence, when the feeling of personal invulnerability is maximal. As many as 3 million teenagers smoke, and as many as 3000 youngsters start smoking every day. The inevitable toxicity is not appreciated until the smoker reaches middle age.

The health-related costs of cigarette smoking in the United States were greater than $50 billion in 1993. This figure includes direct medical costs (hospital, doctors, medication, home health care, and nursing homes) for smokers who suffer from smoking-induced illnesses. This figures translates into an average medical cost of $2.06 for each pack of cigarettes smoked. In addition, another $47 billion was wasted in lost productivity. Finally, more than 420,000 deaths occur yearly as a result of smoking.

Given these facts and statistics, what should be our educational, legislative, and enforcement response? Satcher and Eriksen list six ways to prevent and control tobacco use:[41]

1. prevent the onset of tobacco use

2. treat nicotine addiction

3. protect nonsmokers from exposure to environmental tobacco smoke

4. promote nonsmoking messages while limiting the effect of tobacco advertising and promotion on young people

5. increase the price of tobacco products (with proceeds going to treatment and prevention programs so that the government does not profit from the increase in taxation)

6. regulate tobacco products

Former U.S. Surgeon General Antonia Novello urges the following steps:[34]

1. expose the seduction of our children by the tobacco industry and work proactively to counter its messages and techniques

2. spur legislation that will limit minors' access to tobacco, including the banning of cigarette vending machines and the sale of single cigarettes, and the restriction of cigarette sales to closely controlled outlets (Klonoff and coworkers demonstrate how easily minors can buy cigarettes, especially in minority neighborhoods.[42])

3. speak out against the seduction of women by the tobacco industry

4. alert the public about the dangers of environmental tobacco smoke

5. control the widespread use of smokeless or "spit" tobacco as a "safe" alternative to smoking

6. recognize the importance of price in controlling tobacco use, especially in youth

7. document, assess, and change society's attitudes and practices regarding tobacco use, especially where our children are concerned

8. strengthen and harness our tools for controlling tobacco: legislation, taxation, and individual and public health education

9. become personally involved in prevention and control

Although these suggestions will not remove cigarettes from our culture, they might prepare adults to live cigarette-free in a society where cigarettes are readily available.

Alcohol

In addition to cigarettes, we should be equally concerned about alcohol. Alcohol is the direct cause of death for more than 31,000 Americans each year and an indirect cause of more than 37,000 deaths by accident or violence. Fifty percent of our highway deaths involve alcohol, and the drug is a factor in 70 percent of homicides.

Every year the average American consumes the equivalent of three gallons of pure alcohol. This amount of alcohol is equivalent to 591 twelve-ounce cans of beer, 115 fifths of table wine, or 35 fifths of 80-proof liquor. Samson and Harris reference government estimates that in the United States the cost of alcohol-related problems was about $136 billion in 1990 and could easily exceed $150 billion by 1995.[43] These problems include medical treatment of alcoholism; alcohol-related illness; fetal alcohol syndrome; loss of life, productivity, and property (including fire losses); crime; motor vehicle accidents; and social costs (for courts, jails, law enforcement, etc.). One out of four families is troubled by a family member who drinks alcohol—the highest incidence of problem drinking in 37 years. An estimated 10 million adults in the United States are alcoholics, and 7 million adults are problem drinkers. Alcohol-associated deaths account for at least 25 times more deaths than those caused by all the illegal drugs combined.

Especially devastating are the injuries and fatalities among youths:

1. More than 40 percent of teenage deaths result from automobile accidents, and more than half of them involve alcohol.

2. Alcohol-related motor vehicle crashes are the number one public health problem among young people.[44]

3. Approximately 10 youths between 15 and 19 years of age die each day from alcohol-related traffic accidents.

4. Youths between 15 and 24 years of age account for 37 percent of all alcohol-related traffic deaths.

5. A yearly cost of over $6 billion is incurred by teenage drivers who cause automobile accidents while under the influence of alcohol.

6. More than 30 percent of high school seniors report recent binge drinking. Junior and senior high school students consume 1.1 billion cans of beer each year, which translates into more than $200 million in revenues for the beer industry alone.[44]

By a 1987 estimate, an 18-year-old has seen more than 100,000 beer commercials.[45] Thus, teenagers are repeatedly exposed to alcohol advertising, but the influence of such advertising on youth has only recently been addressed. Quite clearly, this advertising has a powerful impact on our society and particularly on children, their peer groups, and their families.

Grube and Wallack[46] and Madden and Grube[47] documented that televised sports programming is saturated with beer advertising, especially in sports associated with a high risk of traumatic injury. Youth are particularly likely to watch such shows. By interview, the researchers determined that alcohol advertising has a powerful influence over youths' drinking beliefs and intentions, predisposing young people to drink:

> Children who were more aware of beer advertisements held more favorable beliefs about drinking, intended to drink more frequently as adults, and had more knowledge of beer brands and slogans. The findings provide support for the hypothesis that awareness of alcohol advertising influences children's drinking beliefs, knowledge, and intentions.[48]

Obviously, millions of dollars would not be spent on youth-targeted beer advertising if it did not effectively recruit new drinkers. Mosher concludes that beer advertising has a powerful impact on society, particularly on children.[44] Also, the beer industry's refusal to reform its marketing practices reflects a fundamental lack of concern for public safety and the health of our youth. Needed is new legislation to curtail youth-targeted alcohol and tobacco advertising.

To limit the numbers of persons who are harmed by alcohol, society should implement the following general policies:

1. Eliminate alcohol promotion to minors, and limit youth-targeted advertising.

2. Strictly enforce minimum-age drinking laws.

3. Teach people responsible methods of drinking for those occasions when they feel it is necessary, or socially appropriate, to drink.

4. Enforce drunk driving laws more strictly. Reduce the legal blood alcohol limit to 0.08 percent for adults and to 0.00 (zero) percent for drivers under 18 years of age.

5. Educate judges so that they understand the need for harsh penalties and rehabilitation when they are sentencing intoxicated drivers.[49] Any driver found with a blood alcohol level above the legal limit should have his or her driver's license suspended.

6. Educate people so that they dissociate the drinking of alcoholic beverages from the smoking of cigarettes. Most long-term drinkers are smokers, and some toxicities are additive.

7. Discourage all advertising that associates the use of alcohol with socializing.[45]

We often seem to have become desensitized to the deaths, illnesses, traffic accidents, family traumas, social havoc, and dollar costs associated with the use of alcohol. At a minimum, we must teach people to make conscious decisions about the use of alcohol. For example, we all know that alcohol interferes with a person's ability to drive an automobile, yet people who drink alcohol continue to drive. Few people seem to understand the relationship between drinking alcohol, the blood levels of alcohol that result, and the impairment of driving ability that follows.

In many states, a blood alcohol concentration (BAC) of 0.10 percent indicates "intoxication," and a person who drives with a BAC of 0.10 percent or greater may be charged with "driving while under the influence of alcohol." Thus, many people assume that a level of 0.09 percent is acceptable but a level of 0.11 percent is not. However, the behavioral effects of alcohol are not all or none; alcohol (like all sedatives) progressively impairs a person's ability to function. Thus, the 0.10-percent blood level is only a legally established, arbitrary value. Driving ability is minimally impaired at a BAC of 0.01 to 0.04 percent. However, at 0.05 to 0.09 percent, a driver has increasingly impaired judgment and reactions and becomes less inhibited; as a result, the risk of an accident quadruples. The deterioration of a person's driving ability continues at a BAC of 0.10 to 0.14 percent, leading to a sixfold to sevenfold increase in the risk of having an accident. At 0.15 percent and higher, a person is 25 times more likely to become involved in a serious accident.

Figure 15.5 illustrates the correlation between alcohol and driving impairment. To use this chart, first glance at the left margin and find the number that is closest to your body weight in pounds. Then, look

Blood Alcohol Concentration—a guide

Drinks   One drink equals 1 ounce of 80 proof alcohol; 12 ounce
bottle of beer; 2 ounces of 20% wine; 3 ounces of 12% wine.

Weight (lb)	1	2	3	4	5	6	7	8	9	10
100	.029	.058	.088	.117	.146	.175	.204	.233	.262	.290
120	.024	.048	.073	.097	.121	.145	.170	.194	.219	.243
140	.021	.042	.063	.083	.104	.125	.146	.166	.187	.208
160	.019	.037	.055	.073	.091	.109	.128	.146	.164	.182
180	.017	.033	.049	.065	.081	.097	.113	.130	.146	.162
200	.015	.029	.044	.058	.073	.087	.102	.117	.131	.146
220	.014	.027	.040	.053	.067	.080	.093	.106	.119	.133
240	.012	.024	.037	.048	.061	.073	.085	.097	.109	.122

CAUTION	DRIVING IMPAIRED	LEGALLY DRUNK

Alcohol is "burned up" by your body at .015% per hour, as follows:

No. hours since starting first drink	1	2	3	4	5	6
Percent alcohol burned up	.015	.030	.045	.060	.075	.090

Calculate your BAC

Example: 180 lb man—8 drinks in 4 hours is .130% on chart.
Subtract .060% burned up in 4 hours. BAC equals .070%—DRIVING IMPAIRED.

FIGURE 15.5   Relation between blood alcohol concentration, body weight, and the number of drinks ingested. See text for details. Wallet-sized copies of this table are available from the Washington State Liquor Control Board, Capitol Plaza Building, Olympia, Washington 98504. [Data developed by Richard Zylman, Center for Alcohol Studies, Rutgers University, New Brunswick, N.J.]

across the columns to the right and find the column that shows the number of drinks that you have consumed. By matching your body weight with the number of drinks that you have ingested, you can find your BAC. From this number, subtract the amount of alcohol that has been metabolized (remember from Chapter 4 that approximately 1 ounce of hard liquor is metabolized in 1 hour). The final figure is your approximate BAC. By calculating this number, you can predict the degree to which your driving ability is impaired.

The following examples illustrate how to use the chart in Figure 15.5. Consider a 140-pound man who takes 6 drinks in 2 hours. The chart value for the blood alcohol concentration is 0.125 percent. Subtract 0.030 percent for metabolism (0.015 percent × 2 hours). His resulting BAC is 0.095 percent, which is not legally intoxicating (in most states) but is enough to impair his driving ability. Next, consider a 120-pound woman who also takes 6 drinks in 2 hours. The chart value is 0.145 percent. Subtract the same 0.030 percent for metabolism. Her resulting BAC is 0.115 percent, which is a legally intoxicating value.

As mentioned in Chapter 5, the presence of another sedative in the body will potentiate the effects of alcohol. Such potentiation is not

included in Figure 15.5. Thus, the person who has ingested other sedatives as well as alcohol will be more impaired than the chart in Figure
15.5 indicates.

Nosology of Drug Abuse

Drug abuse is difficult to define.[50] In general, it seems to imply the use
of any drug for reasons other than its assigned purposes. Does it refer
to use only in medical treatment? Is any use of drugs for reasons other
than the treatment of medically diagnosed disorders abuse? Are there
no legitimate uses of drugs for nonmedical, recreational pursuits? The
history of the use of psychoactive drugs (including alcohol) clearly indicates that psychoactive drugs may be used for recreation, relaxation,
or escape when one feels that there are no better alternatives.

Figure 15.6 presents a continuum of use and abuse of psychoactive
drugs. *Legitimate uses* of psychoactive drugs, listed in Table 15.1, are
not all medical and cannot be dictated by law. Thus, some drugs can be
used legitimately for recreation and as a means of experiencing altered
states of consciousness. As noted above, the public health approach to
managing drug abuse accepts the centuries-old concept of recreational
drug use, while attempting to minimize the possible dangers to the individual and to society.

Drug misuse is the use of any drug (legal or illegal) for a medical
or recreational purpose when other alternatives are available, practical, or warranted or when drug use endangers either the users or
others who are around them. In medicine, drug misuse applies to seeking, prescribing, or using of any drug for any purpose other than the
prevention or treatment of diagnosed disease or the alleviation of
physical or mental discomfort. A physician who prescribes a mild
sedative (such as a benzodiazepine) for a patient merely because the
patient requested it or to terminate the interview with a patient may be
allowing the patient to misuse a drug. A recreational drug is misused
when it impedes the user's social functioning, when it results in a

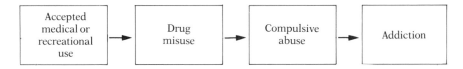

FIGURE 15.6   A continuum of the use and abuse of psychoactive drugs.

TABLE 15.1 Medical and recreational uses of psychoactive drugs.

Medical
1. Treatment or prevention of diagnosed disease
2. Alleviation of physical or mental discomfort

Recreational
1. Relief from anxiety
2. Achievement of a state of disinhibition or euphoria
3. Achievement of altered states of consciousness
4. Expansion of creative abilities
5. Attempt to gain interpersonal or external insight
6. Escape from uncomfortable or oppressive surroundings
7. Experience of altered states of mood

preoccupation with drug use, or when it endangers the physical or mental health of the user or others (harmful use).

Compulsive abuse is an extension of misuse. It refers to the state where a person uses a drug despite adverse social or medical consequences. In compulsive abuse, the user has developed an intense reliance on the effects of self-administered drugs.

Addiction is a further extension of drug use. It refers to the state where a person is overwhelmingly involved with using a drug and securing its supply. The addicted person has a high tendency to relapse after the drug has been withdrawn. Drug use thus pervades the user's life and controls his or her behavior.

The vagueness of the terms *misuse* and *abuse* led the World Health Organization to abandon these terms and to replace them with the following:

1. Unsanctioned Use: Use of a drug not approved by a society or a group within that society. Who disapproves should be made clear when the term is used. The term implies the acceptance of disapproval without having to determine or justify its basis.

2. Hazardous Use: Use of a drug that will probably lead to harmful consequences for the user.

3. Dysfunctional Use: Use of a drug that leads to impaired psychological or social functioning (e.g., loss of job or marital problems).

4. Harmful Use: Use of a drug that is known to have caused the particular person tissue damage or mental illness.[50]

Drug education and treatment must consider the extent of a person's behavioral and physiological involvement with psychoactive drugs. Although educational programs and alternatives to drug use may be useful approaches, formal treatment programs are necessary for those persons who are compulsive abusers or addicts. As stated by Jaffe:

> The indications for treatment vary with the drugs being used as well as with the social and cultural factors determining the particular pattern of drug use. Some patterns of drug use, such as weekly use of [less reinforcing drugs such as] marijuana, do not require treatment any more than does the occasional smoking of tobacco or the social use of alcohol. Such casual use is not without hazard, and it may jeopardize vocational status. . . . However, such patterns of use do not necessarily constitute a treatable disorder. It is likely that changing views about drug use will continue to create gray areas where the indications for treatment are unclear. However, there is general agreement that treatment is appropriate for the adverse consequences of drug use and for the compulsive drug user who voluntarily seeks help.[51]

Alternatives to Drugs

Society must not only teach cognitive-behavioral decision-making skills to combat drug misuse but also provide suitable alternatives to the drug experience to reduce the reliance on the recreational use of drugs. These alternatives to using drugs must be matched to the type of experience that a drug user is seeking and the motives for seeking that experience. Provision of nondrug, natural highs, for example, might replace drug-induced altered states of consciousness. New experiences might be achieved by high-energy activities (athletics, dance, and so on), creative endeavors (photography or business training), interpersonal activities (for example, Outward Bound), and spiritual and self-worth training (religious retreats and experiences), to name only a few.

Implementing these alternatives should be a high priority for family, community, and society. Almost 25 years ago, Beecher remarked:

> These and other "alternatives to the drug experience" are gaining favor among young people because they are superior to drugs, not because they are safer than drugs. An experienced drug user . . . often finds that some form of meditation more effectively satisfies his desire to get high. One sees a great many drug takers give up drugs

for meditation, but one does not see any meditators giving up meditation for drugs. Once you have learned from a drug what being high
really is, you can begin to reproduce it without the drug; all persons
who accomplish this feat testify that the non-drug high is superior.[52]

General Policies for the 1990s and the Twenty-first Century

To conclude, we list a few policies that will be necessary to address our
current drug abuse problem:

1. As noted above, we must consider drug addiction and drug
dependence as primarily a public health problem.[22] Harm reduction
to the individual and to society should be the central strategy of this
approach.

2. Crime, whether or not it is drug related, is primarily a law
enforcement problem. Law enforcement personnel rarely need to deal
with the majority of drug-addicted individuals; they only need address
the actual crime committed. Noting this fact will separate public
health problems from the enforcement of the law.

3. All drugs must be evaluated by their potential to cause harm,
regardless of legal status. Such an evaluation will further keep the
function of public health and legal agencies separate.

4. Punitive measures to eliminate the supply of drugs has failed in
the past and is failing now. Thus, preventive measures must be aimed
at reducing the demand for drugs. Education, alternatives to drug use,
curtailment of advertising, treatment, relapse prevention, and other
measures are intended to reduce the demand, regardless of available
supply. Jonas states that "the drug problem is caused primarily by
demand for drugs and those factors which create demand."[22]

5. We need to address the problem of youth-oriented advertising
of cigarettes and alcohol, as discussed above.

6. We need to address the problem of birth defects and other fetal
damage induced by maternal use of psychoactive drugs. Nothing is
more disastrous than the harm done to an innocent victim by drugs
consumed by a pregnant woman.

7. We must address the spread of AIDS by intravenous drug users.

These approaches should

reduce the use and abuse of all the recreational drugs; reduce the
tremendous pressure on and corruption of the criminal justice and
law-enforcement systems created by the present approach, freeing

them to focus on other criminal behaviors; and largely pay for itself through taxes on recreational drug sales, use, advertising, and profits. Its major political downside is that it requires a major assault on the tobacco and alcohol industries. But it can be done. Based on the record achieved by public health so far, it will meet with success.[53]

Study Questions

1. What is meant when a particular psychoactive drug is called a "behavioral reinforcer"?
2. Why might the evaluation of drug reinforcing properties in animals be valuable in the assessment of human experiences?
3. Is a propensity to abusing drugs caused by a psychopathological process in the user, or is it a property of the drug in particular? Defend your position.
4. On a physiological level, what might explain the lack of self-reinforcing action of phenothiazines or tricyclic antidepressants?
5. What is the mechanism that underlies the behavioral reinforcing properties of certain psychoactive drugs?
6. List several key principles that underlie a positive approach toward drug abuse education.
7. Where has drug education failed? How might drug education be used successfully?
8. List, from the most harmful to the least harmful, the classes of psychoactive drugs that have been presented in this text. Defend your choices.
9. How do the entries in the list made in the previous question correlate in terms of social acceptance and current legal status?
10. Should certain drugs be more readily available? How should our legislative efforts be directed?

Notes

1. J. H. Jaffe, "Drug Addiction and Drug Abuse," in A. G. Gilman, T. W. Rall, A. S. Nies, and P. Taylor, eds., *Goodman and Gilman's The Pharmacological Basis of Therapeutics*, 8th ed. (New York: Pergamon, 1990), p. 522.
2. E. L. Gardner, "Brain Reward Mechanisms," in J. H. Lowinson, P. Ruiz, R. B. Millman, and J. G. Langrod, eds., *Substance Abuse: A Comprehensive Textbook*, 2nd ed. (Baltimore: Williams & Wilkins, 1992), p. 70.
3. D. L. Dunner, ed., "Psychopharmacology II," *The Psychiatric Clinics of North America* 16, no. 4 (December 1993).
4. A. Goldstein, *Addiction: From Biology to Drug Policy* (New York: W. H. Freeman and Company, 1994), p. 9.

5. B. D. Johnson and J. Muffler, "Sociocultural Aspects of Drug Use and Abuse in the 1990s," in J. H. Lowinson, P. Ruiz, R. B. Millman, and J. G. Langrod, eds., *Substance Abuse: A Comprehensive Textbook,* 2nd ed. (Baltimore: Williams & Wilkins, 1992), pp. 118–137.

6. Goldstein, *Addiction,* p. 6.

7. G. F. Koob, "Drugs of Abuse: Anatomy, Pharmacology, and Function of Reward Pathways," *Trends in Pharmacologic Sciences* 13 (1992): p. 177.

8. I. Stolerman, "Drugs of Abuse: Behavioral Principles, Methods, and Terms," *Trends in Pharmacological Sciences* 13 (1992): p. 171.

9. C.-E. Johanson, "Behavioral Studies of the Reinforcing Properties of Cocaine," in D. Clouet, K. Asqhar, and R. Brown, eds., *Mechanisms of Cocaine Abuse and Toxicity,* NIDA Research Monograph 88 (Rockville, Md.: National Institute on Drug Abuse, 1988), p. 110.

10. Jaffe, "Drug Addiction and Drug Abuse," p. 524.

11. R. L. Bolster, "Pharmacological Effects of Cocaine Relevant to Its Abuse," in D. Clouet, K. Asqhar, and R. Brown, eds., *Mechanisms of Cocaine Abuse and Toxicity,* NIDA Research Monograph 88 (Rockville, Md.: National Institute on Drug Abuse, 1988), pp. 1–13.

12. C.-E. Johanson, "Assessing the Reinforcing Properties of Drugs," in L. S. Harris, ed., *Problems of Drug Dependence, 1989,* NIDA Research Monograph 95 (Rockville, Md.: National Institute on Drug Abuse, 1990), p. 136.

13. N. S. Miller and M. S. Gold, "A Hypothesis for a Common Neurochemical Basis for Alcohol and Drug Disorders," *Psychiatric Clinics of North America* 16 (1993): 105–117.

14. R. R. Griffiths, G. E. Bigelow, and I. A. Liebson, "Reinforcing Effects of Caffeine in Coffee and Capsules," *Journal of the Experimental Analysis of Behavior* 52 (1989): 127–140.

15. K. Battig and H. Welzl, "Psychopharmacological Profile of Caffeine," in S. Garattini, ed., *Caffeine, Coffee, and Health* (New York: Raven Press, 1993), pp. 213–253.

16. Gardner, "Brain Reward Mechanisms," p. 71.

17. Ibid., pp. 76–77.

18. Koob, "Drugs of Abuse," p. 178.

19. Gardner, "Brain Reward Mechanisms," p. 78.

20. Ibid., p. 86.

21. Stolerman, "Drugs of Abuse," p. 174.

22. S. Jonas, "Public Health Approach to the Prevention of Substance Abuse," in J. H. Lowinson, P. Ruiz, R. B. Millman, and J. G. Langrod, eds., *Substance Abuse: A Comprehensive Textbook,* 2nd ed. (Baltimore: Williams & Wilkins, 1992), p. 936.

23. Office of National Drug Control Policy, *National Drug Control Strategy* (Washington, D.C.: U.S. Government Printing Office, 1989), p. 13.

24. Jonas, "Public Health Approach," p. 930.

25. Ibid., p. 929.

26. M. S. Forbes, "Fact and Comment," *Forbes* (1 December 1986), p. 25.

27. J. Shedler and J. Block, "Adolescent Drug Use and Psycho-logical Health," *American Psychologist* 45 (1990): 612–630.

28. Office of National Drug Control Policy, Executive Office of the President, *Understanding Drug Prevention* (Washington, D.C.: U.S. Government Printing Office, 1992), p. 16.

29. Goldstein, *Addiction*, pp. 208–209.

30. Office of National Drug Control Policy, *Understanding Drug Prevention*, p. 17.

31. Institute of Medicine, *Treating Drug Problems: A Study of the Evolution, Effectiveness, and Financing of Public and Private Drug Treatment Systems*, vol. 1 (Washington, D.C.: National Academy Press, 1990).

32. B. J. Primm, "Future Outlook: Treatment Improvement," in J. H. Lowinson, P. Ruiz, R. B. Millman, and J. G. Langrod, eds., *Substance Abuse: A Comprehensive Textbook*, 2nd ed. (Baltimore: Williams & Wilkins, 1992), p. 624.

33. Jonas, "Public Health Approach," p. 938.

34. A. C. Novello, "From the Surgeon General, U.S. Public Health Service," *Journal of the American Medical Association* 270 (1993): 806.

35. C. Eliopoulos and others, "Hair Concentrations of Nicotine and Cotinene in Women and Their Newborn Infants," *Journal of the American Medical Association* 271 (1994): 621–623.

36. J. E. Fielding, "Smoking and Women: Tragedy of the Majority," *New England Journal of Medicine* 317 (1987): 1343-1345.

37. J. P. Pierce, L. Lee, and E. A. Gilpin, "Smoking Initiation by Adolescent Girls, 1944 through 1988," *Journal of the American Medical Association* 271 (1994): 608–611.

38. A. A. Skolnick, "Kid Stuff," *Journal of the American Medical Association* 271 (1994): 578–579.

39. A. Blum, "The Marlboro Grand Prix. Circumvention of the Television Ban on Tobacco Advertising," *New England Journal of Medicine* 324 (1991): 913–917.

40. U.S. Department of Health and Human Services, *Preventing Tobacco Use among Young People: A Report of the Surgeon General* (Atlanta, Ga.: U.S. Department of Health and Human Services, Public Health Service, Centers for Disease Control and Prevention, National Center for Chronic Disease Prevention and Health Promotion, Office on Smoking and Health, 1994).

41. D. Satcher and M. Eriksen, "The Paradox of Tobacco Control," *Journal of the American Medical Association* 271 (1994): 627–628.

42. E. A. Klonoff, J. M. Fritz, H. Landrine, R. W. Riddle, and L. Tully-Payne, "The Problem and Sociocultural Context of Single-Cigarette Sales," *Journal of the American Medical Association* 271 (1994): 618–620.

43. H. H. Samson and R. A. Harris, "Neurobiology of Alcohol Abuse," *Trends in Pharmaceutical Science* 13 (1992): 206–211.

44. J. F. Mosher, "Alcohol Advertising and Public Health: An Urgent Call for Action," *American Journal of Public Health* 84 (1994): 180–181.

45. N. Postman, C. Nystrom, L. Strate, and C. Weingartner, *Myths, Men and Beer: An Analysis of Beer Commercials on Broadcast Television, 1987* (Falls Church, Va.: AAA Foundation for Traffic Safety, 1988).

46. J. W. Grube and L. Wallack, "Television Beer Advertising and Drinking Knowledge, Beliefs, and Intentions among Schoolchildren," *American Journal of Public Health* 84 (1994): 254–259.

47. P. A. Madden and J. W. Grube, "The Frequency and Nature of Alcohol and Tobacco Advertising in Televised Sports, 1990 through 1992," *American Journal of Public Health* 84 (1994): 297–299.

48. Grube and Wallack, "Television Beer Advertising," p. 257.

49. M. Colquitt, P. Fielding, and J. F. Cronan, "Drunk Drivers and Medical and Social Injury," *New England Journal of Medicine* 317 (12 November 1987): 1262–1266.

50. H. D. Kleber, "The Nosology of Abuse and Dependence," *Journal of Psychiatric Research* 24, Suppl. 2 (1990): 57–64.

51. Jaffe, "Drug Addiction and Drug Abuse," pp. 559–560.

52. E. M. Beecher and Consumer Reports editors, *Licit and Illicit Drugs* (Mt. Vernon, N.Y.: Consumers Union, 1972), p. 510.

53. Jonas, "Public Health Approach," p. 941.

CHAPTER 16

INTEGRATION OF DRUGS AND PSYCHOTHERAPY IN TREATING MENTAL DISORDERS

Donald E. Lange and Robert M. Julien

> Since no illness occurs in a vacuum, medications should never be prescribed as the sole treatment. There is a fluid interaction between an individual and that individual's illness (e.g., life situations may aggravate the illness and vice versa).[1]

This chapter describes the role of psychopharmacotherapy in the overall care of patients, a topic that is unavoidably intertwined with the topic of psychotherapy.* In particular, this chapter

1. describes the roles of medication and psychotherapy in the treatment of patients with mental disorders and describes the thorough assessment and accurate diagnosis vital to appropriate treatment

2. provides an overview of the standard classification system used in mental health, the fourth edition of the *Diagnostic and Statistical Manual of Mental Disorders* (DSM-IV)[2]

3. discusses the major categories of mental disorders that require an integrated treatment approach

Role of Medication

The use of psychoactive drugs in treating psychological illness is termed *psychopharmacotherapy*.[3] Only rarely do medications cure the

---

*As used in this chapter, the term *psychotherapy* covers a wide range of modalities, from education and supportive counseling to insight-oriented, dynamically based therapy.

presenting problem. For example, if a patient is experiencing hallucinations as a result of a schizophrenic disorder, neuroleptics (Chapter 11) can reduce some of the symptoms. However, the patient will not be cured—the medication will not eliminate the underlying process that is producing the hallucinations.

In addition to treating the symptomatology of mental disease, medication may serve a prophylactic function, preventing the onset of a symptom complex (e.g., reducing the frequency of recurrence of symptomatology). Thus, drugs can be used to ameliorate debilitating symptoms of acute or chronic conditions and to prevent the development of additional symptoms, thus allowing the introduction of nonpharmacological therapies.

Rarely are psychoactive drugs the only answer to a psychological problem. One large study found no difference between the effectiveness of antidepressant drugs and psychotherapeutic interventions when either treatment was used alone. However, in combination, they provided a synergistic effect that significantly decreased the time to recovery.[4,5] Thus, judicious use of drugs, while important in the successful treatment of many mental disorders, serves primarily as an adjunct to psychological therapies.

Role of the Treatment Team

No single health care provider is a sole caregiver. Usually a team of caregivers with members from several disciplines assists in the treatment of the patient.* One team member may be a clinician with prescription privileges. Another clinician who does not prescribe medication may have responsibility for psychotherapeutic interventions. However, the actions and side effects of the medications will affect the delivery of—and even the ability to deliver—treatment. Each team member must continually evaluate changes in symptomatology caused by the medication. This assessment includes the interrelationships between drug effects, psychotherapeutic effects, and the patient's overall goals in treatment. Team members should assess how a particular drug affects the treatment strategy and, conversely, how psychotherapy affects the intended therapeutic effects of prescribed medications.

Besides the prescribing clinician and the psychotherapist, other caregivers may include nurses, pharmacists, counselors, vocational

---

*In the outpatient setting, the individual under treatment is referred to as the "client"; in the hospital setting, this same individual is referred to as the "patient."

rehabilitation counselors, physical or occupational therapists, dieticians, pastoral counselors, psychiatric, occupational, or recreational assistants, and family members. Team rapport is improved if each member perceives that his or her input is accepted and appreciated. Each member must be an involved, active participant, addressing the patient's needs from the member's own frame of reference, which, in turn, affects the team member's perception of treatment or training needs. Thus, medication is an important variable in process intervention strategies and in psychotherapeutic outcomes.

All members of the treatment team need to know which drugs their clients are taking and which effects should be expected. All must monitor for both positive and negative effects. All must be sensitive to the meaning that medications have to the clients. Indeed, effective psychotherapy depends on the ability of patients to comply with treatment requirements. Thus patients must have at least a threshold level of concentration, cooperation, and motivation and must be free of incapacitating symptomatology.

Psychotropic medication is frequently used to help achieve these prerequisite conditions. Although the drug is prescribed for its beneficial effects, some side effects may reduce the patient's concentration or cooperation, thus hindering the patient's progress in psychotherapy. Similarly, inadequate doses of medication may decrease therapeutic effectiveness. Therefore, levels of the drug in blood may be monitored, especially when there is either an inadequate response to the drug or when side effects become prominent.[6]

Regardless of their individual roles, all team members share certain basic functions. Most important is that of evaluation and assessment. For a clinical psychologist, this function may involve the administration of various psychometric instruments. A mental status examination frequently assists in establishing a tentative diagnosis. The purpose of assessment is to obtain a clear, objective report of the patient's signs and symptoms and, as much as possible, to relate these to possible causes. A psychological assessment may include a formal diagnosis, or it may be a description of the development of the patient's behavior. Either type of assessment should address both the strengths and weaknesses of the patient. An assessment that also includes the etiology of the problem is most beneficial.

The clinician may list all possible explanations for the observed behaviors in a comprehensive format called the *differential diagnosis,* from which the causes may be determined. Frequently further assessment is necessary to rule out some of the possible causes. Usually less plausible causes can be readily eliminated. The differential diagnosis then guides further assessment and treatment. Different possible causal factors in the differential diagnosis often have markedly different treatments. Consequently, an accurate assessment and diagnosis of the causes of the patient's behavior must precede any treatment planning or therapeutic intervention.

Evaluation by mental health professionals is often formalized into a standard diagnostic format. Most often used is the diagnostic system of the DSM-IV.

DSM-IV Classification of Mental Disorders

Diagnosis is the practice of distinguishing one disease from another. In clinical psychology, diagnosis is based on the signs and symptoms of a mental disorder, regardless of the morbid changes producing them. DSM-IV defines a mental disorder as

> a clinically significant behavior or psychological syndrome or pattern that occurs in a person and that is associated with present distress (e.g., a painful symptom) or disability (i.e., impairment in one or more important areas of functioning) or with a significantly increased risk of suffering death, pain, disability, or an important loss of freedom. In addition, this syndrome or pattern must not be merely an expected and culturally sanctioned response to a particular event, for example, the death of a loved one. Whatever its original cause, it must currently be considered a manifestation of a behavioral, psychological, or biological dysfunction in the individual. Neither deviant behavior (e.g., political, religious, or sexual) nor conflicts that are primarily between the individual and society are mental disorders unless the deviance or conflict is a symptom of a dysfunction in the individual, as defined above.[7]

The DSM-IV classification provides a shorthand description of the patterns of behavior that can be expected with each disorder.

> DSM-IV is a categorical classification that divides mental disorders into types based on criteria sets with defining features. . . . In DSM-IV there is no assumption that each category of mental disorder is a complete discrete entity with absolute boundaries dividing it from other mental disorders or from no mental disorder. There is also no assumption that all individuals described as having the same mental disorder are alike in all important ways. This outlook allows more flexibility in the use of the system, encourages more specific attention to boundary cases, and emphasizes the need to capture additional clinical information that goes beyond diagnosis.[8]

Thus, the DSM-IV provides a set of guidelines for describing and characterizing clinical symptoms. Its categories also help in defining the etiology of the disorders. Thus, it provides information about the context in which infrequently observed, abnormal behaviors occur as well as a description of the actions themselves.

In the DSM-IV classification system, each individual being diagnosed is not merely assigned a single diagnostic category (for example, bipolar disorder). Instead, he or she is characterized by clinically relevant factors that are grouped into five "axes":

Axis I: primary classification (diagnosis) of the major problem requiring attention (for example, alcohol dependence)

Axis II: mental retardation and personality disorders generally believed to begin in childhood or adolescence and persisting into adult life

Axis III: any physical disorder that seems relevant to a case and that may have implications for present treatment (for example, asthma that is exacerbated by psychological factors)

Axis IV: psychosocial and environmental problems that may affect the diagnosis, treatment, and prognosis of the mental disorders listed under Axes I and II (for example, illiteracy or unemployment)

Axis V: global assessment of psychological functioning, social relationships, and occupational activities (includes ratings of both the current level of functioning and the highest level of functioning during the past year)

In emergencies, a preliminary classification must often be made even though much information is lacking. In such situations, any assessment is considered tentative and subject to revision as additional medical, psychological, and psychosocial assessments are made.

The first three axes constitute official diagnostic categories of the American Psychiatric Association. Axes IV and V are regarded as supplementary categories for use in clinical and research settings. However, it is common practice to describe a case using all five axes. The major categories of Axis I classification are listed in Table 16.1.

Here we consider 3 of the 16 Axis I categories: mood disorders, schizophrenia, and anxiety disorders. These three were chosen because they are so prevalent[9-11] and because they are the disorders most frequently treated with a combination of medication and psychotherapy.

Forty-four million Americans are identified as having a psychological disorder (Table 16.2). Of these, 1.7 million are identified as having schizophrenia, 15 million a mood disorder, and at least 20 million an anxiety disorder. Another 15 million are reported to have a substance

TABLE 16.1 DSM-IV Axis I categories.

Category	Examples
Disorders usually first diagnosed in infancy, childhood, or adolescence	Attention deficit and disruptive behavior disorders, learning disorders, certain eating disorders
Delirium, dementia, and amnestic and other cognitive disorders	Transient or permanent brain dysfunction attributable to such factors as aging, dementia due to head trauma or Alzheimer's, and amnestic disorders (memory loss)
Substance-related disorders	Disorders related to alcohol, all chemical withdrawal syndromes, and some disorders related to or caused by substances such as substance-induced psychotic disorders
Schizophrenia and other psychotic disorders	Chronic disorganized behavior and thought of psychotic proportions (delusions, hallucinations), incoherence, and social isolation; disorders that are well-organized systems of delusions without the incoherence, bizarreness, and other social isolation seen in schizophrenia
Mood disorders	Depression and bipolar disorder
Anxiety disorders	Anxiety, tension, and worry without psychotic features (delusions, hallucinations); post-traumatic (reactive, stress caused) disorders, whether brief or chronic
Somatoform disorders	Physical symptoms for which no medical causes can be found (symptoms apparently not under voluntary control and linked to psychological factors or conflicts)
Factitious disorders	Physical or behavioral symptoms that are voluntarily produced by the individual, apparently in order to play the role of patient and often involving chronic, blatant lying

abuse disorder (drugs or alcohol), which is often found along with one of the other three disorders. Patients with one of these four disorders are the most frequent users of the mental health delivery system.

Regier and coworkers reported that only about half of the 44 million Americans with a mental health disorder received mental health services over the 12-month period of study; providers of these health services were equally split between specialists and general medical providers. Regier and others suggested that more individuals should be receiving treatment for their disorders. Only 64 percent of the individuals diagnosed with schizophrenia received treatment; the

TABLE 16.1 DSM-IV Axis I categories *(continued)*.

Category	Examples
Dissociative disorders	Sudden, temporary change in the normal functions of consciousness (for example, loss of memory, sleepwalking)
Sexual and gender identity disorders	Deviant sexual thoughts and behavior that are either personally anxiety provoking or socially maladaptive
Eating disorders	Disorders of eating such as anorexia nervosa
Sleep disorders	Insomnia or difficulty in going to sleep or staying asleep, excessive daytime sleeping, complaints of sleep disturbance without objective evidence, impairment of respiration during sleep, disturbance of sleeping schedule, sleepwalking, sleep terrors
Impulse control disorders, not classified elsewhere	Maladaptations characterized by failure to resist impulses (for example, pathological gambling, chronic stealing of desired objects, habitual fire setting)
Adjustment disorders	Maladaptive reactions to identifiable life events or circumstances that are expected to lessen and cease when the stressor ceases; reactions may be dominated by depressed mood, anxiety, withdrawal, conduct disorder such as truancy, or a lessening in work or job performance
Mental disorders due to general medical condition, not classified elsewhere	Disorders that may be due to a medical condition, such as a psychotic disorder that emerges in response to renal failure
Other conditions that may be a focus of clinical attention	Includes such things as medication-induced movement disorders such as tardive dyskinesia or partner or parent/child relational problems

Abstracted from DSM-IV, pp. 13–24.

corresponding figures for individuals with a mood disorder or an anxiety disorder were 45 percent and 32 percent, respectively.[11]

Similar findings reported by Mandersheid and coworkers[9] and by Narrow and coworkers[10] confirm that many individuals diagnosed with mental and addictive disorders do not receive treatment or, if they do receive treatment, it is not in a mental health setting. Therefore, it is important for therapists in clinical settings to become familiar with the assessment, treatment, and diagnosis of common mental disorders, including the pharmacology of the medications that their patients and clients may be taking.

TABLE 16.2 Prevalence of mental disorders in combined community and institutionalized population over 18 years of age.

Disorder	1-year prevalence	No. of persons[a]
Any DIS ADM disorder	28.1 ± 0.5	44,679,000
Any DIS disorder except alcohol or drug	22.1 ± 0.4	35,139,000
Any mental disorder with comorbid substance use	3.3 ± 0.2	5,283,000
Any substance use disorder	9.5 ± 0.3	15,054,000
Any alcohol disorder	7.4 ± 0.3	11,766,000
Any drug disorder	3.1 ± 0.2	4,929,000
Schizophrenic/schizophreniform disorders	1.1 ± 0.1	1,749,000
Affective disorders	9.5 ± 0.3	15,143,000
Any bipolar	1.2 ± 0.1	1,908,000
Unipolar major depression	5.0 ± 0.2	7,950,000
Dysthymia	5.4 ± 0.2	8,586,000
Anxiety disorders	12.6 ± 0.3	20,034,000
Phobia	10.9 ± 0.3	17,331,000
Panic disorder	1.3 ± 0.1	2,067,000
Obsessive-compulsive disorder	2.1 ± 0.1	3,339,000
Somatization disorder	0.2 ± 0.0	365,000
Antisocial personality disorder	1.5 ± 0.1	2,385,000
Cognitive impairment (severe)	2.7 ± 0.1	4,293,000

Adapted from Regier and coworkers,[11] tab. 2, p. 88.
[a]The combined community and institutional civilian adult population was 159 million in 1980, 167 million in 1983, and 184 million persons in 1990. A 16.5 percent population increase from 1980 to 1990 is an adjustment factor that may be applied to these data to estimate the number of persons with disorders or service use in 1990. For example, the 44,679,000 persons with any mental or addictive disorder in 1980 would be increased to 52,051,000 in 1990.

DIS, diagnostic interview schedule; ADM, alcohol, drug, and mental. Rates are standardized to the age, sex, and race distribution of the 1980 institutionalized and noninstitutionalized population of the United States aged 18 years and older. Data are mean ± standard error.

Integrated Treatment of Major Disorders

Mood Disorders

The term *mood* refers to a perceptual bias that alters how one views the world. Mood disorders may include major depressive, manic, or hypomanic episodes or alternating recurrences of one or more such moods. All of us experience mood shifts, such as mild anxiety, depression, sadness, and grief, in response to difficult life events. These responses are natural and certainly do not constitute a mood disorder.

The DSM-IV classification of mood disorders pertains to distinct, severe processes that interfere with daily activities. These dysfunctional processes are, however, amenable to treatment.[12]

General medical conditions may be a causal factor, as may drug use. A normal course of bereavement due to environmental factors (for example, death of a loved one) is not classified as a mood disorder, even though it may temporarily incapacitate the individual.

In general, mood disorders are subclassified by type and duration of the mood episode. For example, two weeks of severely depressed mood (as indicated by a specific set of four additionally related symptoms) is required for a diagnosis of a major depressive episode.[13] Two years of mildly depressed mood and the presence of two related symptoms is required for diagnosis of dysthymic disorder.[14] The DSM-IV groups mood disorders into depressive disorders, bipolar disorders, substance-induced mood disorders, and mood disorders due to general medical conditions.

The following features common to some mood disorders do not by themselves indicate any specific condition:

1. pathological change in mood from despair to elation or vice versa

2. a change in interests or in the ability to obtain pleasure; greatly diminished or excessive involvement in pleasurable activities

3. vegetative changes (changes in sleep, energy level, appetite, or libido)

4. deviations in mannerisms that suggest changes in self-concept; such altered patterns may suggest worthlessness or a sense of great self-worth

5. diminished ability to think, focus, concentrate, and/or make decisions

6. recurrent suicidal ideation, suicidal plans, or suicide attempts

Chapters 8 and 9 describe both the continuum of mood episodes and their pharmacological treatment.

Assessment and Diagnosis   Careful assessment of psychological disorders is the initial step in effective treatment planning, whether the planned treatment is pharmacological, psychological, or a combination of both. Thorough assessment assists in distinguishing between functional and organic causes. In other words, not only do we need to develop a DSM-IV classification of symptom-based behavioral dysfunction, but we also need to make a differential diagnosis of all possible causative factors for the observed behaviors.[15] This list is then narrowed to one or perhaps a few possibilities so that the likely cause can be identified and more effectively treated.

Development of a differential diagnosis can be quite difficult. Consider a 19-year-old student who had been the "perfect" son. When initially seen, he was reporting delusions, had pressured speech, and was making psychotic verbalizations. It was established that he had been abusing alcohol, marijuana, and stimulant drugs. A differential diagnosis included both bipolar illness and polysubstance abuse. During a one-week period of hospitalization, his symptoms remitted. He subsequently did well for three weeks, until his friends provided him with alcohol and drugs. He was arrested after a bar fight and began displaying his prior delusional symptoms and psychotic verbalizations. Two weeks later, during a second period of hospitalization, the symptoms again subsided. Recovery after discharge went well for about a month. Then he was arrested one evening when he was found directing traffic while naked. Hospitalized a third time, he strongly denied any drug or alcohol use. Finally, diagnosis of bipolar disorder was made after hypomanic symptoms returned in the absence of drug abuse. Without a valid differential diagnosis, effective treatment, which included the use of lithium carbamate (Chapter 9), could not have been initiated.

A thorough assessment also includes an investigation of social and psychological factors that may contribute to pathology.[16] Other sociopsychological conditions may exacerbate existing physical or psychological problems.

Relieving symptoms through prescribed drugs fails to treat the root of the mood disorder, especially if the disorder results from a nonbiological, exogenous source. In such a case, long-term resolution of symptomatology can be achieved only through a comprehensive treatment of the total person.

Treatment The biological, psychological, and social factors in mood disorders must be addressed in a comprehensive treatment plan. Studies have shown that treatment combining medication and psychotherapy is more effective than either treatment alone.[3,5,6,17–22] Even reactive (exogenous) depression and adjustment mood disorders have a biological component that may require intervention with pharmacological agents along with psychotherapy.[23] Furthermore, with the most refractory mood disorders, a psychological or psychotherapeutic approach is made more effective with medication; both approaches work together to increase efficacy and prevent relapse. Medication often reduces symptoms arising from biochemical dysfunction to a level that allows the introduction of psychological interventions.

An individual's basic perceptual beliefs, cognitive and intellectual processing, and experiences affect that person's interaction with the environment and with other individuals. Eventually one develops a sense of how that self interacts with others. Individuals suffering from a mood disorder learn a pattern of behavior that may cause their problems to become worse and make the disorder resistant to treatment and intervention.

Psychological therapies can change that pattern of behavior. There are many techniques, "from simple education to supportive counseling to insight-oriented dynamically based therapy."[24] Cognitive therapy (or cognitive-behavioral therapy) is one frequently used therapeutic intervention. It is designed to analyze the patterns of cognition that perpetuate dysfunctional thoughts and behaviors. Although medication may elevate mood, promote sleep, reduce anxiety, and help the patient achieve pleasure from daily activities, the patient must learn to perceive and respond to the world differently. Thus, psychotherapy may address feelings of loss of control and inadequacy, making the patient an active participant in the treatment and thus enhancing compliance.[25] "If there are more complicated problems or persistent personal issues, then formal psychotherapy may be indicated."[25]

In 1993, as part of a government program to establish clinical standards of practice for commonly encountered disorders, the Agency for Health Care Policy and Research (AHCPR) published a two-volume set of guidelines for the detection, diagnosis, and treatment of major depression.[26,27] These volumes were carefully reviewed by Clinton, McCormick, and Besteman,[28] by Schulberg and Rush,[29] and by Munoz and coworkers.[30] The last authors state:

> The AHCPR guidelines suggest that any of several time-limited psychotherapies may be useful in the treatment of depression, particularly the cognitive-behavioral and the interpersonal psychotherapies. According to the guidelines, psychotherapy is a viable alternative to pharmacotherapy for patients with depressions of mild to moderate severity, although pharmacotherapy is to be preferred for patients with more severe disorders. . . . Combining drugs and psychotherapy enhances the breadth of response by retaining the different advantages possessed by either single modality.[31]

This statement is consistent with the conclusion of Miller, Norman, and Keitner that adding cognitive-behavioral therapy to standard antidepressant pharmacotherapy cuts the rate of relapse of depression by about one-half during the year following treatment termination.[32] Schulberg and Rush state:

The most evaluated depression-specific psychotherapy is cognitive therapy that aims at symptom removal by identifying and correcting the patient's distorted, negatively biased thinking and at preventing relapse-recurrence by identifying and correcting silent assumptions. ... Short-term therapies targeting affective symptoms or psychosocial problems related to a mild or moderate depression have an efficacy rate of approximately 50%, and these therapies are more similar than different in their efficacy.[33]

Regarding combination therapy, Schulberg and Rush go on to say that "it is thought that persons with more severe or chronic depression and partial responders to either treatment alone [psychotherapy or medication] may benefit from the combination."[34]

Individuals who work with patients with major depressive disorder are urged to read the AHCPR reports. Finally, as noted in Chapter 9, similar practice guidelines have been published for the treatment of bipolar disorder (see reference 51, page 232).

Schizophrenia

The term *schizophrenia* is often thought of as being synonymous with *psychosis* or *major mental illness*. The formal DSM-IV definition of schizophrenia is presented in Table 16.3. The symptoms of schizophrenia include hallucinations, delusions, disorganized speech, and bizarre behavior. These are often referred to as the "positive" symptoms of schizophrenia. "Negative" symptoms include impaired social interactions, impoverished and blunted affect, an absence of motivation, and significant social withdrawal (Chapter 11). The disorder often begins in adolescence or young adulthood, frequently following a progressively deteriorating course with few patients making a complete recovery.

Because schizophrenia was once so broadly defined, most patients displaying even moderate psychotic symptoms were incorrectly diagnosed as schizophrenic and inappropriately medicated with neuroleptic drugs. We now know that psychosis may be a part of another mental disorder or condition, such as a bipolar illness or polysubstance abuse.

Regier and coworkers reported that 1.1 percent of the adult U.S. population, or 1.7 million individuals, have been diagnosed with symptoms attributable to schizophrenia.[11] This figure agrees with the worldwide incidence of about 1 percent. The reported incidence tends to be slightly higher in lower socioeconomic classes. However, this is due to "social drift": Schizophrenics of higher socioeconomic classes become members of the lower socioeconomic classes as a result of

TABLE 16.3 DSM-IV categories of schizophrenia and related disorders.

Schizophrenia is a disturbance that lasts for at least 6 months and includes at least 1 month of active-phase symptoms (i.e., two [or more] of the following: delusions, hallucinations, disorganized speech, grossly disorganized or catatonic behavior, negative symptoms). Definitions for Schizophrenia subtypes (Paranoid, Disorganized, Catatonic, Undifferentiated, and Residual) are also included in this section.

Schizophreniform Disorder is characterized by a symptomatic presentation that is equivalent to Schizophrenia except for its duration (i.e., the disturbance lasts from 1 to 6 months) and the absence of a requirement that there be a decline in functioning.

Schizoaffective Disorder is a disturbance in which a mood episode and the active-phase symptoms of Schizophrenia occur together and were preceded or are followed by at least 2 weeks of delusions or hallucinations without prominent mood symptoms.

Delusional Disorder is characterized by at least 1 month of nonbizarre delusions without other active-phase symptoms of Schizophrenia.

Brief Psychotic Disorder is a psychotic disturbance that lasts more than 1 day and remits by 1 month.

Shared Psychotic Disorder is a disturbance that develops in an individual who is influenced by someone else who has an established delusion with similar content.

In **Psychotic Disorder due to a General Medical Condition,** the psychotic symptoms are judged to be a direct physiological consequence of a general medical condition.

In **Substance-Induced Psychotic Disorder,** the psychotic symptoms are judged to be a direct physiological consequence of a drug of abuse, a medication, or toxin exposure.

Psychotic Disorder Not Otherwise Specified is included for classifying psychotic presentations that do not meet criteria for any of the specific Psychotic Disorders defined in this section or psychotic symptomatology about which there is inadequate or contradictory information.

Reproduced with permission from DSM-IV, pp. 273–274.

their impaired functioning. The disorder affects males and females equally, although the onset of symptoms in females tends to occur an average of six years later than in males.

Individuals diagnosed with schizophrenia often present with a variety of bizarre behaviors, illogical or tangential thought, and shallow, blunted, or inappropriate affect. The so-called first-rank (or positive) symptoms typical of schizophrenia include such events as the following:[35]

1. audible thoughts, where voices speak the patient's thoughts out loud
2. voices commenting on the patient's behavior
3. voices that argue and sometimes refer to the patient in the third person
4. somatic passivity imposed by outside forces
5. thoughts from outside forces when the patient feels as if his mind were empty
6. thought insertions, where outside forces place thoughts in the patient's mind
7. thought broadcasting, where a patient's thoughts seem to escape his mind and are overheard by others
8. the feeling that impulses, volitional acts, or feelings that are not the patient's own are forced on the patient by outside forces
9. delusional perceptions, where the patient attributes delusional meaning to normal perceptions

Antipsychotic Medication   The use of the phenothiazines and other neuroleptic drugs to reduce the positive symptoms of the person diagnosed with schizophrenia is universally accepted:

> All of the symptoms associated with schizophrenia are affected to some degree by neuroleptics. Positive symptoms including hallucinations, delusions, and disorganized thoughts, are more responsive to drug treatment than are negative symptoms, such as blunted affect, emotional withdrawal, and lack of social interest. Frequently, positive symptoms will be eliminated by drug treatment, whereas negative symptoms are only modestly improved and continue to impair the patient's social recovery. A substantial proportion of schizophrenic patients—about 10% to 20%—fail to demonstrate substantial improvement when they are treated with neuroleptics. This subgroup of treatment-refractory schizophrenic patients often requires long-term institutionalization in state hospitals and similar facilities. Clozapine and other atypical antipsychotic drugs may be particularly effective for these patients.[36]

Clozapine is the first of a second generation of antipsychotic drugs (Chapter 11). These newer agents are effective in at least 30 percent of those individuals who are severely disabled by negative symptoms. Prior to these drugs, the symptomatology in these individuals could not be relieved. Chapter 11 discusses the limitations associated with the use of these latter agents.

Psychotherapy and Rehabilitation The development of anti-psychotic drugs established the usefulness of psychotropic therapy in treating mental disorders. Similarly, the limits of medication demonstrate the need for concomitant psychotherapy and other rehabilitative procedures. While psychotropic medication frequently relieves symptomatology, the addition of psychotherapy can be important, particularly in an outpatient setting.

> Having established the primary role of antipsychotics, there is evidence that psychosocial therapies, when administered with these agents, improve long-term prognosis. Because chronically psychotic patients have difficulties with social adjustment, reason dictates that they and their families could benefit from such interventions. Regardless of theoretical orientation, it is clear that practitioners should provide psychosocial therapy as part of a comprehensive treatment strategy.[37]

In general, most cost–benefit studies find that the addition of psychological therapies in an outpatient setting encourages drug compliance. Indeed, therapeutic interventions are more appropriate for outpatients.[38] Such interventions improve social skills and assist in the rehabilitation of cognitive functions. Psychological therapy in conjunction with drug therapy also extends relapse time and reduces the intensity of relapse episodes.

Typically, the most beneficial strategy is a sociopsychological therapy emphasizing self-esteem, social skills, and cognitive rehabilitation. This emphasis addresses the interaction between the client's symptoms and their social and psychological consequences. These strategies develop and rehabilitate cognitive functions, resulting in a more positive self-image and more effective social and cognitive functioning. Medication addresses the biophysical component of the disorder. Social therapy, with structured or supported living, teaches and reinforces social skills. Psychological therapy addresses the intrapsychic and psychodynamic issues. Vocational rehabilitation is important in developing self-esteem and establishing financial independence.

Functions of the Treatment Team The treatment team should teach the client the positive and negative effects of any prescribed drugs; in addition, it should answer any questions and relieve any doubts that a patient has about any medication. Helping the client remain drug compliant is important in reducing the rate of relapse. Indeed, monitoring of drug levels in plasma can provide important information, improve drug effectiveness, and reduce unwanted side effects.[36] The client should also understand the limitations of his or her medication. A team member should help the client understand that motivation, medication, and psychological therapy are all important in stabilization and recovery.

Anxiety Disorders

Symptoms of anxiety are normal and serve as an early-warning system that helps one avoid potentially dangerous situations. Excessive anxiety, however, may be a source of significant suffering and require intervention. Because anxiety touches everyone, it becomes a disorder only when it is objectively uncomfortable or is perceived to be out of control. At such times, the usual feelings of anxiety increase and interfere with one's normal functioning. Severe symptoms of anxiety require assessment and treatment.

Understanding the underlying causes and formulating a differential diagnosis will help the clinician determine which drugs and which psychological interventions will be the most effective. What we continue to discover is not only the subtlety of anxiety but also its pervasiveness:

> Anxiety accompanies almost every psychiatric disorder and is a common component of numerous organic disorders as well (e.g., hypothyroidism, hypoglycemia, pheochromocytoma, complex partial seizures, pulmonary disorders, acute myocardial infarction, caffeine intoxication, and substance abuse).[39]

Regier and coworkers (see Table 16.2) reported a one-year prevalence of all anxiety disorders of 12.6 percent in the U.S. adult population (20 million persons).[11] Most of these individuals had a phobic disorder (10.9 percent or 17 million persons) while 1.3 percent had panic disorder and 2.1 percent had obsessive-compulsive disorder. Indeed, anxiety disorders had the highest prevalence rate of the major DSM-IV diagnostic groups.

Added to these 20 million persons are individuals who have *generalized anxiety disorder* (GAD), most of whom are undiagnosed. It is likely that mental health workers have not been aware of people with GAD because they perceive the symptoms, especially the worry, as part of their clients' daily lives. The exact incidence of GAD is unknown, although estimates run as high as 5 percent of the adult population.[40] However, awareness is increasing, and more cases of GAD are reported every year. GAD is also becoming recognized as a condition responsive to medication (see the discussion of buspirone, Chapter 4) and to psychological intervention.

The chronicity of anxiety disorders is similar to that of mood disorders—more enduring than that of substance abuse disorders but less deep-seated than that of the schizophrenias. Only about 30 percent of individuals with anxiety disorders receive treatment,[11] a percentage that is even lower if GAD is included. Thus a high percentage of mental health and addictive disorders are actually anxiety disorders, but many of these disorders go completely untreated or are not treated by mental health specialists.

Characteristic of anxiety disorders are the symptoms of anxiety and avoidance behavior. Anxiety is a complex response that includes subjective feelings of dread, apprehension, fear, tension, and related psychomotor responses. The last may include motor tension, increases in autonomic responses, vigilance, and scanning. The DSM-IV lists several subcategories of the anxiety disorders,[41] which are listed in Table 16.4.

Using drugs to treat anxiety disorders is controversial. The controversy arises from diagnostic difficulties, the chronic nature of many anxieties, and the addictive potential for the drugs used in therapy. In the 1960s, the benzodiazepines appeared to treat anxiety disorders quickly, effectively, and safely. However, over time, the potential addictiveness of benzodiazepine therapy became evident. Similarly, clinicians noted that anxiolytics, which reduced the outward symptoms of anxiety, could be counterproductive in some cases. As our knowledge of the causal factors of the anxiety disorders grew, our sophistication in diagnosing and treating them similarly expanded.

> It is imperative for clinicians to become knowledgeable about the basic pharmacology of these drugs, along with their appropriate clinical indications, dosages, and duration of usage. **Most importantly, their limitations must receive as much attention as their assets.**[42]

Accurate assessment and diagnosis is especially vital in planning the appropriate treatment for anxiety disorders. Generally, more diffuse and severe anxiety symptoms require some initial pharmacological intervention. Less severe, more circumscribed symptoms of phobias may be more responsive to cognitive and behavioral therapy; in such cases, it is often unnecessary to prescribe the potentially addictive anxiolytics.

Panic Disorder   Panic disorder is one of the most common anxiety disorders for which people seek treatment, and it is also the most disabling.[43] Comprehensive therapy reduces the severity of its course and enhances outcome. Medications typically used to relieve the symptoms of panic disorder include the antidepressants (Chapter 8)

TABLE 16.4 DSM-IV categories of anxiety disorders.

A **Panic Attack** is a discrete period in which there is the sudden onset of intense apprehension, fearfulness, or terror, often associated with feelings of impending doom. During these attacks symptoms such as shortness of breath, palpitations, chest pain or discomfort, choking or smothering sensations, and fear of "going crazy" or losing control are present.

Agoraphobia is anxiety about, or avoidance of, places or situations from which escape might be difficult (or embarrassing) or in which help may not be available in the event of having a Panic Attack or panic-like symptoms.

Panic Disorder without Agoraphobia is characterized by recurrent unexpected Panic Attacks about which there is persistent concern. **Panic Disorder with Agoraphobia** is characterized by both recurrent unexpected Panic Attacks and Agoraphobia.

Agoraphobia without History of Panic Disorder is characterized by the presence of Agoraphobia and panic-like symptoms without a history of unexpected Panic Attacks.

Specific Phobia is characterized by clinically significant anxiety provoked by exposure to a specific feared object or situation, often leading to avoidance behavior.

Social Phobia is characterized by clinically significant anxiety provoked by exposure to certain types of social or performance situations, often leading to avoidance behavior.

Obsessive-Compulsive Disorder is characterized by obsessions (which cause marked anxiety or distress) and/or by compulsions (which serve to neutralize anxiety).

Post-Traumatic Stress Disorder is characterized by the reexperiencing of an extremely traumatic event accompanied by symptoms of increased arousal and by avoidance of stimuli associated with the trauma.

Acute Stress Disorder is characterized by symptoms similar to those of Post-Traumatic Stress Disorder that occur immediately in the afterrnath of an extremely traumatic event.

Generalized Anxiety Disorder is characterized by at least 6 months of persistent and excessive anxiety and worry.

Anxiety Disorder Due to a General Medical Condition is characterized by prominent symptoms of anxiety that are judged to be a direct physiological consequence of a general medical condition.

Substance-Induced Anxiety Disorder is characterized by prominent symptoms of anxiety that are judged to be a direct physiological consequence of a drug of abuse, a medication, or toxin exposure.

Anxiety Disorder Not Otherwise Specified is included for coding disorders with prominent anxiety or phobic avoidance that do not meet criteria for any of the specific Anxiety Disorders defined in this section (or anxiety symptoms about which there is inadequate or contradictory information).

Because Separation Anxiety Disorder (characterized by anxiety related to separation from parental figures) usually develops in childhood, it is included in the "Disorders Usually First Diagnosed in Infancy, Childhood, or Adolescence" section. Phobic avoidance that is limited to genital sexual contact with a sexual partner is classified as Sexual Aversion Disorder and is included in the "Sexual and Gender Identity Disorders" section.

Reproduced with permission from DSM-IV, pp. 393–394.

and the anxiolytics (Chapter 4). Antidepressant drugs appear to be the pharmacological treatments of choice[43] except for patients also experiencing severe agitation. For those patients, an anxiolytic, such as a benzodiazepine, appears to be more effective on a short-term basis.[43]

Of the antidepressants, the SSRIs (such as fluvoxamine, fluoxetine, and clomipramine) appear to be superior to the standard tricyclic antidepressants (such as imipramine) and to alternative agents such as maprotiline (Chapter 8).[43] Of the benzodiazepines, alprazolam (Xanax) is the most widely studied for treating panic disorder. Other benzodiazepines that have been studied include lorazepam (Ativan) and clonazepam (Clonopin). Finally, the monoamine oxidase inhibitors have been shown to be effective in treating panic disorder, particularly in patients who do not respond to more traditional antidepressant compounds.[44]

For all antidepressant medications, treatment should continue for six to twelve months. Doses of medication should be gradually tapered as the patient becomes free of symptoms.

In some clinical situations, cognitive and behavioral psychotherapeutic interventions are also indicated. These interventions should target avoidance behaviors that patients have learned over time to reduce the frequency of panic attacks. One part of the cognitive-behavioral approach is teaching the patient specific relaxation and stress management techniques.

Panic disorder appears to be a chronic condition. Attention must be given to preventing relapse. Helping patients to examine stressors in their lives and to learn adaptive responses to such stressors is an important part of treatment. When stress is severe, a panic attack may be averted or substantially reduced as the result of such treatment.

Indeed, Janicak, Davis, Preskorn, and Ayd state that "Non-drug approaches found to be beneficial [in the treatment of panic disorder] include: exposure therapy, cognitive therapy, and applied relaxation."[45] The combination of antidepressants and cognitive-behavioral therapy appears superior to either treatment alone.[44] Further analysis of such therapies must await the publication of a forthcoming report of the AHCPR,[46] scheduled for publication in 1995.

Generalized Anxiety Disorder Individuals with generalized anxiety disorder (GAD) constantly seem to be anxious, nervous, or worried. To others, this worry appears irrational, illogical, excessive, and unrealistic. But worry is usually a part of the life of sufferers from a very early age. For some clients, symptoms are so well integrated that they appear to be a natural part of clients' lives. Many clinicians believe that the milder forms of GAD are best treated with psychotherapy in which the patient is taught strategies for anxiety management. "In some patients, careful listening, astute questioning, and appropriate advice may be the best form of intervention. . . . Some psychotherapies have been reported effective to teach techniques for coping with and/or reducing anxiety."[47]

For example, cognitive-behavioral therapies teach clients to examine how their unrealistic thoughts and ruminations affect their behavioral functioning. Relaxation therapy, biofeedback, and stress management are used to teach these patients how to relax even under stress.

Many anxious people worry about being unable to cope. They fear losing control, "going crazy," or being publicly embarrassed. As a consequence, these fears increase anxiety, causing a vicious cycle: anxious thoughts increase anxiety symptoms, which, in turn, generate even more anxious thoughts. Cognitive-behavioral techniques help patients break this cycle by allowing them to deal appropriately with anxious thoughts and their related behavioral expressions.

Patients diagnosed with GAD who have been on long-term benzo-diazepine therapy (to control the symptoms of anxiety) require much more intensive psychotherapy than do other anxious or depressed patients. Indeed, Kushner, Sher, and Beitman conclude that GAD may often be a manifestation of masked or occult alcoholism.[48] GAD may also be a prodromal phase or a subclinical form of various other psychological disorders, such as depression, panic, and obsessive-compulsive disorder.

In acutely anxious individuals, anxiolytic drugs (e.g., benzo-diazepines) are unquestionably effective. Anxiolytics rapidly reduce symptomatology, especially in the first weeks of therapy.[49] Because of the risk of developing drug dependence, most authorities agree that anxiolytics should be prescribed at the lowest possible dose for the shortest possible period of time.

As discussed in Chapter 4, buspirone has recently become available for treating GAD, especially for long-term therapy. Indeed, buspirone is now considered to be the drug of first choice in situations where a slow onset of action is acceptable and the drug may be required for a prolonged time.

> Because it [buspirone] has no abuse liability, no [deleterious] effects on cognitive or psychomotor functioning, and does not result in a withdrawal syndrome when abruptly discontinued, it also has major advantages over benzodiazepines for the long-term treatment of generalized anxiety disorder. Nonetheless, because it has a slower onset of effect with initial response not occurring for several weeks, it may be less useful for syndromes requiring acute and rapid anxiolysis.[50]

Antidepressant medications, particularly those that effectively treat anxiety (e.g., imipramine) or ruminations (e.g., clomipramine) have also been shown to be helpful. The newer selective serotonin reuptake inhibitor (SSRI) antidepressants have not been well studied in double-blind trials but appear to be effective.

Because GAD is often chronic, both acute efficacy and long-term prevention of relapse must be considered when choosing both drug and psychotherapeutic interventions. Rickels and Schweitzer reported that buspirone-treated patients had significantly fewer long-term relapses than did benzodiazepine-treated patients.[51] Also, any psychotherapeutic intervention should begin before medication is discontinued in order to minimize the likelihood of relapse.

Specific Phobia and Social Phobia   The phobias are characterized by extreme anxiety about a specific object (specific phobia) or a generalized or discrete social situation (social phobia). Patients with social phobias are at high risk for developing mood or anxiety disorders and schizophrenia.[52] Wolpe presented a model for the acquisition of phobic behavior based on the experimental and theoretical literature of the psychology of learning.[53] According to this theory, organisms will select that behavior which moves them from a state of stress to a state in which the stress is reduced. Wolpe reasoned that if a conditioned stimulus were repeatedly presented in such a manner that it did not produce a conditioned emotional response, then the original association would be extinguished.

The object of therapy based on this reasoning (termed *targeted exposure therapy*) is to pair fear-evoking incidents with relaxation training in a sequence that finally leads to the presentation of the original fear-inducing or anxiety-arousing stimulus. Targeted exposure to the object of the phobia, either in the presence of the object or through mental imagery, is an accepted behavioral treatment for phobias.[54]

This therapy may be administered through *client-active systematic desensitization*. Here the clients have more control over and responsibility for their own treatment.[55] Cognitive and behavioral therapies usually span a few months, with maintenance sessions to enhance confidence.

When the patient with a phobia displays severe anxiety symptoms, anxiolytics may be administered to treat acute symptoms. For longer-term pharmacological management, antidepressant agents are indicated, especially those with anxiolytic properties. Alprazolam (Xanax) can be quite effective, as are serotonin-specific antidepressants and the MAO inhibitors (Chapter 8). Fluoxetine and other SSRIs also appear to be efficacious,[56,57] as does buspirone.[58]

Obsessive-Compulsive Disorder Obsessive-compulsive disorder (OCD) is characterized by recurrent and disturbing thoughts and/or repetitive behaviors that the individual feels driven to perform but recognizes as irrational or excessive.

> Although traditionally viewed as resistant to a variety of therapeutic interventions, recent advances have been made in the psychopharmacologic and behavioral therapy of OCD. In particular, the clear efficacy of serotonin reuptake inhibitors, such as clomipramine, fluvoxamine, fluoxetine, and sertraline, has been established in double-blind studies in patients with OCD. Consistent with these drug response data are the hypotheses that changes in serotonin function are critical to the treatment of OCD and perhaps involved in the pathophysiology of at least some patients with the disorder.[59]

In a recent multicenter study, Tollefson and coworkers reported on the efficacy of fluoxetine in treating OCD.[60] Currently clomipramine is the only agent specifically approved by the U.S. Food and Drug Administration for treating OCD, and it has been shown to be effective in approximately 40 to 60 percent of OCD patients.[59,61] For the many individuals unresponsive to serotonin reuptake inhibitor therapy, drugs such as tryptophan, fenfluramine, lithium, and buspirone have been tried, either alone or in combination with the serotonergic agents.

Dager favors a combination of medication and behavioral therapy.[61] He believes that in some cases behavioral conditioning can be useful as the primary intervention for compulsions, although the approach appears to be less effective for obsessional thinking. Systematic desensitization or cognitive-behavioral therapy is also used.

A paradoxical behavioral approach known as exposure therapy is sometimes used to treat OCD. In exposure treatment, the client is asked to experience the stimuli that produced the obsessional thinking or compulsive behavior. For example, a client who obsesses about the prospect of throwing up in public may be asked to go to a public place and attempt to regurgitate. As another example, a person who obsesses about the doors in the house being locked and who must repeatedly check them may be asked to repeatedly go around the house and open them up.

Although cognitive-behavioral therapies have been quite useful, other types have not. "Psychoanalysis and psychodynamically-oriented psychotherapy have been particularly unsuccessful in treating OCD,"[61] Dager notes. Janicak, Davis, Preskorn, and Ayd summarize: "Because significant OCD symptoms often remain or recur, even when there is substantial improvement with a specific therapy, a combined complementary approach seems to be the optimal strategy for most patients."[62]

Post-Traumatic Stress Disorder Krystal and coworkers have suggested that transient and long-lasting neurological alterations may underlie acute and long-term neuronal responses to traumatic stress.[63] Comorbidity is frequent; individuals with post-traumatic stress disorder (PTSD) experience a high incidence of GAD, phobias, depression, and substance abuse.[64] Thus, the treatment of PTSD must be comprehensive and individualized, utilizing carefully balanced pharmacotherapeutic and psychotherapeutic interventions that address both the PTSD and any comorbid disorder. According to Vargas and Davidson, "Symptom relief provided by pharmacotherapy enables the patient to participate more thoroughly in individual, behavioral, or group therapy."[65]

Most drugs that are effective for PTSD are also useful for treating major depression and panic disorder.[66] Thus, numerous drugs have been tried, including tricyclic antidepressants, MAO inhibitors, carbamazepine, benzodiazepines, serotonin reuptake inhibiting antidepressants, and others. Clinical studies suggest that "a serotonergic action is necessary for good clinical effect in PTSD, analogous to the situation in OCD."[67] Some clinicians advocate the use of hypnotic techniques to facilitate working through the traumatic events. This approach is based on the frequently observed interrelationship between dissociative reactions and physical trauma.[66]

Therapeutic Alliance in Anxiety Disorders

Nowhere is the term *therapeutic alliance* so well illustrated as in the treatment of the anxiety disorders. Because anxiety is common to so many disorders, one can easily make a wrong diagnosis. One must therefore guard against any quick judgment to avoid missing an underlying etiology. To focus only on the anxiety without examining other symptoms or causes may lead to misdiagnosis and mistreatment.

Once a diagnosis is made, all caregivers must determine the course of treatment. In acutely anxious patients, an anxiolytic can be highly effective. However, the specific drug and the duration of administration will vary according to the specific anxiety disorder as well as the presence of any comorbid disorders. For instance, an individual with a dual diagnosis of panic disorder and alcoholism presents a challenging situation. Prescribing potentially addicting drugs (such as the benzodiazepines), even for short-term use, must be done with great care. This difficult circumstance was recently addressed in a study that reported the beneficial effects of individualizing benzodiazepine therapy for alcohol withdrawal.[68,69]

By general consensus, an appropriate course of therapy for individuals with anxiety disorders employs anxiolytic medication to treat acute symptoms for a short period of time, followed by psychotherapy and support to change the learned behavior. Especially in disorders involving avoidance, such as the social and specific phobias, the use of psychotherapy—particularly systematic desensitization, cognitive-behavioral, or behavioral therapy—is a crucial element. Anxiolytic medications may reinforce the avoidance of therapy and therefore perpetuate the anxiety, placing the patient at risk for developing a drug dependence. For individuals suffering from GAD, the same benzodiazepine limitations apply, and the first choice of treatment is psychotherapy.

It is important for both the psychotherapist and the patient to understand that in most anxiety disorders (except those in which there is a clear biochemical dysfunction), medication temporarily reduces the anxiety but does not change the pattern of learning that perpetuates the anxiety. Behavioral therapy and cognitive-behavioral therapy have described this process well, and highly effective treatment procedures are available.[70,71] Unfortunately, these therapeutic techniques do not reduce the anxiety quickly. On the other hand, they provide the client the power of self-control and the opportunity for real changes in behavior in the long run.

In treatment, emphasis should be on the partnership, with the therapist providing support while the patient gains behavioral control over the anxiety symptoms. Some degree of anxiety is unavoidable, but it is possible to learn how to control its frequency and intensity.

This chapter has not covered the pharmacological and psychotherapeutic interventions for a variety of other DSM disorders, including anorexia nervosa, bulimia nervosa, insomnia and related sleep disorders, and borderline states. Reviews relevant to these subjects have been recently published.[72-74]

Notes

1. P. G. Janicak, J. M. Davis, S. H. Preskorn, and F. J. Ayd, *Principles and Practice of Psychopharmacotherapy* (Baltimore: Williams & Wilkins, 1993), p. 268.
2. American Psychiatric Association, *Diagnostic and Statistical Manual of Mental Disorders*, 4th ed. (Washington, D.C.: American Psychiatric Association, 1994).

3. A. S. Bellack, M. Hersen, and J. M. Himmelhoch, "A Comparison of Social-Skills Training, Pharmacotherapy, and Psychotherapy for Depression," *Behavioral Research and Therapy* 21 (1983): 101–107.

4. I. Elkin and others, "NIMH Treatment of Depression Collaborative Research Program: General Effectiveness of Treatments," *Archives of General Psychiatry* 46 (1989): 971–982.

5. M. T. Shea and others, "Course of Depressive Symptoms over Follow-up: Findings from the National Institute of Mental Health Treatment of Depression Collaborative Research Program," *Archives of General Psychiatry* 49 (1992): 782–787.

6. S. H. Preskorn, M. J. Burke, and G. A. Fast, "Therapeutic Drug Monitoring: Principles and Practice," *Psychiatric Clinics of North America* 16 (September 1993): 611–641.

7. American Psychiatric Association, *Diagnostic and Statistical Manual*, pp. xxi–xxii.

8. Ibid., p. xxii.

9. R. W. Mandersheid, D. S. Rae, W. E. Narrow, B. Z. Locke, and D. A. Regier, "Congruence of Service Utilization Estimates from the Epidemiologic Catchment Area Project and Other Sources," *Archives of General Psychiatry* 50 (1993): 108–114.

10. W. E. Narrow, D. A. Regier, D. S. Rae, R. W. Mandersheid, and B. Z. Locke, "Use of Services by Persons with Mental and Addictive Disorders: Findings from the National Institute of Mental Health Epidemiologic Catchment Area Program," *Archives of General Psychiatry* 50 (1993): 95–107.

11. D. A. Regier, W. E. Narrow, D. S. Rae, R. W. Mandersheid, B. Z. Locke, and F. K. Goodwin, "The de Facto U.S. Mental and Addictive Disorders Service System: Epidemiologic Catchment Area Prospective 1-Year Prevalence Rates of Disorders and Services," *Archives of General Psychiatry* 50 (1993): 85–94.

12. American Psychiatric Association, *Diagnostic and Statistical Manual*, p. 317.

13. Ibid., p. 320.

14. Ibid., p. 345.

15. Janicak, Davis, Preskorn, and Ayd, *Principles and Practice of Psychopharmacotherapy*, pp. 187–201.

16. D. L. Dunner, "Diagnostic Assessment," *Psychiatric Clinics of North America* 16 (September 1993): 431–441.

17. A. J. Rush, A. T. Beck, M. Kovacs, and S. D. Hollon, "Comparative Efficacy of Cognitive Therapy and Pharmacotherapy in the Treatment of Depressed Outpatients," *Cognitive Therapy Research* 1 (1977): 17–37.

18. A. T. Beck, S. D. Hollon, J. E. Young, R. C. Bedrosian, and D. Budenz, "Treatment of Depression with Cognitive Therapy and Amitriptyline," *Archives of General Psychiatry* 42 (1985): 142–148.

19. L. Covi and R. S. Lipman, "Cognitive-Behavioral Group Psychotherapy Compared with Imipramine in Major Depression," *Psychopharmacological Bulletin* (1987): 173–176.

20. S. D. Hollon and others, "Cognitive Therapy and Pharmacotherapy for Depression: Singly and in Combination," *Archives of General Psychiatry* 49 (1992): 774–781.

21. D. J. Kupfer and others, "Five-Year Outcome for Maintenance Therapies in Recurrent Depression," *Archives of General Psychiatry* 49 (1992): 769–773.

22. K. B. Wells, M. A. Burnam, W. Rogers, R. Hays, and P. Camp, "The Course of Depression in Adult Outpatients: Results from the Medical Outcomes Study," *Archive of General Psychiatry* 49 (1992): 788–794.

23. E. Richelson, "Treatment of Acute Depression," *Psychiatric Clinics of North America* 16 (September 1993): 461–478.

24. Janicak, Davis, Preskorn, and Ayd, *Principles and Practice of Psychopharmacotherapy,* p. 268.

25. Ibid., p. 269.

26. Depression Guideline Panel, *Depression in Primary Care,* vol. 1, *Diagnosis and Detection,* Clinical Practice Guideline No. 5, AHCPR Publication 93-0550 (Rockville, Md.: Department of Health and Human Services, Public Health Service, Agency for Health Care Policy and Research, 1993).

27. Depression Guideline Panel, *Depression in Primary Care,* vol. 2, *Treatment of Major Depression,* Clinical Practice Guideline No. 5, AHCPR Publication 93-0551 (Rockville, Md.: Department of Health and Human Services, Public Health Service, Agency for Health Care Policy and Research, 1993).

28. J. J. Clinton, K. McCormick, and J. Besteman, "Enhancing Clinical Practice: The Role of Practice Guidelines," *American Psychologist* 49 (1994): 30–33.

29. H. C. Schulberg and A. J. Rush, "Clinical Practice Guidelines for Managing Major Depression in Primary Care Practice: Implications for Psychologists," *American Psychologist* 49 (1994): 34–41.

30. R. F. Munoz, S. D. Hollon, E. McGrath, L. P. Rehm, and G. R. VandenBos, "On the AHCPR *Depression in Primary Care* Guidelines," *American Psychologist* 49 (1994): 42–61.

31. Ibid., pp. 49–50.

32. I. Miller, W. Norman, and G. Keitner, "Cognitive-Behavioral Treatment of Depressed Inpatients: Six- and Twelve-Month Follow-up," *American Journal of Psychiatry* 146 (1989): 1274–1279.

33. Schulberg and Rush, "Clinical Practice Guidelines," p. 38.

34. Ibid., p. 39.

35. M. A. Taylor, "Schneiderian First-Rank Symptoms and Clinical Prognostic Features in Schizophrenia," *Archives of General Psychiatry* 26 (1972): 64–67.

36. S. R. Marder, A. Ames, W. C. Wirshing, and T. Van Putten, "Schizophrenia," *Psychiatric Clinics of North America* 16 (September 1993): 567–588.

37. Janicak, Davis, Preskorn, and Ayd, *Principles and Practice of Psychopharmacotherapy,* pp. 158–159.

38. Ibid., p. 162.

39. Ibid., p. 406.

40. D. Cowley, "Generalized Anxiety Disorder," in *Psychopharmacology 1993* (Menlo Park, Calif.: Healthline, 1993), pp. 11–12.

41. American Psychiatric Association, *Diagnostic and Statistical Manual,* pp. 393–444.

42. Janicak, Davis, Preskorn, and Ayd, *Principles and Practice of Psychopharmacotherapy,* p. 405.

43. P. Roy-Byrne, D. Wingerson, D. Cowley, and S. Dager, "Psychopharmacologic Treatment of Panic, Generalized Anxiety Disorder, and Social Phobia," *Psychiatric Clinics of North America* 16, no. 4 (December 1993): 721.

44. M. R. Lebowitz and others, "Phenelzine vs. Atenolol in Social Phobia: A Placebo Controlled Trial," *Archives of General Psychiatry* 49 (1992): 290–300.

45. Janicak, Davis, Preskorn, and Ayd, *Principles and Practice of Psychopharmacotherapy,* pp. 458–459.

46. Anxiety and Panic Disorder Guideline Panel, *Diagnosis and Treatment of Anxiety and Panic Disorder in the Primary Care Setting,* Clinical Practice Guideline No. 21, AHCPR Publication (Rockville, Md.: Department of Health and Human Services, Public Health Service, Agency for Health Care Policy and Research, in preparation).

47. Janicak, Davis, Preskorn, and Ayd, *Principles and Practice of Psychopharmacotherapy,* p. 419.

48. M. G. Kushner, K. J. Sher, and B. D. Beitman, "The Relation between Alcohol Problems and the Anxiety Disorders," *American Journal of Psychiatry* 147 (1990): 685–695.

49. Janicak, Davis, Preskorn, and Ayd, *Principles and Practice of Psychopharmacotherapy,* p. 416.

50. P. Roy-Byrne, D. Wingerson, D. Cowley, and S. Dager, "Psychopharmacologic Treatment of Panic, Generalized Anxiety Disorder, and Social Phobia," *Psychiatric Clinics of North America* 16, no. 4 (December 1993): 727.

51. K. Rickels and E. Schweitzer, "The Clinical Course and Long-Term Management of Generalized Anxiety Disorder," *Journal of Clinical Psychopharmacology* 10 (1990): 1015–1105.

52. P. Roy-Byrne, D. Wingerson, D. Cowley, and S. Dager, "Psychopharmacologic Treatment of Panic, Generalized Anxiety Disorder, and Social Phobia," *Psychiatric Clinics of North America* 16, no. 4 (December 1993): 730.

53. J. Wolpe, *Psychotherapy by Reciprocal Inhibition* (Stanford, Ca.: Stanford University Press, 1958).

54. I. Marks and G. O'Sullivan, "Drugs and Psychological Treatments for Agoraphobia/Panic and Obsessive-Compulsive Disorders: A Review," *British Journal of Psychiatry* 153 (1988): 650–658.

55. D. Lange and F. A. C. Wright, *Client-Active Systematic Desensitization in Dentistry* (Winnipeg, Canada: Hyperion Press, 1978).

56. B. Black, T. W. Uhde, and M. E. Taylor, "Fluoxetine for the Treatment of Social Phobia," *Journal of Clinical Psychopharmacology* 12 (1992): 293–295.

57. F. R. Schneier and others, "Fluoxetine in Social Phobia," *Journal of Clinical Psychopharmacology* 12 (1992): 61–64.

58. D. J. Munjack, J. Brun, and P. L. Baltazar, "A Pilot Study of Buspirone in the Treatment of Social Phobia," *Journal of Anxiety Disorders* 5 (1991): 87–88.

59. C. J. McDougle, W. K. Goodman, J. F. Leckman, and L. H. Price, "The Psychopharmacology of Obsessive Compulsive Disorder: Implications for Treatment and Pathogenesis," *Psychiatric Clinics of North America* 16, no. 4 (December 1993): 749.

60. G. D. Tollefson and others, "A Multicenter Investigation of Fixed-Dose Fluoxetine in the Treatment of Obsessive-Compulsive Disorder," *Archives of General Psychiatry* 51 (1994): 559–567.

61. S. Dager, "Obsessive Compulsive Disorder," in *Psychopharmacology 1993* (Menlo Park, Ca.: Healthline, 1993), pp. 2–4.

62. Janicak, Davis, Preskorn, and Ayd, *Principles and Practice of Psychopharmacotherapy,* p. 471.

63. J. H. Krystal and others, "Neurobiological Aspects of PTSD: Review of Clinical and Preclinical Studies," *Behavioral Therapy* 20 (1989): 177–198.

64. J. R. T. Davidson and others, "Post-Traumatic Stress Disorder in the Community: An Epidemiological Study," *Psychological Medicine* 21 (1991): 713–721.

65. M. A. Vargas and J. Davidson, "Post-Traumatic Stress Disorder," *Psychiatric Clinics of North America* 16, no. 4 (December 1993): 745.

66. Janicak, Davis, Preskorn, and Ayd, *Principles and Practice of Psychopharmacotherapy,* p. 477.

67. M. A. Vargas and J. Davidson, "Post-Traumatic Stress Disorder," *Psychiatric Clinics of North America* 16, no. 4 (December 1993): 743.

68. R. Saity, M. F. Mayo-Smith, M. S. Roberts, H. A. Redmond, D. R. Bernard, and D. R. Calkins, "Individualized Treatment for Alcohol Withdrawal: A Randomized Double-Blind Controlled Trial," *Journal of the American Medical Association* 272 (17 August 1994): 519–523.

69. R. K. Fuller and E. Gordis, "Refining the Treatment of Alcohol Withdrawal," *Journal of the American Medical Association* 272 (17 August 1994): 557–558.

70. D. Meichenbaum, *Cognitive-Behavior Modification: An Integrative Approach* (New York: Plenum Press, 1977).

71. D. Meichenbaum, *Stress Inoculation Training* (New York: Pergamon Press, 1985).

72. L. Hoffman and K. Halmi, "Psychopharmacology in the Treatment of Anorexia Nervosa and Bulimia Nervosa," *Psychiatric Clinics of North America* 16 (December 1993): 767–778.

73. W. B. Mendelson, "Insomnia and Related Sleep Disorders," *Psychiatric Clinics of North America* 16 (December 1993): 841–852.

74. J. R. Brinkley, "Pharmacotherapy of Borderline States," *Psychiatric Clinics of North America* 16 (December 1993): 853–884.

BASIC ANATOMY OF THE CENTRAL NERVOUS SYSTEM

Because the brain is the most complex of all biological structures, any discussion about its anatomy and function is necessarily complicated. Still, a relatively uncomplicated outline of the anatomy and physiology of the brain can be given that will help explain the effects of psychoactive drugs on brain function as well as on behavior.

The *central nervous system* (CNS) consists of all the nerve cells (neurons) in the brain and the spinal cord (Figure I.1). The brain is a collection of some 20 billion neurons, along with their dendrites and axons, that are contained entirely within the skull. The lower part of the brain, which is attached to the upper part of the spinal cord, is referred to as the *brain stem*. The brain stem is situated entirely within the skull. All the impulses that are conducted in either direction between the spinal cord and the brain must, of necessity, go through the brain stem, which is also important in the regulation of vital body functions.

As the upper part of the spinal cord enlarges, it separates into three distinct segments, which are referred to as the *medulla*, the *pons* (or bridge), and the *midbrain*. These three segments form the *brain stem*. Behind the midbrain is a large bulbous structure, which is called

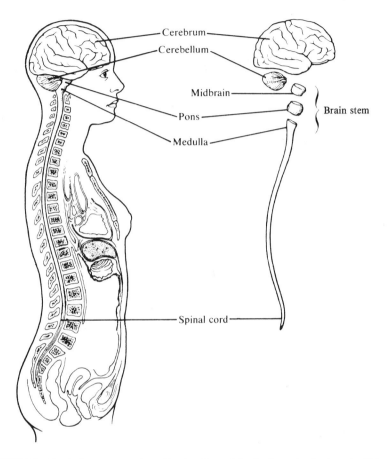

FIGURE I.1 Central nervous system. The location of the brain and spinal cord within the body is shown at the left and the principal components of the central nervous system at the right.

the *cerebellum*. The area immediately above the brain stem and covered by the cerebral hemispheres is the *diencephalon* (Figure I.2). This area includes the hypothalamus, the pituitary gland, various fiber tracts (bundles of axons that travel as a group from one area to another), and the thalamus. The region below the thalamus is referred to as the *subthalamus*. Finally, almost completely covering the brain stem and the diencephalon are the left and right hemispheres of the cerebrum.

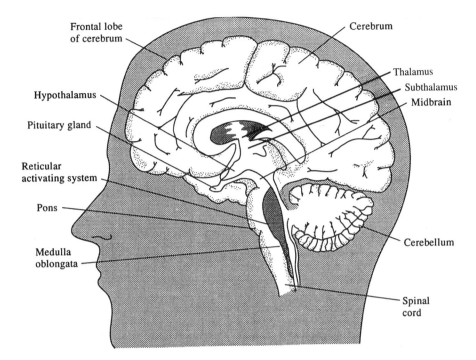

FIGURE I.2   Midline section of the brain illustrating several structures lying below the cerebral cortex and thus not visible in Figure I.1.

Spinal Cord

The spinal cord extends from the lower end of the medulla to the upper levels of the sacral vertebrae. It consists of a mass of neurons and fiber tracts. The spinal cord is involved in (1) carrying sensory information from skin, muscles, joints, and internal body organs to the brain, (2) organizing and modulating the motor outflow to the muscles (to produce coordinated muscle responses), (3) modulating sensory input, and (4) providing autonomic (involuntary) control of vital body functions.

The neurons of the spinal cord both communicate with higher centers in the brain and exert local control over spinal reflexes. Such local control is vitally important, for example, in the modulation of painful impulses and in the action of opioid narcotics (Chapter 10). Also, neurons in the spinal cord are strongly influenced by information received from the brain. For example, drugs that cause behavioral sedation decrease the flow of information from the brain to the spinal cord. Such drugs are used as muscle relaxants because they decrease the spinal cord's control over muscle tone by indirectly decreasing the activity of the motor neurons.

Brain Stem

The brain stem connects the spinal cord with the cerebral hemispheres and the diencephalon. The brain stem is the direct continuation of the spinal cord in the skull. All ascending and descending fiber tracts that connect the brain and the spinal cord pass through the structures of the brain stem. Also present are centers that largely control respiration, blood pressure, heart rate, gastrointestinal functioning, and the states of sleep and wakefulness. The brain stem is also involved in behavioral alerting, attention, and arousal responses through a so-called reticular activating system. Depressant drugs (such as the barbiturates, Chapter 3) depress this brain stem activating system; such action probably underlies much of their hypnotic action.

The major biological amine-containing neurons that project to the cerebrum are also found in the brain stem. These regions are also the primary relay areas for sensory information that enters the CNS from the face, head, and most visceral organs.

Cerebellum

The cerebellum is a large, highly convoluted structure that is situated immediately behind the brain stem, to which it is connected by large fiber tracts. The cerebellum is necessary for the proper integration of movement and posture. Some drugs exert noticeable effects on cerebellar activity. Drunkenness, which is characterized by loss of coordination, staggering, loss of balance, and other deficits, appears to be caused largely by an alcohol-induced depression of cerebellar function.

Diencephalon

The diencephalon is situated above the brain stem but below and between the right and left cerebral hemispheres. The diencephalon may be subdivided into several areas, four of which will be discussed: the thalamus, the hypothalamus, the subthalamus, and the limbic system.

Thalamus

The thalamus, the largest structure of the diencephalon, is actually a group of many smaller structures. It lies in the center of the brain, beneath the cerebral hemispheres and basal ganglia and just above the hypothalamus. The thalamus is often referred to as a way station, where incoming sensory pathways, which travel up the spinal cord and through the brain stem, synapse before they pass into the various areas of the cerebral cortex. Thus, the thalamus may be thought of as one of the primary relay stations of the brain.

Various subdivisions of the thalamus receive projections from specific sensory organs; in turn, the neurons in these subdivisions relay information to specific areas of the cerebral cortex that are associated with the particular senses involved. Other areas of the thalamus, which are not well defined, are referred to as *association areas*. These areas integrate incoming information and relay it to the association areas of the cerebral cortex. Still other areas of the thalamus connect caudally with the reticular formation, the hypothalamus, and the limbic system. These areas form the *diffuse thalamic projection system*. Electrical stimulation of the diffuse thalamic projection system yields behavioral alerting reactions that are similar to those that follow stimulation of the reticular activating system. This diffuse thalamic projection system may therefore be an extension of the brain-stem-activating areas.

Subthalamus

The subthalamus is a small area underneath the thalamus and above the midbrain; it contains a variety of small structures that, together with the basal ganglia, constitute one of our motor systems, the *extrapyramidal system*. Patients who have Parkinson's disease—a disorder that is characterized by exaggerated motor movements—have a deficiency of the neurotransmitter dopamine in the terminals of their nerve axons, which originate from cell bodies in the substantia nigra (one of the subthalamic structures). Administration of levodopa to these patients replaces the dopamine and ameliorates the symptoms. The subthalamic structures, together with the cerebellum, are important in the coordination of motor activity.

Hypothalamus

The hypothalamus is a collection of neurons in the lower portion of the brain that is near the junction of the midbrain and the thalamus. Thus it is located near the base of the skull, just above the pituitary

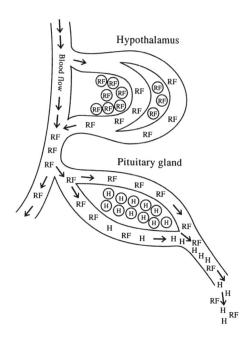

FIGURE I.3 Blood flow enters the hypothalamus, carrying hypothalamic releasing factors (RF) as it leaves the structure. The releasing factor induces the release of pituitary hormones (H), which are released into the blood that leaves the gland.

gland (the function of which it largely modulates). The hypothalamus is the principal center in the brain responsible for the integration of our entire autonomic (involuntary or vegetative) nervous system. Thus it helps control such vegetative functions as eating, drinking, sleeping, the regulation of body temperature, sexual behavior, blood pressure, emotion, and water balance. In addition, the hypothalamus closely controls hormonal output of the pituitary gland. Neurons in the hypothalamus produce substances called *releasing factors,* which travel to the nearby pituitary gland (Figure I.3). There they induce the production and secretion of hormones that act on our sex organs to regulate menstrual cycling and ovulation in females and sperm formation in males.

The hypothalamus is a site of action for many psychoactive drugs, either as a site for the primary action of the drug or as a site responsible for side effects associated with the use of a drug.

Limbic System

Closely associated with the hypothalamus is the limbic system, the major components of which are the *amygdala,* the *hippocampus,* the *mammillary bodies,* and a variety of other smaller structures. These structures exert primitive types of behavioral control; they integrate emotion, reward, and behavior with motor and autonomic functions. Because the limbic system and the hypothalamus interact to regulate emotion and emotional expression, these structures are logical sites for the study of psychoactive drugs that alter mood, affect, emotion, or responses to emotional experiences. The classical notion that the limbic system is important in learning and memory tasks has prompted investigations of both this structure and the hypothalamus as sites of action for compounds that affect these functions.

The hypothalamic and limbic areas contain structures important in psychopharmacology and the abuse potential of drugs. Included here are the *limbic reward centers* (the self-stimulation and behavior-reinforcing centers) that involve the ventral tegmental area, the median forebrain bundle, the nucleus accumbens, and the limbic system (Figure I.4). These centers contain dopamine-secreting neurons, which modulate specific types of reward and avoidance behaviors. The activity of these *dopaminergic neurons* is under the influence of opioid, GABAergic, and other neuronal influence. Throughout this text, this reward system is discussed as a site of the behavior-reinforcing action of psychoactive drugs that are subject to compulsive abuse.

Cerebral Cortex

In humans the cerebrum is the largest portion of the brain. It is separated into two distinct hemispheres, left and right. Numerous fiber tracts interconnect the two hemispheres both above the thalamus and through the multisynaptic pathways in the brain stem. Because skull size is limited and the cerebrum is so large, the outer layer of the cerebrum, the cerebral cortex, is deeply convoluted and fissured. Like other portions of the brain, the cerebral cortex is divided by function; that is, it contains centers for vision, hearing, speech, sensory perception, and emotion.

The regions of the cerebral cortex can be classified in several ways. The most useful classification for our purposes is a subdivision by the type of function or sensation that is processed (Figure I.5). The anterior (front) and posterior (back) portions of the cerebral cortex can be divided by a lateral longitudinal groove, which is called the *central sulcus.* The area of cortex that is immediately in front of the central

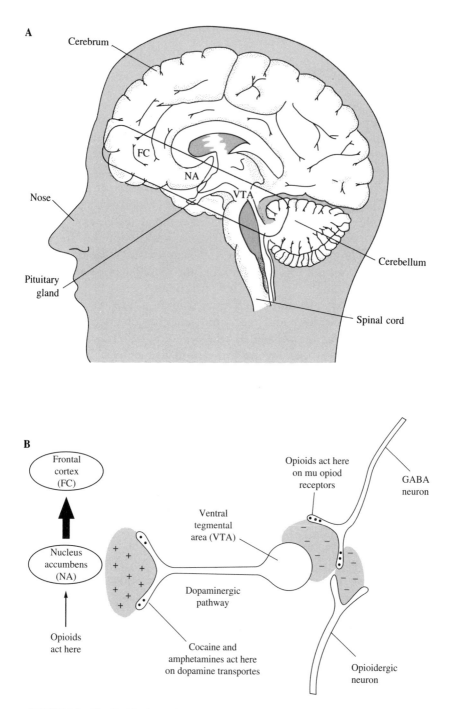

FIGURE I.4 The limbic dopaminergic reward pathway. (**A**) Human brain sliced open lengthwise, showing the relevant midbrain and forebrain area, outlined by an oval, with ventral tegmental area (VTA), nucleus accumbens (NA), and frontal cortex (FC) labeled. (**B**) Cartoon diagram of the area outlined in (**A**). Heavy dots, stored neurotransmitter at nerve endings; +, excitatory neurotransmitter; –, inhibitory neurotransmitter. [From A. Goldstein, *Addiction: From Biology to Drug Policy* (New York: W. H. Freeman and Company, 1994), p. 55, with permission.]

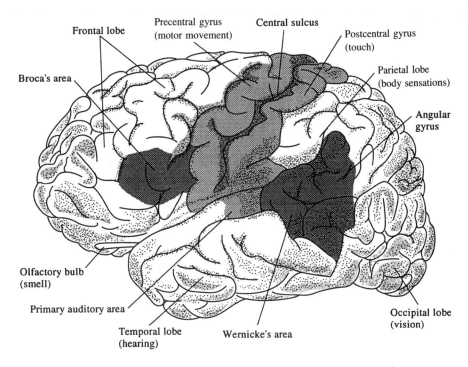

FIGURE I.5 Surface structure of the brain, showing major areas of the cerebral cortex. [Modified from N. Geschwind, "Specializations of the Human Brain," in *The Brain, a Scientific American* book (San Francisco: W. H. Freeman and Company, 1979), p. 111.]

sulcus is called the *precentral gyrus.* The precentral gyrus is involved in the control of motor movement. The area behind the central sulcus is the *postcentral gyrus,* which is the major processing center for the sensation of touch. Posterior to the postcentral gyrus lie the *parietal* and *occipital lobes,* which process body sensation and vision, respectively. In front of the precentral gyrus lies the *frontal lobe,* which is involved in behavior, reward, learning, memory, visceral sensations, abstract thought, and other specialized functions. Finally, below the central sulcus lies the *temporal lobe,* which is primarily involved in hearing and the integration of hearing with speech, which is controlled by Broca's area and Wernicke's area.

The central nervous system is extremely complex in structure and function, and the cerebral cortex represents the ultimate development of this complexity. Only now are we beginning to understand something of the brain's precise functioning and how it relates to the actions of psychoactive drugs.

PHYSIOLOGY OF
THE NEURON

To understand the effects of drugs on the nervous system, the structure and function of the nerve cell (neuron), which is the basic component of the nervous system, must be described. Neurons have special properties that distinguish them from all other cells in the body. The first is their ability to conduct electrical impulses over long distances. The second is their ability to carry out specific input and output relations with other nerve cells and with other tissues of the body, the functions of which the neurons may control. These input/output connections determine the function of a particular neuron and thus the patterns of behavioral response that neuronal activity may elicit.

The human brain contains about 100 billion neurons, most of which share common structural and functional characteristics (Figure II.1).

A typical neuron consists of the *soma* (cell body), which contains the nucleus of the cell. Extending from the soma are many short fibers, called *dendrites* (consisting of hundreds or thousands of widely branched extensions), which connect with the axons of other neurons to receive impulses through receptor sites located on the dendritic membrane. An electrical current is generated and travels down the dendrite to the soma. Extending from the soma is an elongated process called an *axon*, which varies in length from as short as a few millimeters to as long as a meter (for example, the axons that project down the spinal cord and the axons that run from the motor neurons of the

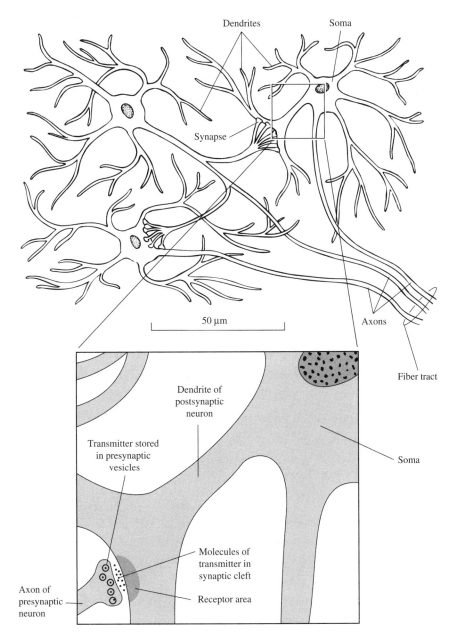

FIGURE II.1 Schematic representation of three nerve cells, showing the major subdivisions of such cells and the interactions between them.

spinal cord out to the muscles that they innervate). The axon, in essence, transmits activity from the soma to other neurons or to muscles, organs, or glands of the body. Normally, the axon conducts impulses in one direction only: from the soma, down the axon, to a specialized structure that, together with one or more dendrites from another neuron, forms a complex microspace called a *synapse* (Figure II.2).

A synapse is a minute space that exists between the presynaptic membrane (which is the axon terminal) of one neuron and the post-synaptic membrane (which is usually located on a dendrite*) of the receiving neuron. The presynaptic terminal contains numerous structural elements, the most important of which (for our purposes) are the small synaptic vesicles, each of which contains several thousand molecules of neurotransmitter chemical. These vesicles, therefore, store the transmitter, which is available for release (Figure II.3). Through a process called *exocytosis,* molecules of transmitter are released into the synaptic cleft itself. The transmitter substance diffuses across the synaptic cleft and attaches to *receptors* on the dendrite of the next neuron, thereby transmitting information chemically from one neuron to another. Because the neurons do not physically touch each other, synaptic transmission is a chemical rather than an electrical process.

Usually only one axon arises from the soma, but, in its projection, the axon may give off many side branches, sending pulses to hundreds or thousands of other neurons (causing a *divergence of information*). On the other hand, several dendrites can arise from one soma. The dendrites branch profusely and receive several thousand contacts from other cells (which results in the *convergence of information).* The dendrites then process the impulses and passively transmit electrical activity to the soma. The soma, in turn, actively transmits the impulses down the axon to as many as 10,000 other neurons. Thus, thousands of neurons converge on a single neuron, which, in turn, spreads its own impulses to thousands of other neurons.

---

*In this introductory discussion, we discuss most synapses as occurring between axon terminals of one neuron and postsynaptic receptors located on dendrites of a second neuron. Axon terminals are also located on the soma of the second neuron, in which instance the transmitter substance most often exerts a profound inhibitory effect on neuronal function. In addition, some axons synapse directly onto the axon terminals of a second neuron. Again, these are usually inhibitory in nature. In this instance, the process is termed *presynaptic inhibition.* Such synapses are thought to function in a type of negative feedback inhibition, since the discharge of the second neuron causes the release of inhibitory neurotransmitter directly on the presynaptic terminal of the first neuron, limiting its ability to release further amounts of transmitter.

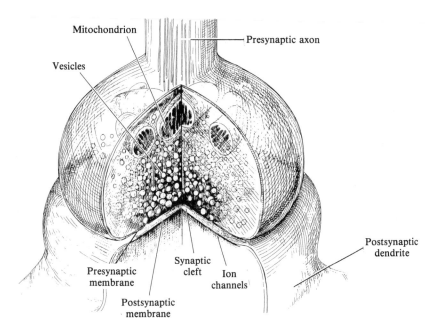

FIGURE II.2 A synapse is the relay point at which information is conveyed by chemical transmitters from one neuron to another. A synapse consists of two parts: the knoblike tip of an axon terminal at the presynaptic side and the receptor region on the dendritic surface of another neuron at the postsynaptic side. The membranes are separated by a synaptic cleft some 200 nanometers across. Molecules of chemical transmitter, stored in vesicles in the axon terminal, are released into the cleft by arriving nerve impulses. The transmitter changes the electrical state of the receiving neuron, making it either more likely or less likely to fire an impulse. [From C. F. Stevens, "The Neuron," in *The Brain,* a *Scientific American* book (San Francisco: W. H. Freeman and Company, 1979), p. 11.]

As a consequence of this convergence and divergence of electrical activity, neurons tend to group together and form circuits. The properties of these circuits determine how information is handled in the nervous system. Traditionally one distinguishes those areas of the brain where cell bodies are concentrated (areas referred to as *nuclei*) from those regions that consist mainly of bundles of axons that project from one group of neurons to another (*fiber tracts*). In the peripheral nervous system (that is, outside the brain and spinal cord), these fiber tracts are referred to as *nerves*. Thus, the *sciatic nerve* is actually a bundle of axons, the somas of which are located in the spinal cord (*motor neurons*), the dorsal root ganglia (*sensory neurons*), or autonomic ganglia.

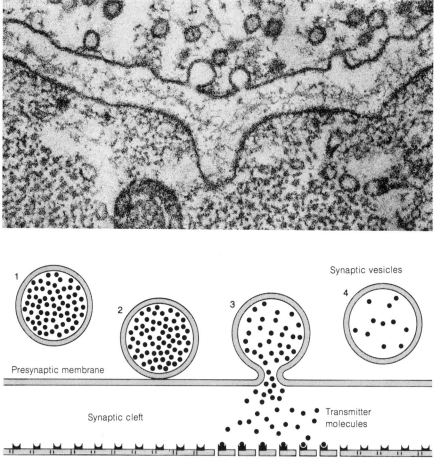

FIGURE II.3 Transmitter is discharged into the synaptic cleft at the synaptic junction between neurons by vesicles that open up after they fuse with the axon's presynaptic membrane, a process called exocytosis. This electron micrograph, made by Heuser, has caught the vesicles in the terminal of an axon in the act of discharging acetyl-choline into the neuromuscular junction of a frog. The structures that appear in the micrograph are enlarged some 115,000 diameters. Synaptic vesicles are clustered near the presynaptic membrane. The diagram shows the probable steps in exocytosis. Filled vesicles move up to the synaptic cleft, fuse with the membrane, discharge their contents, and are reclaimed, re-formed, and refilled with transmitter. [From C. F. Stevens, "The Neuron," in *The Brain,* a *Scientific American* book (San Francisco: W H. Freeman and Company, 1979), p. 24.]

In the brain, nuclei tend to congregate to form yet larger structures (such as the *thalamus, hypothalamus, amygdala,* and *hippocampus*). The fiber tracts connecting neurons of different discrete nuclei are given names that indicate the areas of the brain that they link. For example, the bundle of sensory axons that runs from the spinal cord to the thalamus is referred to as the *spinothalamic tract.*

In addition to neurons, other types of cells are also found in the brain. The most conspicuous of these are the *glial cells,* which make up more than half the volume of the brain. One type of glial cell, the *astrocyte,* surrounds blood capillaries in the brain to form part of the blood–brain barrier (Chapter 2). Other glial cells provide structural support for the brain and metabolic support for the neurons in a fashion that has not yet been well identified.

C. R. Stevens well summarizes the structure of the brain:

> The brain, then, is an immense number of spidery nerve cells, interconnected in a complex net, and embedded in a supporting and protecting meshwork of neuroglia. Dendrites spring from the neuron cell body, branch profusely, and along with the soma receive myriads of axon terminals, making it possible for a single nerve cell to gather information from hundreds of others. Furthermore, cell bodies are collected into groups, the nuclei, and these, in turn, into clusters. Running back and forth between nuclei, or between collections of nuclei, are fiber tracts, the main channels of communications between one part of the brain and another. Altogether, these structures are arranged in an orderly way to form the brain of the animal and to provide the anatomical basis for neural function. [From "The Neuron," in *The Brain,* a *Scientific American* book (San Francisco: W. H. Freeman and Company, 1979), p. 25.]

S. Cohen adds:

> It is reasonable to think of the brain as a symphony of almost infinite orchestration with assemblies of instrumentations evoking an infinite ensemble of informational responses. The brain, vast and adaptable, is capable of providing for all the subtleties of sensing, integrating and responding. . . . The neuron is the basic information processor and transmitter. [From *The Chemical Brain* (Irvine, Calif.: Care Institute, 1988), p. 8.]

Relevant to this anatomy, and critical to the study of neuropsychopharmacology, is the fact that psychoactive drugs exert their behavioral effects by altering the synaptic function of neurons located within specific areas of the brain, usually by either potentiating or inhibiting the process of chemical transmission.

Axon

As discussed previously, the neuron consists of three main elements: the dendrites, the soma, and the axon. In brief, electrical impulses originate in the dendrites, are integrated in the soma, and are transmitted down the axon to the synapse. Unlike the dendrites and the soma, the axon is specialized solely for the reliable conduction of electrical activity, which occurs in the form of electrical impulses called *action potentials.* All action potentials are conducted down a given axon rapidly and without alteration. The only way to change the content of information relayed by an axon is to alter the number of action potentials that are conducted each second. The axon is not a major site of action for psychoactive drugs, but it is the site of action for local anesthetics, such as lidocaine (Xylocaine). Here, the local anesthetic blocks the propagation of impulses down the axon. Synaptic processes are not involved.

Dendrites

How do action potentials (which are conducted down the axon) influence the activity of other neurons? The distal terminals of an axon align themselves at the synapse with one or more of the dendrites or the soma of the next neuron. Dendrites are specialized structures containing *receptors* that are sensitive to transmitter released from other neurons. When action potentials have been conducted down the axon of a neuron and transmitter has been released from that neuron, the receptors on the dendrites of the postsynaptic neuron exhibit an electrical change, the magnitude of which is proportional to the amount of transmitter released by the presynaptic neuron (Figure II.4). To accomplish this, when action potentials reach the synapse, a chemical transmitter is released. As described above, molecules of transmitter diffuse across a small, fluid-filled gap (the synaptic cleft) and attach to the postsynaptic receptors.

What exactly are these receptors? Most receptors appear to be membrane-spanning, transmitter-activated ("ligand-gated") cylindrical channels, formed by large proteins that array themselves such that a pore or channel runs down through the middle and opens to both the inside (cytoplasmic side) and the outside (synaptic side) of the neuronal membrane (Figure II.5).

These receptor–protein complexes exist in two states, open and closed. In their resting state, the channel is closed, and ions (which are electrically charged atoms, usually of calcium, sodium, chloride, or

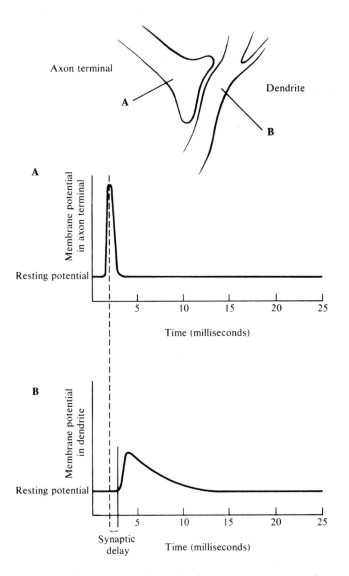

FIGURE II.4 Transmission of impulses from one neuron to another at a synapse. Graph (**A**) is a recording of electrical activity in the axon terminal as an action potential arrives at the synapse. Graph (**B**) is a recording of electrical activity in the dendrite of the next neuron, showing the postsynaptic activity resulting from the transmission of impulses across the synapse. [Modified from C. F. Stevens, *Neurophysiology: A Primer* (New York: Wiley, 1966), fig. 3.2, p. 35.]

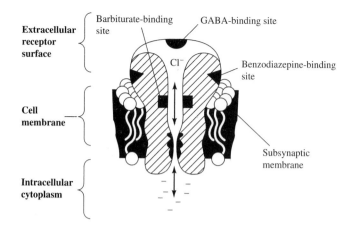

FIGURE II.5 GABA$_A$ receptor in a perpendicular section through the membrane. The localization of the various binding sites is purely hypothetical. [From W. E. Haefely, J. R. Martin, J. G. Richards, and P. Schoch, "The Multiplicity of Actions of Benzodiazepine Receptor Ligands," *Canadian Journal of Psychiatry* 38, Suppl. 4 (1993): 5102–5107, with permission.]

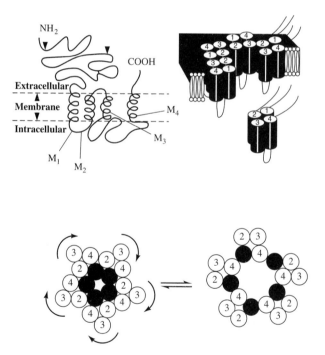

FIGURE II.6 Presumed topology of the GABA$_A$ receptor. *Top left:* Single subunit with its large extracellular terminal part, and the four transmembrane domains (M1 to M4) with their intracellular connecting stretches. *Top right:* Arrangement of the transmembrane domains of five subunits to form a central channel. Bottom: The transmembrane domains in a transverse section through the membrane when the channel is closed (left) and open (right). [From W. E. Haefely, J. R. Martin, J. G. Richards, and P. Schoch, "The Multiplicity of Actions of Benzodiazepine Receptor Ligands," *Canadian Journal of Psychiatry* 38, Suppl. 4 (1993): 5102–5107, with permission.]

potassium) cannot pass through the pores to reach the cytoplasm of the cell. When a transmitter chemical attaches to the receptor protein (on the synaptic side), the configuration of the membrane-spanning protein complex rotates and moves slightly apart, enlarging the pore and allowing ions to enter the postsynaptic cell (Figure II.6).

This inflow of ions alters intracellular mechanisms; as a result, action potential can be generated or inhibited, or intracellular enzymes can be affected that alter the biochemical functioning of the cell. The chemical transmitter that diffuses across the synaptic cleft and attaches to the receptor is called the *first messenger*; the cytoplasmic proteins that are altered, thus affecting the function of the postsynaptic cell, are referred to as the *second messengers* (see Appendix III).

If the first messenger affects receptor function so that positively charged ions enter the postsynaptic neuron, the membrane becomes depolarized and the neuron becomes more excitable (see Figure II.4). This depolarizing current produces what is known as an *excitatory postsynaptic potential* (EPSP). Note in Figure II.4 that a slight delay (approximately 0.5 millisecond) occurs between the arrival of an action potential at a nerve terminal and the EPSP in the postsynaptic (dendritic) membrane. This time lag, called the *synaptic delay,* is the time required for the transmitter substance released by the axon to reach the dendrite of the next cell.

Some neurotransmitters (such as gamma-aminobutyric acid, GABA), instead of depolarizing the dendrites, *hyperpolarize* the dendritic membrane through the inflow of negatively charged ions (primarily chloride ions). The resulting hyperpolarization is referred to as an *inhibitory postsynaptic potential* (IPSP). This IPSP opposes the action of the EPSP, stabilizing the neuron and tending to prevent the generation of action potentials.

All neurons in the CNS receive impulses from both excitatory and inhibitory synapses and are held in a balance between excitation and inhibition. Indeed, the exquisite beauty of the nervous system is maintained by this delicate balance. Because they affect synaptic transmission, psychoactive drugs upset this balance by acting on different types of receptors. This alteration of excitability within specific areas of the nervous system leads to drug-induced alterations in behavior, as we repeatedly discuss throughout this text.

Soma

The dendrites and soma (Figure II.7) receive input from other neurons through synapses and respond by becoming either depolarized or hyperpolarized. The net effect is reflected in the excitability of the

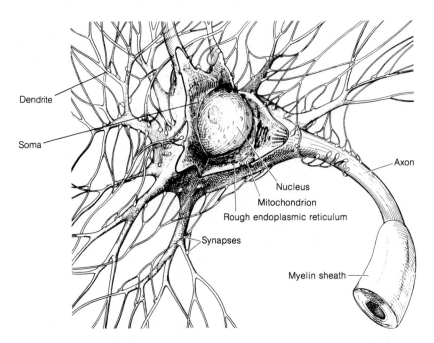

FIGURE II.7 The cell body of a neuron contains the genetic material and complex metabolic apparatus common to all cells. Unlike most other cells, however, neurons do not divide after embryonic development; an organism's original supply must serve a lifetime. Projecting from the cell body are several dendrites and a single axon. The cell body and dendrites are covered by synapses—knoblike structures where information is received from other neurons. Mitochondria provide the cell with energy. Proteins are synthesized on the endoplasmic reticulum. A transport system moves proteins and other substances from the cell body to sites where they are needed. [From C. F. Stevens, "The Neuron," in *The Brain,* a *Scientific American* book (San Francisco: W. H. Freeman and Company, 1979), p. 17.]

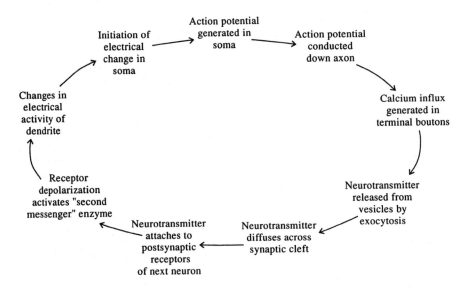

FIGURE II.8 Sequence of the transmission of information between neurons.

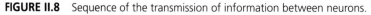

soma. If the influence of excitatory synapses is greater than the influence of inhibitory synapses, the soma responds by producing an action potential that is propagated through its axon and conducted to the next synapse. If, instead, the influence of inhibitory synapses predominates, the soma hyperpolarizes and the neuron becomes less excitable.

Figure II.8 summarizes the steps in transfering information from one neuron to another. Appendix III focuses on the process of synaptic transmission, the chemical substances involved, the protein structure of representative receptors, and some concepts that relate to drug-induced alterations of synaptic transmission.

SYNAPTIC TRANSMISSION, NEUROTRANSMITTERS, AND INFORMATION TRANSFER IN THE CNS

In Appendix II, we discussed the neuronal electrical phenomena that are the basis of nervous system function. All information transfer in the brain occurs through a two-step interaction between two neurons: (1) the liberation of a chemical transmitter (the first messenger) into the synaptic cleft between the neurons and (2) subsequent activation of intracellular processes or enzymes (the second messenger) that alters the function of the postsynaptic neuron.

The concept of chemical transmission in the CNS has developed slowly over the past 75 years. Today this theory is well accepted, and the actions of most psychoactive drugs can be interpreted in terms of alterations in the steps of synaptic transmission. Recent studies have provided insights into how chemical transmission ultimately affects the functioning of postsynaptic neurons.

This appendix focuses on specific chemical substances known to function in the CNS as synaptic transmitters. Also, the role of these transmitters both in neuropsychological disorders and in the action of psychoactive drugs is discussed.

Historical Background

Research in the early twentieth century established the concept that neuronal excitation in the peripheral nervous system results in the local release of a chemical substance, which causes specific activity when the substance combines with some constituent of an organ, muscle, or gland. This work led to the identification of acetylcholine and epinephrine as transmitter substances in the peripheral nervous system (nerves that lie outside the brain and spinal cord).

From 1946 through the 1970s, neurochemical research delineated many neurochemical pathways within the CNS and identified acetylcholine, serotonin, norepinephrine, and dopamine as CNS neurotransmitters. Studies of psychedelic drugs supported the hypothesis that behavioral effects occurred as a result of stimulation or blockade of one or more steps in the process of synaptic transmission.

During the 1980s, many more neurotransmitters were shown to exist. Currently about 40 neurotransmitters have been identified; some serve as primary transmitters, while others function as modulators (for example, they presynaptically modulate the release of a primary transmitter) or as a neurohormone (autocoid) that alters the responsiveness of postsynaptic neurons (see the discussion of caffeine in Chapter 7).

It is not clear whether a single neuron liberates only one or several transmitter substances. It was formerly thought that one neuron could manufacture and release only a single neurotransmitter, neuromodulator, or neurohormone. As stated by Cohen:

> It may be that most neurons contain multiple transmitters, for example, an amine or amino acid [as a primary transmitter], along with a neuropeptide to modulate the transmission and sometimes a neurohormone to prolong the transmission. All neurochemical information circuits are widely dispersed and are almost never localized in discrete brain areas. As a corollary, many neurotransmitting systems converge on single brain regions. These features of transmitter function make simple statements about the effects of various transmitters incomplete. Furthermore, the receptors exhibit a considerable self-regulatory capability, changing their sensitivity during excessive or infrequent use.

> Many of the important transmitters are amines and are called biogenic [biological] amines as a group. Most are monoamines; that is, they have a single ammonium (NH_2) radical in their structure. The biogenic amines derived from catechol (dihydrobenzene) are named catecholamines and include dopamine, norepinephrine, and epinephrine. Another monoamine is serotonin (5-hydroxy-tryptamine). Acetylcholine is not an amine. It does not contain an NH_2 group. It can be classified as a choline ester.[1]

Research today is yielding an explosion of information about the structure of receptors and the processes by which neurotransmitters effect biochemical or functional changes within the cytoplasm of postsynaptic neurons.

Steps in Synaptic Transmission

Appendix II introduced the synapse as vital to the functioning of the nervous system and to the action of psychoactive drugs. Here we consider the specific steps in synaptic transmission. Figure III.1 shows a schematic representation of an idealized synapse.

There are about a dozen steps in the synaptic transmission process (numbered in Figure III.1), and each one constitutes a possible site of drug action. Some of these steps occur within the presynaptic terminal, some on the presynaptic membrane, some within the synaptic cleft, some on the postsynaptic membrane, and some within the postsynaptic neuron. Events in the presynaptic terminal and within the synaptic cleft itself can involve long-term cellular adaptive mechanisms (possibly involved in drug tolerance or dependence); they can also involve presynaptic modulation, which controls the amount of transmitter released in response to the calcium influx that follows arrival of an action potential.

Of increasing interest are events that occur on and within the postsynaptic membrane. Modern techniques of gene cloning and molecular biology are providing important insights into the structure and function of postsynaptic receptors. In general, these receptors are large proteins that can be loosely classified into three groups:[2]

   1. transmitter- (ligand-) gated ion channels
   2. transport proteins embedded in cell membranes
   3. membrane-spanning proteins that are configured into a helical array, forming a cylindrical structure without a central pore

Details of the transmitter-gated ion channel are discussed later in this appendix.

All cell membranes (both neuronal and nonneuronal) contain membrane transporters for essential body nutrients such as sugars and amino acids, which are large, molecular-sized substances that normally cannot cross the cell membrane. Such transporters are essential to the survival of cells of the body. Other specific transporters located at axon terminals remove specific neurotransmitters (e.g., norepinephrine, epinephrine, dopamine, and serotonin) from the synapse, providing a mechanism for terminating transmitter action.

One of these transporters (the dopamine transporter, which is selectively blocked by cocaine) has been well characterized, and its structure is illustrated in Chapter 6 (Figure 6.4). As summarized:

> This protein chain (of the transporter) crossed the (presynaptic) cell membrane 12 times, leaving two long tails inside the cell and loops of different sizes outside. Four chains of sugar molecules are attached to the largest loop on the outside of the cell. How such a structure

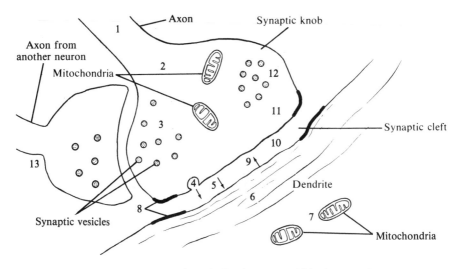

FIGURE III.1 Schematic diagram of an idealized synapse within the central nervous system. The steps in the transmission of information across such a synapse are numbered in this diagram.

1. Conduction of the action potential down the presynaptic axon.
2. Arrival of the action potential at the nerve terminal.
3. Synthesis and storage of transmitter in the synaptic vesicles (this may occur before steps 1 and 2).
4. Release of transmitter from synaptic vesicles (by a process of exocytosis) into the synaptic cleft when an action potential arrives.
5. Diffusion of transmitter across the synaptic cleft.
6. Stimulation of the postsynaptic receptors by transmitter.
7. Postsynaptic cellular response to receptor activation.
8. "Adaptive" or "plastic" processes on presynaptic and postsynaptic membranes in response to excess or deficient amounts of transmitter.
9. Release of transmitter from postsynaptic receptors back into the synaptic cleft.
10. Metabolism of some of the transmitter in the synaptic cleft by extracellular enzymes.
11. Reuptake of some of the transmitter back into the presynaptic nerve terminal.
12. Uptake of transmitter that is free in the intracellular fluid of the presynaptic nerve terminal into the synaptic vesicles, where it is protected from destruction by enzymes located in the cytoplasm.
13. Presynaptic inhibition by an axon.

actually moves a neurotransmitter like dopamine across the neuronal cell membrane and into the inside of the neuron is still a complete mystery. Cocaine binds to this transporter and blocks its function, causing dopamine to accumulate to excessive levels in the synapses.[2]

Finally, the membrane-spanning proteins all belong to what is known as the "superfamily of G-protein-coupled seven-helix receptors," which include the muscarinic acetylcholine receptor, and the $GABA_B$, dopamine, THC, serotonin, and dopamine receptors. As an example of one such receptor, we will examine the structure and function of the *serotonin$_{1A}$* receptor, one of at least 10 subtypes of serotonin receptors, and the receptor upon which buspirone (see Chapter 4) acts to produce its anxiolytic action.

The serotonin$_{1A}$ receptor is a single protein, approximately 420 amino acids long. It is divided into seven membrane-spanning regions of approximately 25 amino acids each, which thread back and forth across the cell membrane (Figure III.2). Four intervening sequences face the extracellular space, while four others face the cytoplasm. The long cytoplasmic loop (shown in Figure III.2) is the most diverse genetically and is thought to interact with intracellular second-messenger proteins such as adenylate cyclase (discussed later).

Figure III.2 illustrates the serotonin receptor in two dimensions, but in reality the three-dimensional structure resembles a cylinder, somewhat like an ion channel but without a central pore. Instead the extracellular "mouth" forms a pocket that accommodates the specific ligands. When a neurotransmitter becomes attached in the synapse, the helix is probably moved in such a way as to initiate a process we call *signal transduction*.

Attached to the long intracellular loop of the helical structure is a special protein (called a *G-protein*) that, when released from the receptor protein, can either initiate or inhibit other functional proteins within the cell (Figure III.3). Transmitter-induced alteration in the three-dimensional structure of the helix causes release of this G-protein, which then becomes active. In the serotonin$_{1A}$ receptor, the released G-protein inhibits the enzyme adenylate cyclase.[3,4] Other G-proteins regulate the opening or closing of transmembrane ion channels, while still other G-proteins activate (rather than inhibit) intracellular enzymes, such as phospholipase C, shown in Figure III.3.

In the mid-1990s, we are just beginning to understand how the attachment of the neurotransmitter to the receptor leads to alterations in cellular function. Eventually this knowledge will lead to new understanding of the action of agonist and antagonist drugs and of the effects of drugs on second-messenger processes such as G-protein-induced inhibition of adenylate cyclase. As discussed in Chapter 9, alteration of postsynaptic second-messenger systems may underlie the antimanic effect of lithium.[5]

Transmitter Substances

The major neurotransmitter substances in the brain are acetylcholine, norepinephrine, dopamine, serotonin, excitatory and inhibitory amino acids, and the opioid peptides.

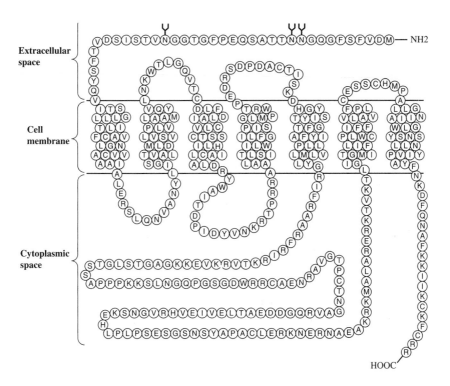

FIGURE III.2 Schematic representation of the primary structure of the rat serotonin$_{1A}$ receptor. [Reproduced with permission from Mestikawy, Fargin, Raymond, Gozlan, and Hnatowich.[3]]

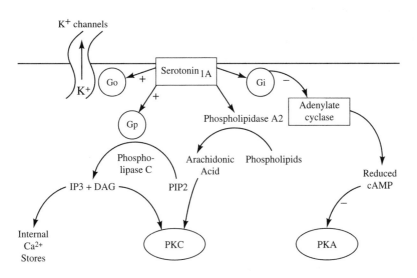

FIGURE III.3 Schematic representation of second-messenger pathways reported to be linked to the serotonin$_{1A}$ receptor. Ca, calcium; cAMP, cyclic adenoside mono-phosphate; DAG, diacylglycerol; Gi, inhibitory GTP-binding protein; Go, GTP-binding protein; GP, phospholipase-C-associated GTP-binding protein; IP3, inositol triphos-phate; K, potassium; PIP2, phosphoinositol bis-phosphate; PKA, cAMP-dependent protein kinase; PKC, protein kinase C. [Reproduced with permission from Harrington, Zhong, Garlow, and Ciaranello.[4]]

Acetylcholine

Acetylcholine (ACh) was first identified as a transmitter chemical in the peripheral nervous system. Large amounts of ACh are also present in brain tissue. Here we discuss the evidence for the role of ACh as a transmitter in the CNS.

The chemical reactions in the nerve terminal that lead to the synthesis of ACh are illustrated in Figure III.4. The dynamics of an ACh nerve terminal (that is, a nerve terminal that releases ACh) are shown in Figure III.5. Following synthesis, ACh is stored inside the nerve terminal within synaptic vesicles. It is released into the synaptic cleft when an action potential arrives from the axon. The ACh then diffuses across the cleft and attaches itself to postsynaptic receptors (presumably a seven-helix complex very similar to that of the serotonin$_{1A}$ receptor shown in Figure III.2). Scopolamine is a psychedelic deliriant drug that blocks the postsynaptic receptors for ACh. Thus, in Chapter 12, it is referred to as an anticholinergic psychedelic drug.

There are two types of ACh receptor: a "nicotinic" receptor (which is a ligand-gated ion channel) and a "muscarinic" receptor (which is part of the seven-helix family). In either case, once ACh has exerted its effect on the postsynaptic dendritic membrane, its action is terminated by the enzyme acetylcholine esterase (AChE). The process is illustrated in Figure III.6. The enzymatic reaction that degrades ACh is important, because many drugs (referred to as *AChE inhibitors*) inhibit this enzyme. Such drugs are quite toxic. Commercially, this toxicity is exploited in agriculture, where AChE inhibitors are used as insecticides,

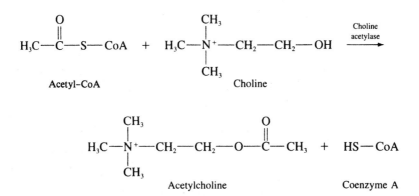

FIGURE III.4 Chemical reactions in the brain that are responsible for the synthesis of acetylcholine (ACh). The acetylcholine is synthesized from acetyl-CoA and choline.

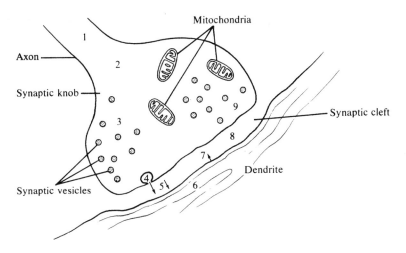

FIGURE III.5 Schematic diagram of an acetylcholine (ACh) synapse. The steps in transmission of information across such a synapse are numbered in this diagram.

1. Conduction of the action potential down the presynaptic axon.
2. Arrival of the action potential at the nerve terminal.
3. Synthesis of ACh (see Figure III.4) and storage of ACh in the synaptic vesicles (this may occur before steps I and 2).
4. Release of ACh from synaptic vesicles into the synaptic cleft when an action potential arrives.
5. Diffusion of ACh across the synaptic cleft.
6. Stimulation of the postsynaptic receptors by ACh.
7. Release of ACh from postsynaptic receptors back into the synaptic cleft.
8. Metabolism of ACh in the synaptic cleft by the enzyme acetylcholine esterase (see Figure III.6).
9. Uptake of choline that was produced by metabolism of ACh into the presynaptic nerve termlnal for the resynthesis of ACh.

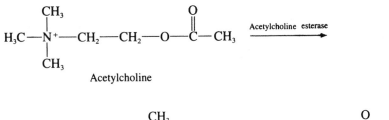

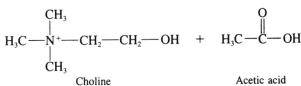

FIGURE III.6 Destruction of acetylcholine by the enzyme acetylcholine esterase (AChE).

and in the military, where they have been stockpiled as lethal nerve gases.

ACh is distributed widely in the brain (Figure III.7). The highest concentrations are found in the caudate nucleus, certain brain stem nuclei, and the cerebral cortex (especially the frontal cortex). High concentrations of ACh are also found in the motor neurons that emerge from the spinal cord, reflecting the fact that ACh is the transmitter at the neuromuscular junction.

In the basal ganglia, ACh-containing neurons persist after dopamine neurons degenerate in patients who have Parkinson's disease; the relatively unopposed action of ACh may be involved in the symptomatology of patients with this disease. In patients who have died of Alzheimer's disease (presenile dementia),[6] acetylcholine receptors in the cerebral cortex are largely absent.[7] Interestingly, scopolamine

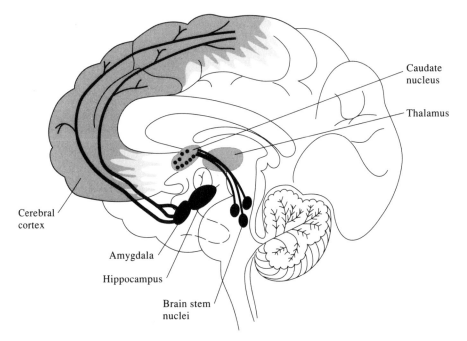

FIGURE III.7 ACh pathways in the human brain. Cell bodies and fiber tracts (axonal projections) are shown in black. Shaded areas show the locations of ACh terminals. [Modified from L. L. Iversen, "The Chemistry of the Brain," in *The Brain,* a *Scientific American* book (San Francisco: W. H. Freeman and Company, 1979), p. 77.]

blocks ACh receptors and is a potent amnestic agent, and amnesia is a prominent symptom of Alzheimer's disease. ACh is also important in mechanisms related to behavioral arousal, learning, memory, attention, energy conservation, mood, and REM activity during sleep. Finally, ACh-secreting neurons located in the hippocampus and cerebral cortex participate in learning, memory formation, and retrieval of memory.

Norepinephrine and Dopamine

The term *catecholamine* refers to three chemically related compounds: epinephrine (Epi), norepinephrine (NE), and dopamine (DA). Epi, a neurotransmitter in the peripheral nervous system, is important in maintaining blood pressure and heart rate. Epi is not commonly found in the brain, but NE and DA are the primary catecholamine neurotransmitters in the brain. Many of the drugs that profoundly affect brain function and behavior exert their effects by altering the synaptic action of NE and DA in the brain. Thus, in many instances, the effects of new drugs on behavior have been predictable, because we knew how they would affect the actions of catecholamine neurotransmitters.

DA and NE are manufactured within catecholamine neurons by the steps shown in Figure III.8. We will confine our study to the step in which the enzyme tyrosine hydroxylase is the catalyst. Inhibition of this enzyme by a drug such as alpha-methyl-para-tyrosine (a clinically useful drug for treating hypertension) reduces the level of catecholamine in the CNS and produces sedation as a side effect. This sedative effect, which results from the inhibition of NE synthesis, implies that the levels and functioning of neurotransmitters within the brain underlie behavior. By similar reasoning, drugs that alter behavior probably produce their effects because they alter the chemical transmission between neurons.

For example, patients who have Parkinson's disease exhibit a level of DA in the caudate nucleus that is lower than the amount normally present. Administration of DA to these patients is not useful therapeutically, because DA does not cross the blood–brain barrier. However, the administration of dopa (the precursor to DA) does increase the level of DA in the caudate nucleus. Dopa can cross the blood–brain barrier into the brain, where it is converted into DA. Thus, the chemical synthesis of a transmitter may be used to clinical benefit.

Metabolic Fate   A transmitter is synthesized, stored, and released; exerts a postsynaptic effect; and then is inactivated. Inactivation can occur by either or both of two processes:

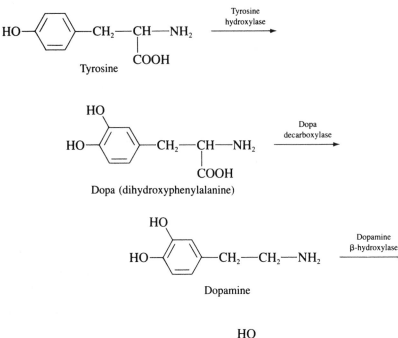

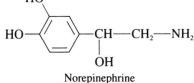

FIGURE III.8 Synthesis of norepinephrine (NE) from tyrosine. Note the intermediate compounds formed in this reaction, dopa and dopamine.

1. enzymatic destruction of the transmitter within the synaptic cleft

2. active reuptake of the transmitter from the synaptic cleft back into the presynaptic nerve terminal

Catecholamines are inactivated by the enzymes monoamine oxidase (MAO) and catechol *O*-methyltransferase (COMT) (Figure III.9). However, these enzymatic inactivations occur too slowly to account for the rapid termination of DA or NE. Thus, the postsynaptic effects of DA or NE are not terminated to any significant extent by enzymes. Rather, the actions of these transmitters are terminated primarily by

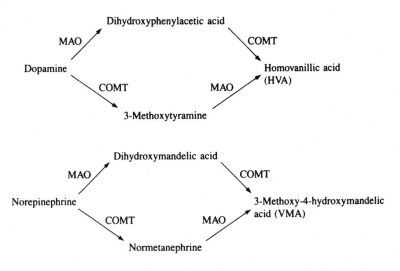

FIGURE III.9 Destruction of dopamine and norepinephrine. The inactivating enzymes are monoamine oxidase (MAO) and catechol O-methyltransferase (COMT).

an active (energy requiring) process of reuptake across the presynaptic nerve membrane back into the nerve endings. When NE or DA is taken up in this way, it is stored again in the synaptic vesicles to be reused later.

The principle of reuptake into the nerve terminal and then into the storage vesicles is crucially important, because certain drugs may block (1) the active uptake process into the nerve terminal (thus prolonging the synaptic action of the transmitter) or (2) the uptake of the transmitter from the intracellular fluid in the nerve terminal back into the synaptic vesicles (thus decreasing the amount of stored transmitter available for release). Cocaine is representative of drugs that block presynaptic reuptake of DA from the synaptic cleft into the nerve terminal; the tricyclic antidepressants are drugs that block presynaptic reuptake into the nerve terminals of NE and serotonin neurons (with the newer antidepressants being more specific for the serotonin transporter); and reserpine is a drug that blocks the uptake of the transmitter back into the vesicle.

Catecholamine Synapse   The dynamics of DA and NE resemble those of other CNS transmitters. A NE synapse is illustrated in Figure III.10. It is similar to the acetylcholine terminal presented in Figure

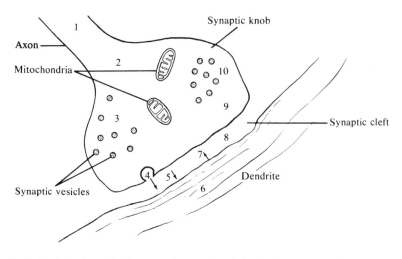

FIGURE III.10 Schematic diagram of a norepinephrine (NE) synapse within the central nervous system. The steps in the transmission of information across such a synapse are numbered in this diagram.

1. Conduction of the action potential down the presynaptic axon.
2. Arrival of the action potential at the nerve terminal.
3. Synthesis of NE (see Figure III.8) and storage of NE in the synaptic vesicles (this may occur before steps 1 and 2).
4. Release of NE from synaptic vesicles into the synaptic cleft when an action potential arrives.
5. Diffusion of NE across the synaptic cleft.
6. Stimulation of the postsynaptic receptors by NE.
7. Release of NE from postsynaptic receptors back into the synaptic cleft.
8. Metabolism of some of the NE in the synaptic cleft by extracellular enzymes.
9. Reuptake of some of the NE back into the presynaptic nerve terminal.
10. Uptake of NE in the presynaptic nerve terminal into the presynaptic vesicles.

III.5; that is, the presynaptic nerve terminal contains mitochondria and small vesicles that contain stored transmitter. However, the DA and NE terminals contain chemical products entirely different from those in an ACh terminal. The amino acid tyrosine (which is obtained from food) is actively taken up into the presynaptic terminal, where it is transformed to dopa, DA, and ultimately NE (see Figure III.8). In those catecholamine nerve terminals in which the enzyme dopamine beta-hydroxylase is not present, DA is not converted to NE and the DA itself serves as the transmitter substance.

After synthesis, the transmitter is stored in the synaptic vesicles. When an action potential arrives at the nerve terminal, this induces a brief influx of calcium, and the transmitter is released by exocytosis from the vesicles (which cluster close to the cleft) into the synaptic cleft. The transmitter then diffuses across this cleft and attaches to its receptors located on the postsynaptic membrane. The transmission process is terminated primarily by the active reuptake of transmitter back into the nerve terminal.

Norepinephrine Pathways and Function The cell bodies of NE neurons are located in the brain stem (Figure III.11). From there, axons project rostrally to nerve terminals in the cerebral cortex, the limbic system, the hypothalamus, and the cerebellum. Axonal projections also travel caudally to dorsal horns of the spinal cord, where they

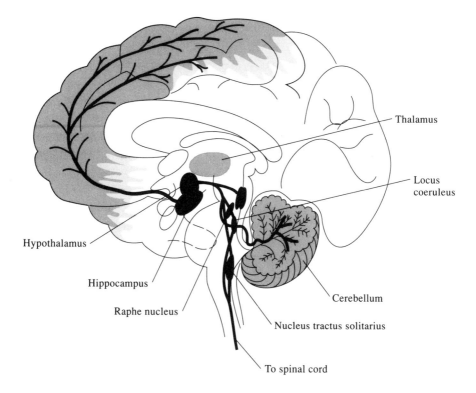

FIGURE III.11 Norepinephrine pathways in the human brain. Cell bodies and fiber tracts are shown in black. Norepinephrine terminals are represented by the shaded areas. [Modified from L. L. Iversen, "The Chemistry of the Brain," in *The Brain,* a *Scientific American* book (San Francisco: W. H. Freeman and Company, 1979), p. 77.

exert an analgesic action by limiting release of substance P (see Chapter 10).

The release of NE produces an alerting, focusing, orienting response (similar to the peripheral fight/flight/fright syndrome), positive feelings of reward, and analgesia, and it regulates blood pressure. A release of NE may also cause basic instinctual behaviors such as hunger, thirst, emotion, and sex.

Dopamine Pathways and Function Large amounts of DA are found in the basal ganglia (a part of the extrapyramidal motor system), the frontal cortex, and the limbic system. The originating cell bodies of these nerve terminals are largely found in a brain stem structure called the substantia nigra (Figure III.12). These cell bodies are also found in other nuclei of the midbrain associated with emotion and reward

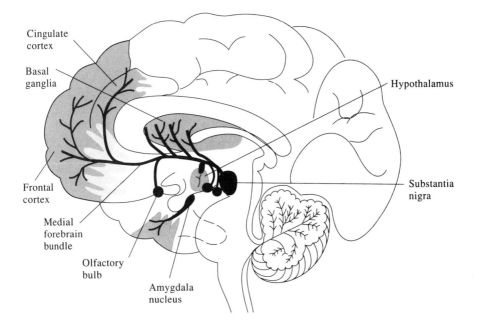

FIGURE III.12 Dopaminergic pathways in the rat brain. Cell bodies and fiber tracts (axonal projections) are shown in black. Dopaminergic terminals are represented by the shaded areas. [Modified from L. L. Iversen, "The Chemistry of the Brain," in *The Brain,* a *Scientific American* book (San Francisco: W. H. Freeman and Company, 1979), p. 77.]

systems that involve the ventral tegmental area and the nucleus accumbens, as discussed in Chapter 15. Those axons that project to the frontal cortex are involved with thought and the integration of emotions.

Two examples of the alteration of DA function involve schizophrenia and parkinsonism. Schizophrenics exhibit an increased sensitivity of DA receptors in the frontal cortex; this fact forms the rationale for treating schizophrenic patients with DA-receptor blockers (see Chapter 11). The parkinsonianlike side effects of phenothiazines reflect a blockade of DA receptors in the basal ganglia (the drugs are not specific for DA receptors located in the frontal cortex).

Similarly, in patients who have Parkinson's disease (see Chapter 11), the neurons in the basal ganglia are devoid of DA, so replacement of DA with levodopa or the administration of drugs that stimulate DA receptors (receptor agonists) can be useful. Finally, the behavioral stimulant and reinforcing properties of cocaine and amphetamine (see Chapters 6 and 15) reflect the activation of DA receptors. Many drugs that affect DA neurons are discussed throughout this text.

Serotonin

Serotonin was first investigated as a CNS neurotransmitter when LSD was found to resemble serotonin structurally. At that time, it was hypothesized that drug-induced hallucinations might be caused by alterations in the functioning of serotonin neurons. In the brain, significant amounts of serotonin are found in the upper brain stem, with a large collection in the pons and the medulla (areas that are collectively called the raphe nuclei). Rostral projections from the brain stem terminate diffusely throughout the cerebral cortex, the hippocampus, the hypothalamus, and the limbic system (Figure III.13).

Because serotonin is an inhibitor of activity and behavior, the rostral projections are thought to function in sleep, wakefulness, mood, temperature regulation, feeding, and sexual activity. Serotonin projections largely parallel those of NE, although serotonin seems to have an effect that is opposite to that of NE (analogously to DA and ACh, whose effects in the basal ganglia are opposing). Caudal projections of serotonin axons from the raphe nuclei inhibit the release of substance P in the spinal cord (see Chapter 10) and modulate spinal reflexes.

Amino Acids

Four amino acids function as CNS neurotransmitters: two (glutamic and aspartic acid) are excitatory to neuronal transmission and two

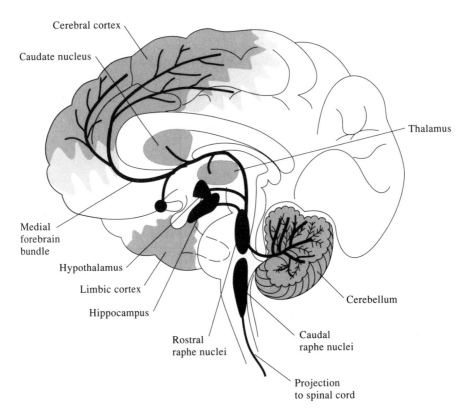

FIGURE III.13 Serotonin pathways in the rat brain. Cell bodies and fiber tracts (axonal projections) are shown in black. Serotenergic terminals are represented by the shaded areas. [Modified from L. L. Iversen, "The Chemistry of the Brain," in *The Brain,* a *Scientific American* book (San Francisco: W. H. Freeman and Company, 1979), p. 77.]

(gamma-aminobutyric acid, or GABA, and glycine) are inhibitory (Figure III.14). In this discussion, we describe GABA as being representative of these transmitters.

GABA is the major inhibitor of neurotransmission in the brain.[8] Drug studies have shown that numerous classes of drugs (benzodiazepines, barbiturates, anesthetics, steroids, alcohol, and others) can bind to various sites on the GABA receptor, enhancing endogenous GABA-mediated inhibition. Probably all neurons of the CNS have GABA receptors embedded in their cell bodies, dendrites, and axon endings and are innervated to greatly varying degrees by

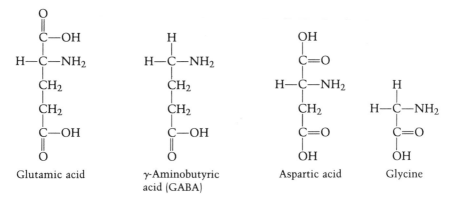

FIGURE III.14 Structures of four amino acid neurotransmitters within the CNS.

GABAergic (GABA secreting) neurons.[9] Therefore, virtually every neuron in the CNS is probably responsive to GABA.

Early research showed that when GABA receptors are activated, chloride permeability increases, thus hyperpolarizing the affected membrane. This type of GABA receptor is now termed a GABA$_A$ receptor. More recently identified is a different type of GABA receptor, the GABA$_B$ receptor, whose activation opens channels to potassium. While activation of GABA$_A$ receptors is responsible for fast inhibitory postsynaptic potentials (Appendix II), activation of GABA$_B$ receptors leads to a much slower, longer-lasting inhibition, the functional significance of which is still largely unclear. Importantly, these two receptor types originate from two separate classes of receptor families. The GABA$_A$ receptor is a ligand-gated ion channel with multiple binding sites for drugs (see Figure II.5 in Appendix II). The GABA$_B$ receptor is a G-protein-coupled receptor, a part of the superfamily of helical receptors similar to the serotonin$_{1A}$ receptor discussed earlier in this appendix).

The GABA$_A$ receptor is complex, composed of several glycoprotein subunits that assemble to form a functional channel with a transmitter (GABA) recognition site (see Figure II.6 in Appendix II). Five noncovalently associated subunits are embedded in the cell membrane and are arranged to form the pore. In the absence of GABA, the channel is closed and is impermeable to chloride ions. Binding of GABA to its binding site leads to a rotational, conformational change in structure, resulting in a pore opening. Chloride ions can then enter from the extracellular fluid and hyperpolarize the membrane. As discussed in

Chapter 4, benzodiazepines bind to adjacent sites and exert a modulatory role that facilitates GABA binding.[9]

Figure III.15 is a diagram of the GABAergic synapse. GABA is synthesized from the amino acid glutamate via the enzyme glutamic acid decarboxylase and stored for release. After release, the transmitter acts on both presynaptic and postsynaptic GABA$_A$ and GABA$_B$ receptors as discussed above. The action is terminated by active reuptake from the synaptic space.

Drugs that facilitate GABAergic neurotransmission (classically the benzodiazepines; see Chapter 4) produce well-known changes in somatic and psychological function. These changes include anxiolytic and antiepileptic properties, sedation, reduced emotional reactivity, reduced vigilance, anterograde amnesia, sleep, muscle relaxation (centrally mediated), and ataxia. The recent clinical introduction of flumazenil, an antagonist of GABAergic neurotransmission, is a signif-

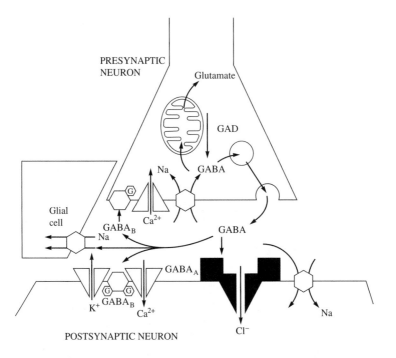

FIGURE III.15   GABAergic synapse, showing synthesis and release from a presynaptic terminal and GABA actions on a postsynaptic neuron. [Reproduced with permission from Tanelian, Kosek, Mody, and MacIver.[8]]

icant advance in the management of patients suffering from benzo-diazepine intoxication.

Of current interest are certain experimental benzodiazepine antag-onists ("partial inverse agonists") with low intrinsic activity that produce an interesting improvement in cognitive functions and an increase in vigilance, both of which may have useful therapeutic appli-cations.[9] Chapter 4 also discusses GABA$_A$ and GABA$_B$ antagonists as cognitive enhancers. The review by Haefely and coworkers lists several other experimental drugs that alter the functioning of GABA$_A$ recep-tors; these drugs may also prove to be therapeutically useful.[9]

Glutamate and aspartate are universally excitatory amino acids.[10] A synthetic derivative of aspartate, N-methyl-D-aspartate (see Chapter 12) is also excitatory. These agents appear to be involved in cellular metabolism by increasing ion conductance across membranes. Chapter 12 discusses the interaction between the psychedelic drug phencyclidine and N-methyl-D-aspartate receptors.

Purines, especially adenine, may function as CNS neurotrans-mitters and possibly as neuromodulators. Chapter 7 describes how the stimulant action of caffeine might result from the antagonism of inhibitory adenosine neuromodulation.

Substance P is a peptide transmitter that is released by nociceptive afferent neurons that synapse in the dorsal horn of the spinal cord. Substance P is discussed further in Chapter 10.

Opioid Peptides

In 1967 it was proposed that chemicals exist in the brain that provide analgesia by acting on specific receptors and that the opioid narcotics might mimic these natural analgesic substances by binding to the same receptors.

In 1973 opioid receptors were identified in localized areas of the brain. First, high concentrations of opioid receptors line the wall of the fourth ventricle in the brain stem. In that area, either morphine or electrical stimulation produces analgesia, which can be blocked by naloxone (Narcan, a pure opioid antagonist). The medial thalamus also has a high concentration of opioid receptors. This area of the brain appears to mediate deep pain that is poorly localized and emo-tionally influenced—the kind of pain most strongly affected by opioids. Opioid receptors are also found in areas of the spinal cord involved with the integration of incoming sensory information. Here, opioids reduce the intensity of painful stimuli. Receptors are also located in a nucleus of the brain stem that receives pain fibers from the face and the hands, as well as in those centers of the brain stem that are involved in the mediation of cough, nausea, and vomiting, maintenance of blood pressure, and control of stomach secretions. Finally, the greatest concentration of opioid receptors in the CNS is located in the limbic system in the amygdala. Although opioids are not thought to exert analgesic actions through these limbic receptors, they probably exert influences through these receptors that affect emotional behavior (see Chapter 10). Very few opioid receptors are found in the cerebral cortex, and none have been found in the cerebellum. Interestingly, opioid receptors are universally present in vertebrates but are not found in invertebrates.

In 1976 three types of opioid receptors were identified: mu, kappa, and sigma. In 1981 a fourth type of receptor (the delta receptor) was added. More recently subtypes of these receptors have been identified, and the existence of the opioid sigma receptor has been disputed.

Mu receptors are located primarily in the brain stem and medial thalamic areas. They appear to mediate morphine-induced analgesia and respiratory depression. Kappa receptors are located primarily in the spinal cord, where they mediate spinal analgesia. In the brain stem, kappa receptors mediate the sedation and miosis (pupil constriction) that are induced by opioids. Delta receptors are thought to be involved in alterations of affective behavior and euphoria. Delta receptors appear to be specific target receptors for the enkephalin peptides (discussed below).

As stated, some opioid receptors are subcategorized. For example, a mu-1 receptor may be associated with analgesia, while a mu-2 receptor may be associated with respiratory depression. In the future, receptor-specific synthetic opioids might be developed so that specific mu-1 or kappa analgesia can be obtained without undesirable delta or mu-2 side effects.

The discovery of opioid receptors did not prove the existence of naturally occurring compounds in the brain that act on these receptors. However, in 1975, researchers isolated crude extracts from the brain that produced actions similar to those produced by morphine in a preparation of small intestines from guinea pigs. In particular, the brain extract inhibited normal intestinal contractions, an action that could be blocked by naloxone. Two proteins were isolated from this crude extract, each of which consisted of five amino acids. These two proteins were named *met-enkephalin* and *leu-enkephalin*. Later these proteins were isolated from pig brain, beef brain, human cerebral spinal fluid, and the pituitary gland of several species. Also isolated from the pituitary gland was a longer protein (called *beta-lipotropin*), within which was found met-enkephalin and other peptides that have opioid activity (Figure III.16).

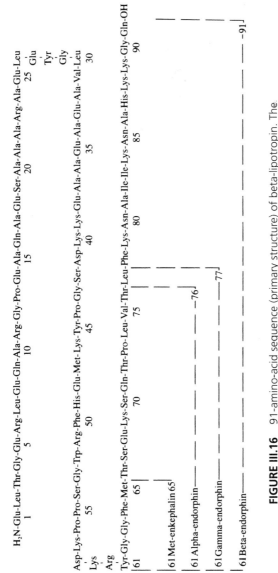

FIGURE III.16 91-amino-acid sequence (primary structure) of beta-lipotropin. The four structures outlined below beta-lipotropin are fragments that are known to exert opioidlike activity.

Several possible functions, including neurotransmission and a role as "natural opioids," have been postulated for the endorphins, dynorphins (pituitary peptides more potent than either beta-endorphin or met-enkephalin), and enkephalins; however, their mechanism of analgesic action is not clear. The question arises concerning the addictive potential of these compounds. Have we finally found a nonaddicting opioid narcotic? Recent work indicates that the answer to this question is no. Physical dependence upon these proteins does develop, and both cross tolerance and cross dependence occur between these proteins and morphine. Therefore, these compounds probably have the same potential for addiction as the opioid narcotics (see Chapters 10 and 15).

A variety of evidence indicates that the enkephalins are physiological neurotransmitters located in specific neuronal systems in the brain. They mediate the integration of sensory inputs related to pain, perception, and emotional behavior. In animals this system is probably relatively inactive; otherwise, pure narcotic antagonists, such as naloxone, would displace them from their receptors and initiate pain (or at least produce an increased responsiveness) to a painful stimulus. Limited investigation into the influence of enkephalins in acupuncture has suggested that these proteins may mediate acupuncture-induced analgesia.

The interesting possibility that enkephalins may play a role in stress responses and in mental illness has been raised. The opioid antagonist naloxone seems to ameliorate the hallucinogenic episodes experienced by chronic schizophrenic patients. Also, in patients who experience chronic pain, naloxone alters enkephalin levels. Certainly, these reports will stimulate additional attempts to clarify the role of enkephalins in various emotional states.

Can enkephalins be involved in the tolerance and dependence that develop to opioid narcotics such as morphine? Administration of narcotic analgesics such as morphine intensely stimulates enkephalin receptors, suppressing the activity of enkephalin neurons through a negative feedback mechanism. As the levels of enkephalins fall, increasing amounts of opioids must be administered to achieve the same effect (i.e., tolerance develops). When the administration of morphine is stopped, neither morphine nor enkephalins are present at the receptor, and withdrawal symptoms appear (i.e., physical dependence develops). The withdrawal symptoms subside only when the enkephalin neurons are reactivated.

In conclusion, research has identified endogenous compounds that exert opioidlike activity.[11–18] The receptors on which these compounds act appear to be the same receptors as those for the opioid narcotics. Whether opioid addiction can be explained by these endogenous substances and what the role of these substances is in certain emotional states remain to be seen.

Notes

1. S. Cohen, *The Chemical Brain: The Neurochemistry of Addictive Disorders* (Irvine, Ca.: Care Institute, 1988), p. 11.
2. A. Goldstein, *Addiction: From Biology to Drug Policy* (New York: W. H. Freeman, 1994), p. 43.
3. S. El Mestikawy, A. Fargin, J. R. Raymond, H. Gozlan, and M. Hnatowich, "The 5-HT$_{1A}$ Receptor: An Overview of Recent Advances," *Neurochemical Research* 16 (1991): 1–10.
4. M. A. Harrington, P. Zhong, S. J. Garlow, and R. D. Ciaranello, "Molecular Biology of Serotonin Receptors," *Journal of Clinical Psychiatry* 53, suppl. (October 1992): 8–27.
5. H. K. Manji, G. Chen, H. Shimon, J. K. Hsiao, W. Z. Potter, and R. H. Belmaker, "Guanine Nucleotide-binding Proteins in Bipolar Affective Disorder," Archives of General Psychiatry 52 (1995): 135–144.
6. P. J. Whitehouse, A. M. Martino, P. G. Antuono, P. R. Lowenstein, J. T. Coyle, D. L. Price, and K. J. Kellar, "Nicotinic Acetylcholine Binding Sites in Alzheimer's Disease," *Brain Research* 371 (1986): 146–151.
7. Cohen, *The Chemical Brain*, pp. 14–16.
8. D. L. Tanelian, P. Kosek, I. Mody, and M. B. MacIver, "The Role of the GABA$_A$ Receptor/Chloride Channel Complex in Anesthesia," *Anesthesiology* 78 (1993): 757–776.
9. W. E. Haefely, J. R. Martin, J. G. Richards, and P. Schoch, "The Multiplicity of Actions of Benzodiazepine Receptor Ligands," *Canadian Journal of Psychiatry* 38, Suppl. 4 (November 1993): S102–S107.
10. D. I. Monaghan, R. J. Bridges, and C. W. Cotman, "The Excitatory Amino Acid Receptors: Their Classes, Pharmacology, and Distinct Properties in the Function of the Central Nervous System," *Annual Review of Pharmacology and Toxicology* 29 (1989): 365–402.
11. S. H. Snyder, "Drug and Neurotransmitter Receptors in the Brain," *Science* 224 (1984): 22–31.
12. O. Civelli, C. Machida, J. Bunzow, P. Albert, E. Hanneman, J. Salon, J. Bidlack, and D. Grandy, "The Next Frontier in the Molecular Biology of the Opioid System. The Opioid Receptors," *Molecular Neurobiology* 1 (1987): 373–391.
13. R. E. Bloom, "Neurotransmitters: Past, Present, and Future Directions," *FASEB Journal* 2 (1988): 32–41.
14. E. J. Simon, "Opioid Receptors and Endogenous Opioid Peptides," *Medicinal Research Reviews* 11 (1991): 357–374.

15. M. Goodman, S. Ro, G. Osapay, T. Tamazaki, and A. Polinsky, "The Molecular Basis of Opioid Potency and Selectivity: Morphiceptins, Dermorphins, Deltorphins, and Enkephalins," *NIDA Research Monograph* 134 (1993): 195–209.

16. T. Reisine and G. I. Bell, "Molecular Biology of Opioid Receptors," *Trends in Neurosciences* 16 (1993): 506–510.

17. G. W. Pasternak, "Pharmacological Mechanisms of Opioid Analgesics," *Clinical Neuropharmacology* 16 (1993): 1–18.

18. D. W. Self and L. Stein, "Receptor Subtypes in Opioid and Stimulant Reward," *Pharmacology and Toxicology* 70 (1992): 87–94.

GLOSSARY

Abstinence syndrome State of altered behavior that follows cessation of drug administration.

Acetylcholine (ACh) Neurotransmitter in the central and peripheral nervous systems.

Additive effect Increased effect that occurs when two drugs that have similar biological actions are administered. The net effect is the sum of the independent effects exerted by the drugs.

Adenosine Chemical neuromodulator in the CNS, primarily at inhibitory synapses.

Adenylate cyclase Intracellular enzyme that catalyzes the conversion of cyclic AMP to adenosine monophosphate.

Affective disorder Type of mental disorder characterized by recurrent episodes of mania, depression, or both.

Agonist Drug that attaches to a receptor and produces actions that mimic or potentiate those of an endogenous transmitter.

Aldehyde dehydrogenase Enzyme that carries out a specific step in alcohol metabolism: the metabolism of acetaldehyde to acetate. This enzyme may be blocked by the drug disulfiram (Antabuse).

Alzheimer's disease Progressive neurological disease that occurs primarily in the elderly. It is characterized by a loss of short-term memory and intellectual functioning. It is associated with a loss of function of acetylcholine neurons.

Amanita muscaria Fly agaric mushroom, used for its psychedelic properties.

Amantadine (Symmetrel) Antiviral drug useful in the treatment of Parkinson's disease.

Amphetamine Behavioral stimulant.

Anabolic-androgenic steroid Testosterone-like drug that acts to increase muscle mass and incurs other masculinizing effects.

Anandamide Andogenous chemical compound that attaches to cannabinoid receptors in the CNS and to specific components of the lymphatic system.

Anandamide receptor Receptor to which anandamide and tetrahydro-cannabinol bind.

Anesthetic drugs Sedative-hypnotic compounds used primarily in doses capable of inducing a state of general anesthesia that involves both loss of sensation and loss of consciousness.

Antabuse Trade name for disulfiram, a drug that interferes with the break-down of alcohol, resulting in the accumulation of acetaldehyde.

Antagonist Drug that attaches to a receptor and blocks the action of either an endogenous transmitter or an agonist drug.

Anticonvulsant Drug that blocks or prevents epileptic convulsions. Many anticonvulsants (e.g., carbamazepine, valproic acid) are also used to treat certain nonepileptic psychiatric disorders.

Antidepressant Drug that is useful in treating mental depression in depressed patients but does not produce stimulant effects in normal persons.

Antipsychotic drugs Class of psychoactive drugs that have the ability to calm psychotic states and make the psychotic patient more manageable.

Anxiolytic Drug used to relieve the symptoms associated with anxiety and related disorders.

Attention deficit hyperactivity disorder Learning and behavioral disability characterized by reduced attention span and hyperactivity. Formerly called *hyperkinetic syndrome, minimal brain disorder,* and *minimal brain dysfunction.*

Autonomic nervous system Portion of the peripheral nervous system that controls or regulates the visceral, or automatic, functions of the body (such as heart rate and blood pressure).

Baclofen (Lioresal) GABA derivative that is useful in the treatment of spasticity.

Barbiturates Class of chemically related sedative-hypnotic compounds that share a characteristic six-membered ring structure.

Basal ganglia Part of the brain that contains vast numbers of dopamine-containing synapses. Forms part of the extrapyramidal system. Parkinson's disease follows dopamine loss in this structure.

Benzodiazepines Class of chemically related sedative-hypnotic agents of which chlordiazepoxide (Librium) and diazepam (Valium) are examples.

Beta-lipoprotein 91-amino-acid protein containing amino acid sequences that have morphine-like activity.

Bipolar disorder Affective disorder characterized by alternating bouts of mania and depression. Also referred to as *manic-depressive illness.*

Blackout Period of time during which one may be awake but memory is not imprinted. It is common in people who have consumed excessive alcohol.

Brain syndrome, organic Pattern of behavior induced when neurons are either reversibly depressed or irreversibly destroyed. Behavior is characterized by clouded sensorium, disorientation, shallow and labile affect, and impaired memory, intellectual function, insight, and judgment.

Brand name Unique name licensed to one manufacturer of a drug. Contrasts with *generic name*, the name under which any manufacturer may sell a drug.

Bufotenin Psychoactive drug found in cohoba snuff, the skin and parotid gland of the toad, and in small amounts in the mushroom *Amanita muscaria*.

Bupropion (Wellbutrin) Nontricyclic second-generation antidepressant.

Buspirone (BuSpar) Nonbenzodiazepine second-generation anxiolytic that exerts a weak agonist effect on serotonin-1A receptors.

C-AMP Cyclic adenosine monophosphate.

Caffeine Behavioral and general cellular stimulant found in coffee, tea, cola drinks, and chocolate.

Caffeinism Habitual use of large amounts of caffeine.

Cannabis Plant that contains marijuana.

Carbamazepine (Tegretol) Antiepileptic drug also used to treat certain psychiatric disorders.

Carbidopa Drug that inhibits the enzyme dopadecarboxylase, allowing increased availability of dopa within the brain. Contained in Sinemet.

Central nervous system (CNS) Brain and spinal cord.

Chlordiazepoxide (Librium) Benzodiazepine sedative-hypnotic drug.

Chlorpromazine (Thorazine) Phenothiazine antipsychotic drug.

Cirrhosis Serious, usually irreversible liver disease. Usually associated with chronic excessive alcohol consumption.

Citalopram Drug that selectively blocks the active reuptake of serotonin into presynaptic nerve terminals.

Clomiphene (Clomid) Ovulation-inducing agent thought to act by blocking the inhibitory (negative-feedback) effect that estrogens exert on the hypothalamus.

Clonazepam (Clonopin) Benzodiazepine anxiolytic useful in the treatment of bipolar disorder.

Clonidine (Catapres) Antihypertensive useful in ameliorating the symptoms of narcotic withdrawal.

Clozapine (Clozaril) Nonphenothiazine atypical antipsychotic drug.

Cocaine Behavioral stimulant.

Codeine Sedative and pain-relieving agent found in opium. Structurally related to morphine but less potent; constitutes approximately 0.5 percent of the opium extract.

Comorbid disorder Psychiatric disorder that coexists with a second psychiatric disorder (e.g., polysubstance abuse in a patient with a major depressive disorder).

Convulsant Drug that produces convulsions by blocking inhibitory neurotransmission.

Crack   Street name for a smokable form of potent, concentrated cocaine.

Cross-dependence   Condition in which one drug can prevent the withdrawal symptoms associated with physical dependence on a different drug.

Cross-tolerance   Condition in which tolerance of one drug results in a lessened response to another drug.

Delirium tremens (DTs, "rum fits")   Syndrome of tremulousness with hallucinations, psychomotor agitation, confusion and disorientation, sleep disorders, and other associated discomforts, lasting several days after alcohol withdrawal.

Dementia   General designation for nonspecific mental deterioration.

Depo-Provera   Long-acting, injectable preparation of progesterone, useful as a long-acting female contraceptive.

Detoxification   Process of allowing time for the body to metabolize and/or excrete accumulations of drug. Usually a first step in drug abuse evaluation and treatment.

Diazepam (Valium)   Benzodiazepine antianxiety drug.

Diethylstilbestrol   Synthetically produced estrogen occasionally used in high doses as a postcoital contraceptive.

Differential diagnosis   Listing of all possible causes that might explain a given set of symptoms.

Dimethyltryptamine (DMT)   Psychedelic drug found in many South American snuffs.

Disinhibition   Physiological state of the central nervous system characterized by decreased activity of inhibitory synapses, which results in a net excess of excitatory activity.

Dopamine transporter   Presynaptic protein that binds synaptic dopamine and transports the neurotransmitter back into the presynaptic nerve terminal.

Dose–response relation   Relation between drug doses and the response elicited at each dose level.

Droperidol (Inapsine)   Antipsychotic drug classified chemically as a butyrophenone.

Drug   Chemical substance used for its effects on bodily processes.

Drug absorption   Mechanism by which a drug reaches the bloodstream from the skin, lungs, stomach, intestinal tract, or muscle.

Drug administration   Procedures through which a drug enters the body (oral administration of tablets or liquids, inhalation of powders, injection of sterile liquids, and so on).

Drug dependence   State in which the use of a drug is necessary for either physical or psychological well-being.

Drug interaction   Modification of the action of one drug by the concurrent or prior administration of another drug.

Drug misuse   Use of any drug (legal or illegal) for a medical or recreational purpose when other alternatives are available, practical, or warranted, or when drug use endangers either the user or others with whom he or she may interact.

Drug receptor   Specific molecular substance in the body with which a given drug interacts to produce its effect.

Drug tolerance   State of progressively decreasing responsiveness to a drug.

DSM-IV   *Diagnostic and Statistical Manual of Mental Disorders,* Fourth Edition (1994), a publication of the American Psychiatric Association.

Electroconvulsive therapy (ECT)   Nonpharmacological treatment used for major depression.

Endorphin   Naturally occurring protein that causes endogenous morphine-like activity.

Enkephalin   Naturally occurring protein that causes morphine-like activity.

Enzyme   Large organic molecule that mediates a specific biochemical reaction in the body.

Enzyme induction   Increased production of drug-metabolizing enzymes in the liver, stimulated by certain drugs, such that use of these drugs increases the rate at which the body can metabolize them. It is one mechanism by which pharmacological tolerance is produced.

Epilepsy   Neurological disorder characterized by an occasional, sudden, and uncontrolled discharge of neurons.

Estrogen   Body hormone secreted primarily from the ovaries of females in response to stimulation by follicle-stimulating hormone (FSH) from the pituitary gland.

Felbamate (Felban)   Recently released antiepileptic drug.

Fentanyl   Potent narcotic analgesic drug.

Fetal alcohol syndrome   Symptom complex of congenital anomalies, seen in newborns of women who ingested high doses of alcohol during critical periods of pregnancy.

Flumazenil (Romazicon)   Benzodiazepine antagonist.

Fluoxetine (Prozac)   Prototype serotonin-specific reuptake inhibitor (SSRI) antidepressant drug.

G-protein   Specific intraneuronal protein.

Gamma-aminobutyric acid (GABA)   Inhibitory amino acid neurotransmitter in the brain.

Generic name   Name that identifies a specific chemical entity (without specifically describing the chemical). Often marketed under different brand names by multiple manufacturers.

Hallucinogen   Psychedelic drug that produces profound distortions in perception.

Haloperidol (Haldol)   Antipsychotic drug classified chemically as a butyrophenone.

Harmine   Psychedelic agent obtained from the seeds of *Peganum harmala.*

Hashish   Extract of the hemp plant (*Cannabis sativa*) that has a higher concentration of THC than does marijuana.

Heroin   Semisynthetic opiate produced by a chemical modification of morphine.

Hypothalamus Structure located at the base of the brain, above the pituitary gland.

Hypoxia State of relative lack of oxygen in the tissues of the body and the brain.

Ibuprofen (Advil, Motrin) Nonnarcotic, nonsalicylate analgesic and anti-inflammatory drug.

ICE Street name for a smokable, free-based form of potent, concentrated methamphetamine.

Ketamine (Ketalar) Psychedelic surgical anesthetic. Acts by blocking ion flows through the NMDA-glutamate receptor.

Levodopa Precursor substance to the transmitter dopamine, useful in ameliorating the symptoms of Parkinson's disease.

Limbic system Group of brain structures involved in emotional responses and emotional expression.

Lithium Alkali metal effective in the treatment of mania and depression.

Lorazepam (Ativan) Benzodiazepine sedative/anxiolytic also useful in the treatment of bipolar disorder.

Lysergic acid diethylamide (LSD) Semisynthetic psychedelic drug.

Major tranquilizer (antipsychotic tranquilizer) Drug used in the treatment of psychotic states.

Mania Mental disorder characterized by an expansive emotional state, elation, hyperirritability, excessive talkativeness, flights of ideas, and increased behavioral activity.

MAO inhibitor (MAOI) Drug that inhibits the activity of the enzyme monoamine oxidase.

Marijuana Mixture of the crushed leaves, flowers, and small branches of both the male and female hemp plant (*Cannabis sativa*).

MDA Synthetically produced derivation of amphetamine.

MDMA Methylene-dioxymethamphetamine; psychedelic drug related to MDA.

Meprobamate (Equanil) Sedative-hypnotic agent frequently used as an antianxiety drug.

Mescaline Psychedelic drug extracted from the peyote cactus (*Lophophora williamsii*).

Methadone (Dolophine) Synthetically produced opiate narcotic.

Methylphenidate (Ritalin) CNS stimulant chemically and pharmacologically related to amphetamine.

Mifepristone (RU-486) Postcoital contraceptive pill that can induce abortion when given in early stages of pregnancy.

Minor tranquilizer Sedative-hypnotic drug promoted primarily for use in the treatment of anxiety.

Mixed agonist–antagonist Drug that attaches to a receptor, producing weak agonist effects but displacing more potent agonists, precipitating withdrawal in drug-dependent persons.

Monoamine oxidase (MAO) Enzyme capable of metabolizing norepin-ephrine, dopamine, and serotonin to inactive products.

Monoamine oxidase inhibitor (MAOI) See MAO inhibitor.

Morphine Major sedative and pain-relieving drug found in opium, compris-ing approximately 10 percent of the crude opium exudate.

Muscarine Drug extracted from the mushroom *Amanita muscaria* that directly stimulates acetylcholine receptors.

Myristin Psychedelic agent obtained from nutmeg and mace.

Naloxone (Narcan) Pure narcotic antagonist.

Naltrexone (Trexan) Long-acting narcotic antagonist.

Neurotransmitter Endogenous chemical released by one neuron that alters the electrical activity of another neuron.

Nicotine Behavioral stimulant found in tobacco; responsible for the psyche-delic effects of tobacco and for tobacco dependence.

Ololiuqui Psychedelic drug obtained from the seeds of the morning glory plant.

Opioid Natural or synthetic drug that exerts actions on the body similar to those induced by morphine, the major pain-relieving agent obtained from the opium poppy (*Papaver somniferum*).

Opioid narcotic Drug that has both sedative and analgesic actions.

Opium Crude resinous exudate from the opium poppy.

Parkinson's disease Disorder of the motor system characterized by involun-tary movements, tremor, and weakness.

Peptide Chemical composed of a chain-link sequence of amino acids.

Pergonal Preparation of follicle-stimulating hormone extracted from the urine of postmenopausal females.

Peyote Cactus that contains mescaline.

Pharmacodynamics Study of the interactions of a drug and the receptors responsible for the action of the drug in the body.

Pharmacokinetics Study of the factors that influence the absorption, distri-bution, metabolism, and excretion of a drug.

Pharmacology Branch of science that deals with the study of drugs and their actions on living systems.

Phencyclidine (Sernyl, PCP) Psychedelic surgical anesthetic. Acts by bind-ing to and inhibiting ion transport through the NMDA-glutamate recep-tors.

Phenothiazine Class of chemically related compounds useful in the treat-ment of psychosis.

Phenytoin (Dilantin) Antiepileptic drug.

Physical dependence State in which the use of a drug is required for a person to function normally. Such a state is revealed by withdrawing the drug and noting the occurrence of withdrawal symptoms (abstinence syndrome). Characteristically, withdrawal symptoms can be terminated by readministration of the drug.

Placebo Pharmacologically inert substance that may elicit a significant reaction largely because of the mental "set" of the patient or the physical setting in which the drug is taken.

Potency Measure of drug activity expressed in terms of the amount required to produce an effect of given intensity. Potency varies inversely with the amount of drug required to produce this effect—the more potent the drug, the lower the amount required to produce the effect.

Progesterone Hormone secreted from the ovaries in response to stimulation by luteinizing hormone (LH) from the pituitary gland.

Progestins Group of synthetically produced progesterones; most frequently found in oral contraceptive tablets.

Psilocybin Psychedelic drug obtained from the mushroom *Psilocybe mexicana.*

Psychedelic drug Drug that can alter sensory perception.

Psychoactive drug Chemical substance that alters mood or behavior as a result of alterations in the functioning of the brain.

Psychological dependence Compulsion to use a drug for its pleasurable effects. Such dependence may lead to a compulsion to misuse a drug.

Psychopharmacotherapy Clinical treatment of psychiatric disorders with drugs.

Psychotherapy Nonpharmacological treatment of psychiatric disorders utilizing a wide range of modalities, from simple education and supportive counseling to insight-oriented, dynamically based therapy.

Receptor Location in the nervous system at which a neurotransmitter or drug binds to exert its characteristic effect.

Remoxipride Experimental nonphenothiazine atypical antipsychotic drug.

Reye's syndrome Rare CNS disorder that occurs in children; associated with aspirin ingestion.

Risk-to-benefit ratio Arbitrary assessment of the risks and benefits that may accrue from administration of a drug.

Risperidone (Risperdal) Recently available nonphenothiazine atypical antipsychotic drug.

Scopolamine Anticholinergic drug that crosses the blood-brain barrier to produce sedation and amnesia.

Second messenger Intraneuronal protein that, when activated by an excitatory G-protein, initiates the neuronal response to the initial neurotransmitter attachment to an extracellular receptor.

Sedative-hypnotic drugs Chemical substances that exert a nonselective general depressant action on the nervous system.

Serotonin (5-hydroxytryptamine, 5-HT) Synaptic transmitter in both the brain and the peripheral nervous system.

Serotonin-specific reuptake inhibitor (SSRI) Second-generation antidepressant drug.

Side effect Drug-induced effect that accompanies the primary effect for which the drug is administered.

Spasticity   State of abnormal increases in muscle tension, resulting in increased resistance of the muscle to stretching.

Tardive dyskinesia   Movement disorder that appears after months or years of treatment with neuroleptic (antipsychotic) drugs. It usually worsens with drug discontinuation. Symptoms are often masked by the drugs that cause the disorder.

Teratogen   Chemical substance that induces abnormalities of fetal development.

Testosterone   Hormone secreted from the testes that is responsible for the distinguishing characteristics of the male.

Tetrahydrocannabinol (THC)   Major psychoactive agent in marijuana, hashish, and other preparations of hemp (*Cannabis sativa*).

Therapeutic drug monitoring (TDM)   Process of correlating the plasma level of drugs with therapeutic response.

Toxic effect   Drug-induced effect either temporarily or permanently deleterious to any organ or system of an animal or person. Drug toxicity includes both the relatively minor side effects that invariably accompany drug administration and the more serious and unexpected manifestations that occur in only a small percentage of patients who take a drug.

Valproic acid (Valproate)   Antiepileptic drug also used in the treatment of bipolar illness.

Verapamil (Calan)   Calcium channel blocker used in the treatment of cardio-vasular diseases. Occasionally used in the treatment of bipolar disorder.

Withdrawal syndrome   Symptoms that occur when one ceases to ingest a drug. Also called *abstinence syndrome.*

Zolpidem (Ambien)   Nonbenzodiazepine sedative-hypnotic drug that acts through stimulation of $GABA_{1A}$ receptors.

BIBLIOGRAPHY: A BASIC PHARMACOLOGY BOOKSHELF

American Medical Association. *Drug Evaluations Annual 1994*. Milwaukee, Wis.: American Medical Association, 1993.

Bloom, F. E., and D. J. Kupfer, eds. *Psychopharmacology: The Fourth Generation of Progress*. New York: Raven Press, 1994.

Cooper, J. R., F. E. Bloom, and R. H. Roth. *The Biochemical Basis of Neuropharmacology*, 6th ed. New York: Oxford University Press, 1991.

Craig, C. R., and R. E. Stitzel, eds. *Modern Pharmacology*, 4th ed. Boston: Little, Brown, 1994.

DiPalma, J. R., and G. J. DiGregorio. *Basic Pharmacology in Medicine*, 3d ed. New York: McGraw-Hill, 1990.

Facts and Comparisons. *Drug Facts and Comparisons*, 1994 Edition, St. Louis: Facts and Comparisons, 1994.

Gilman, A. G., T. W. Rall, A. S. Nies, and P. Taylor, eds. *Goodman and Gilman's The Pharmacological Basis of Therapeutics*, 8th ed. New York: McGraw-Hill, 1990.

Goldstein, A. *Addiction: From Biology to Drug Policy*. New York: W. H. Freeman, 1994.

Goth, A. *Medical Pharmacology*, 13th ed. St. Louis: Mosby, 1992.

Janicak, P. G., J. M. Davis, S. H. Preskorn, and F. J. Aid. *Principles and Practice of Psychopharmacotherapy*. Baltimore: Williams & Wilkins, 1993.

Julien, R. M. *Drugs and the Body*. New York: W. H. Freeman, 1988.

Lowinson, J. H., P. Ruiz, R. B. Millman, and J. G. Langrod, eds. *Substance Abuse: A Comprehensive Textbook*, 2nd ed. Baltimore: Williams & Wilkins, 1992.

Rang, H. P., and M. M. Dale. *Pharmacology*, 2nd ed. Edinburgh: Churchill Livingstone, 1991.

Smith, C. M., and A. M. Reynard. *Textbook of Pharmacology*. Philadelphia: W. B. Saunders, 1992.

Wingard, L. B., T. M. Brody, J. Larner, and A. Schwartz. *Human Pharmacology: Molecular to Clinical*. St. Louis: Mosby Year Book, 1991.

INDEX